THE GREAT PHYSICIAN'S

R_x

for

HEALTH & WELLNESS

Seven Keys to Unlocking Your Health Potential

JORDAN RUBIN

with David Remedios, M.D.

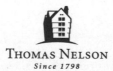

THOMAS NELSON

Since 1798

NASHVILLE   DALLAS   MEXICO CITY   RIO DE JANEIRO   BEIJING

Published in Nashville, Tennessee. Thomas Nelson is a trademark of Thomas Nelson, Inc.

Thomas Nelson, Inc. titles may be purchased in bulk for educational, business, fund-raising, or sales promotional use. For information, please email SpecialMarkets@ThomasNelson.com.

Library of Congress Cataloging-in-Publication Data

Rubin, Jordan.
   The Great Physician's Rx for health and wellness / Jordan Rubin with David Remedios.
      p. cm.
   ISBN: 0-7852-8812-0 (ie)
   ISBN: 0-7852-1352-X (hc)
   ISBN-10: 0-7852-8884-8 (tp)
   ISBN-13: 978-0-7852-8884-8 (tp)
   1. Self-care, Health.   2. Health.   I. Remedios, David.   II. Title.
   RA776.95.R828   2005
   613.2—dc22   2005024890

Printed in the United States of America

07 08 09 10 11 RRD 5 4 3 2 1

I dedicate this book to my son, Joshua Michael. When I hold his tiny hand in mine and look upon him with a breadth of love I didn't know I was capable of feeling, I more fully appreciate the love and sacrifice God made for me over two thousand years ago by sending His only son to die for my sins.

CONTENTS

INTRODUCTION

Offer Your Body as a Living Sacrifice

Whenever I speak at a Sunday worship service, I like to shake things up by springing a pop quiz on the congregation.

"This morning, I want you to turn to the person next to you and tell him or her what you ate for breakfast." No matter how you slice it or serve it, there's something all-American about breakfast, even if it's a meal of French toast, Canadian bacon, and English muffins.

From my vantage point, what happens next is a fascinating display of human behavior. Muffled voices and whispered exchanges emanate from folks clearly embarrassed to reveal what they ate before arriving at church. Perhaps that's because breakfast was an Egg McMuffin snatched up at the drive-thru window, chased with a cup of cream-filled coffee sweetened with several packets of Splenda, or a quick stop at Dunkin' Donuts for sticky treats topped with chocolate and sprinkles.

Others shrug their shoulders, as if to say, *Hey, I had kids to get ready. I didn't have time to eat.* But those who enjoyed a hearty, home-cooked breakfast pridefully regale their captive audience with an enthusiastic description of scrambled eggs with American cheese, crisp bacon, sizzling sausage, and—especially in the South where I live—a heaping helping of grits.

After the conversational buzz dies down, I toss out a second question—one even more penetrating: "How many of you consider what your neighbor ate to be healthy?"

I usually hear nervous laughter and some twittering, and you should see the folks in the pews sit on their hands. After an awkward moment or two, I spot a few arms raised timidly in the air. That's because most people intuitively understand that diving into a plate of high-sugar, high-fat breakfast foods such as, well, French toast made from white bread, with a side order of Canadian bacon, does not constitute healthy eating, and neither does wolfing down a fast-food egg sandwich or chocolate éclairs on the way to church.

People who don't eat healthy are not thriving the way God wants them to, and I'll show you why in *The Great Physician's Rx for Health and Wellness*. Eating healthy and enjoying the fruits of an active lifestyle have been my passion for ten years, and it's a message I love sharing with God's people. It's my strongly held belief that if Christians were healthier than the general population—and we're not, in my estimation—then our churches would be overflowing on Sunday mornings. Why? Because people would be drawn to learn more about why we are so different. I want them to think, *Oh, there are a couple of Christians. Look how healthy and vibrant they are. I want what they have.*

It's my dream that someday every one of the nation's leading TV programs, radio broadcasts, magazines, and newspapers will report that scientific evidence shows that followers of Jesus are three or four or five times healthier than those who don't believe in Jesus—that Christians have less cancer, less heart disease, less diabetes, and less obesity. Wouldn't it be awesome if God's people were so full of good health, so vibrant, that others would notice us from ten or twenty feet away? If that were to happen, our churches wouldn't be big enough to fit the numbers of people rushing to hear about the Great Physician's prescription for their good health. I believe that people from all walks of life would break down the doors to learn more about what God says about living a long and abundant life and ultimately come to know Jesus as their Lord and Savior.

That's my reason for writing *The Great Physician's Rx for Health and Wellness*, and my core message on health can be derived from two Scriptures. The first goes like this: "I urge you, brothers, in view of God's mercy, to offer your bodies as living sacrifices, holy and pleasing to God—this is your spiritual act of worship" (Rom. 12:1).

Are you presenting your physical body as a living sacrifice? Can you say,

"This is the best I have, and I'm giving it to the Lord"? Are you an example of God's best? Can others see your vitality?

They say that if you don't have your health, you ain't got nuthin'. Nothing on earth matters more than your physical well-being because without your health, God cannot use you properly. Since God has great plans for you, He's calling you, one of His children, to present yourself as a living sacrifice today.

Even though I'm only thirty years old, I've attended a few funerals and memorial services in my time, and invariably I'll watch a friend of the deceased ruefully shake his head and say, "I guess it was his time to die."

I heard that exact phrase uttered when someone spoke about the memorial service of an acquaintance of mine—a missions pastor—who died of cancer at the age of thirty-nine. Left behind by this incredible man were a beautiful wife, four wonderful children, and a thriving global ministry. I was scheduled to talk to him about getting on God's health plan shortly before he died, but the call never took place. What if, before the cancer developed, he had followed the Great Physician's prescription for healthy living? Would things have turned out differently? We'll never know because now it's too late.

I believe God designed us to live long and fruitful lives. I believe we can maintain our strength and vigor well into old age by following the Great Physician's prescription for health and wellness.

Think about it: before Moses died, Scripture says that his eyes did not grow dim. The Bible tells us that the eyes are the windows of the soul, the light of the body. If the eyes are good, the whole body is good. In fact, when priests were called upon to diagnose a disease of an Israelite, they looked into the person's eyes. What this means is that Moses did not die of an illness; nor was his body feeble or his mind weak. God was ready to take him home; Moses was simply used up.

Joshua passed away at the age of 110, just months after he came off the battlefield. Caleb was going full bore, battling giants in his late eighties, until the Lord called him home. These heroes of the Bible never spent time in assisted living or nursing homes. They drank the last drop from the cup of life because they followed God's principles of good health found in the Bible. And you can, too, which leads me to my second key passage of Scripture: "Let us make man in our image" (Gen. 1:26).

This means you were created in the image of God. You were made in God's image for a reason, and that's to be a reflection of God to the world for His glory. Think about it: Do you properly reflect His image? Are you healthy? Or do you think you're healthy simply because there's an absence of a grave disease in your life? Maybe you consider yourself healthy because you're not hacking away with a cough, running a 103-degree fever, or dying in a hospital. But is that really the definition of being healthy?

Good health is a lot more than the absence of disease in your life. Good health is waking up in the morning feeling rested and ready to attack the day. Good health is having the energy to keep up with those kids you're raising. Good health is having something left in the tank after you've put in a full day of work. Good health is thriving, not merely surviving.

God wants to use you, but He also needs you at your physical, spiritual, and emotional best. My challenge to you is that by the time you reach the end of *The Great Physician's Rx for Health and Wellness* and the end of this seven-week health plan, you'll say, "Yes, I am a living sacrifice, someone who is causing those who don't know God to want what I have."

MY STORY

I've made the commitment to offer my body as a living sacrifice, but it's been a long road, as I'll explain. I grew up as the older son of Herb and Phyllis Rubin. My father studied to become a naturopathic physician and chiropractor, and in his chiropractic practice, he sought a more natural approach in treating patients and their aches and pains.

Dad and Mom were ahead of their time, even in the 1970s when I was born. Mom eschewed conventional medicine when it came time to deliver me; she gave birth at home with four naturopathic students assisting in the delivery. Her cupboards were filled with jars of raw honey, wheat germ oil, and nearly every supplement and vitamin known to man; our refrigerator stored homemade soy milk, sprouts, and tofu. We were vegetarians for the first four years of my life, but then we started eating meat—mainly chicken and fish—when I turned four, based on my mother's cravings when she was pregnant with my sister, Jenna.

You could say that I was a granola kid growing up. My neighborhood friends often complained that we didn't have any "real food" in the house, but from a young age I knew that Cheetos, Oreos, and their salty and sugary cousins were bad for me. Mom and Dad were determined to raise me and Jenna with an all-natural diet that didn't rely on processed foods like white bread or pastas or sweets made with white sugar. In their view, anything processed or containing preservatives—such as Pop-Tarts or Frosted Flakes—wasn't worth bringing home. "The more natural, the better," my parents always said.

As for my spiritual upbringing, I was definitely raised in a Christian home. In case you're wondering, though, Rubin is a Jewish name, and my parents became messianic Jews when I was two years old. A messianic Jew believes that Jesus is the chosen Messiah who came and will return again. I can't point to a specific time that I "accepted" Jesus as my Lord and Savior, but I knew and believed that Jesus came to this earth to die for my sins by the time I was five years old.

When I reached high school, living in Palm Beach Gardens on Florida's Gold Coast north of Miami, I became actively involved with the youth group at First Baptist Church in West Palm Beach. The teen years were good to me: I grew into a healthy, athletic young man, and I can remember only two or three times when I had a cold or the flu that required any medication. I hardly ever missed school, where I earned good grades and became a national honors student.

Following high school graduation, I was off to a large, secular college campus where football was king—Florida State University, home of the Seminoles. My tuition bills were covered by an academic scholarship. Just before my freshman year, I tried out and earned a spot on the Florida State cheerleading squad and a place on the stadium floor whenever the 'Noles played at home. I called myself a college athlete, although the football players had a different name for us.

Another thing I did immediately upon enrollment was to join the college ministry at First Baptist Church in Tallahassee, which numbered more than one thousand students each Sunday and was the second-largest college ministry in the United States at that time. I quickly joined a traveling musical group as a soloist and was on the ministry's praise team.

Everything was lining up my way. I saw myself playing an evangelistic role on the Tallahassee campus, home to thirty thousand students, so when some other like-minded guys at First Baptist talked about rushing one of the fraternity houses—and being a light in an area of darkness—that sounded like a great idea to me. We decided to pledge at Pi Kappa Alpha—the Pikes—who had been kicked off campus five years earlier and were applying for reinstatement as they came off probation. The chance to impact a party-minded fraternity for God excited me.

I was elected chaplain of Pi Kappa Alpha, which meant that I had a pretty full plate my freshman year. Like any living-life-to-the-max student, I loved the freedom of being on my own, but college life brought a whole new level of stress. I hadn't nailed down my major yet, although I was thinking that pre-ministerial communications would be my path of study. By the end of my freshman year, I felt a strong call to ministry, not knowing if it would be the pastorate, youth ministry, music—or maybe even the missions field. I was so on fire for God that I can remember praying, "Lord, please put somebody in my path today with whom I can share the gospel."

I was always running from one thing to another—attending class, participating in daily Bible studies, going to cheerleading practice, playing intramural football, and traveling to perform at concerts. With so much coming at me, I sometimes cut corners and grabbed something quick to eat—like a softball-sized blueberry muffin in the morning or a burger and fries at lunchtime, topped off with some soft-serve, high-sugar frozen yogurt.

One morning before breakfast, I was reading my Bible when a feeling of sadness—almost grief—came over me. The sorrowful sensation caused me to write down the following notation in my journal: "Lord, I know You're about to do something huge in my life. And I'm scared."

I couldn't overcome the feeling that something bad would happen to me. That feeling became a reality during the summer. I was a counselor at a summer camp when I began having what people would euphemistically call "health challenges." I'm talking nausea, stomach cramps, and horrible digestive problems. I even had these nasty sores in my mouth that bothered me so much I couldn't sleep through the night. I began feeling run-down, and when I'd get on the camp bus for a ride to our next activity, I'd fall fast asleep in the middle of the afternoon. "Jordan, wake up!" my campers would scream. I'd shake the cobwebs from my head, and then they'd laugh, but I couldn't shake the sensation that something was deeply wrong with me.

Toward the end of the summer, despite my health difficulties, I traveled to a different weeklong church-sponsored youth camp as a counselor. The worst part about feeling horrible was dealing with the camp's primitive bathrooms (think glorified outhouse). For instance, I would be helping out on the ropes course when suddenly I would have to sprint to the hole-in-the-floor toilet. My energy was sapped by the constant diarrhea. A combination of eating camp chow, drinking sugary iced tea by the gallon, and working all day under a blazing Florida sun caused me even more problems. I lost twenty pounds in six days!

I didn't want to come to grips with my deteriorating health, but after a week of painful cramps, violent diarrhea, and a high fever, even I knew something was very wrong. I asked a friend to drive me home to Palm Beach Gardens, where my family doctor poked and prodded my abdomen, then ran a battery of tests for every virus in the book—including HIV. The tests came back negative, which didn't surprise me since I had never tried drugs, had a blood transfusion, or been sexually active. But just before leaving the examination room, my doctor wrote me a prescription for two antibiotics. "You'll be okay," he promised. "I don't see any reason why you can't go back to school this fall."

That's what I wanted to hear because I was desperate to get back to Florida State University. Isn't that where God had called me to share my faith while I studied for my degree in preministerial communications? I returned to Tallahassee for the fall semester of my sophomore year, but I didn't feel any better, since the antibiotics failed to help me. In my weakened state, I had to jettison any strength-sapping activities. I quit the Florida State cheerleading team and said good-bye to my buddies at Pi Kappa Alpha.

I moved into a house with seven other guys who had to hear me get up several times a night when 104-degree fevers racked my body. Many mornings, I struggled to get out of bed, and my condition worsened to the point where one day, while I was walking to my music class, my right hip cracked, as if I had broken it and dislocated it at the same time. Painful! I popped the hip back into the socket, but it left me with a limp.

My bigger worry, though, was the location of the bathrooms. No matter where I was on campus, my eyes darted this way and that, always in search of the universal symbol for the male restroom. I wasn't any fun to hang out with, especially if the activity involved a long drive.

Midway through the fall semester, I leveled with my parents. "Mom, I'm not getting any better," I whispered over the phone, trying to keep panic from overtaking my voice. After my confession, I couldn't hold back the tears.

Mom didn't have any answers for me, but when she suggested that I come home, I didn't argue. We agreed that I should temporarily leave Florida State and return to Palm Beach Gardens, where I could seek medical attention and concentrate on getting well. With great disappointment, I boarded a flight for West Palm Beach and left Tallahassee, believing I would be back very soon.

My parents were shocked by my appearance, and I shivered uncontrollably—a sure sign of a high-grade fever. Dad took my temperature, which revealed that my body was fighting a 105-degree fever. He immediately stepped into action, filling our bathtub with ice and cold water, and I gently eased my fever-ridden body into the chilly water. I was talking gibberish in my confusion and delirium, not making any sense at all.

Dad knew it was a life-threatening situation. "My God, I don't want my son to die," he cried out just before calling the hospital. He and Mom rushed me to St. Mary's Hospital in West Palm Beach, where I would spend the next two weeks submitting to various medical tests, including a humiliating one known as a sigmoidoscopy.

Let me tell you: being "scoped" in the rear end wasn't like spending a day at

Daytona Beach. Nor was the barium swallow something to write home about. For that test, I was asked to drink a milk-shake-like liquid that was radioactive so that the medical technicians could watch the barium as it progressed through my digestive tract. They also took a series of X-rays that allowed doctors to examine the condition of my intestinal tract and look for any irregularities.

When the results came back, my doctor delivered a stunning verdict: I was suffering from a digestive disorder known as Crohn's disease. I had never heard of this malady, but everything made sense when my doctor described its symptoms: vomiting, fever, night sweats, loss of appetite, general feeling of weakness, severe abdominal cramps, and diarrhea—often bloody. Crohn's disease, I learned, could affect any portion of the digestive tract, but most patients were affected in the small intestine and/or the colon.

"Crohn's disease is something we don't know a whole lot about, and at the moment, there is no known cure," said my gastroenterologist, Dr. David Wenger. "I'm afraid you're going to have to learn to live with this."

And if I can't? I wondered.

"I'm prescribing several strong medications, including prednisone, which is a powerful anti-inflammatory drug, and you'll likely be on medications for the rest of your life. If your condition worsens, you'll be looking at surgery."

I was afraid to ask what kind of surgery, but I mustered the courage anyway. My doctor rattled off words like *resection* and *colectomy* and *ostomy*, but none of those foreign-sounding words sounded good to me.

"We will go the surgical route only as a last resort," said Dr. Wenger. "The worst-case scenario would be the surgical removal of the colon, in which case we would have to create openings in the abdominal wall known as stomas. Then you would have to wear an appliance to collect fecal waste."

Whoa. That sounded awful—and at the age of nineteen, a fate worse than death. I couldn't imagine going through life like that. Like any young man my age, I believed I was immortal. This nightmare couldn't be happening to me. Didn't God have great plans for my life?

In an effort to avoid surgery at all costs, I embarked on a two-year odyssey to regain my health. All told, my parents spent more than $150,000 in an all-out effort to get me well. I was seen by seventy doctors and medical practitioners (ranging from traditional to alternative), including Dr. Robert Atkins—yes, the doctor behind *The Atkins Diet*—and Barry Sears, Ph.D., author of *The Zone*. I read more than three hundred books on health and tried every dietary plan under the sun, from raw food vegetarianism and macrobiotics to metabolic typing, but none of them worked. Many of these diets had solid underpinnings, but something was just missing.

Meanwhile, I clung to Jeremiah 29:11: "I know the plans I have for you . . . plans to prosper you and not to harm you, plans to give you hope and a future"—but at that point I really wondered what my future would be. A low quality of life? Years of suffering, followed by premature death?

That's the way it looked from my bedroom as I struggled to feel better. As if Crohn's disease weren't enough, my doctors were also treating me for diabetes, arthritis, anemia, and chronic fatigue syndrome. After months of wasting away, I looked like a skeleton.

TURNING A CORNER

After I medically withdrew from college, my life was relegated to a lonely existence. Being cooped up in my old bedroom certainly gave me plenty of time to think. It slowly sank in that I would not be returning to Florida State any time soon.

I couldn't understand why my life had been flipped upside down. When I asked the Lord, "What am I to do?" God whispered two words to me with His still, small voice: *Trust Me.*

One day as I was reading the Bible, I came upon a Scripture that has now become my life verse—Hebrews 11:1 (NKJV), which says, "Now faith is the substance of things hoped for, the evidence of things not seen."

It was my great hope to be cured, but I'm telling you, I had trouble keeping the faith. While my belief in God never wavered, I lacked faith that everything would turn out okay. Looking back, I can see where God was calling on me to rely on Him while I walked through the "valley of the shadow of death," as the verse says in Psalm 23 (NKJV).

I came closest to dying about eighteen months into my health struggles. During one hospitalization, fever spikes ravaged my body, and I couldn't keep anything down. My weight plummeted to 104 pounds, and my heart beat like a Florida State drum major—more than 200 beats per minute. I lifted my hospital gown and looked at my chest, and what I saw horrified me. I could see my heart pounding violently against the chest wall. When a nurse attempted to poke an IV into my arm so that I could get some sustenance, she couldn't get any blood to return. Several nurses and doctors dropped by to investigate. The problem was that my veins were too dry and tapped out, but after two hours of jabbing my outstretched arm, they managed to insert an IV.

My nurse, clearly disturbed, left my room. I heard her crying in the hall and telling another nurse, "This young man is not going to make it through the night."

My situation was becoming *really* serious. I closed my eyes, and with a resigned heart, I talked to God: "Lord, I'm ready to go home. I've had a great life so far, but now I just want to be with You. I don't want to be in this body if life is going to be like this."

I fell asleep, not sure if I would wake up in the morning. After I survived the night, my morning nurse had some good news for me: I had gained ten pounds in water weight from the intravenous fluids.

Now I had my rally cap on, and even though it was the bottom of the ninth with two outs, I was still in the batter's box. I took my last swing. "Lord," I prayed, "while it's my great desire to be physically well, I also want what You have planned for my life. I would like You to heal me, Lord. When that happens, I'll spend the rest of my life helping Your children by leading them out of the bondage that is sickness and disease."

I meant my vow. In fact, I viewed it as a covenant with the Lord. Several days later I was discharged from the hospital and put on a half-dozen medications. All I could do was curl up in bed, rest, and, of course, make dozens of trips to the bathroom. Anytime I ate anything, I immediately felt sick to my stomach, as if sharp knives were constantly stabbing me in the gut.

One afternoon, something happened that changed my life forever. I was sitting up in bed, and I remember reading my Bible and finding myself staring again at Hebrews 11:1, hearing the Lord whisper to me, *Jordan, you need to act on Hebrews 11:1.*

I responded by saying, "Okay, Lord, when I get well, I'm going to proclaim Your goodness to anyone who will listen. When I get well, I'll tell all my friends at the college ministry. When I get well, I'll proclaim Your glory to the world."

In the next moment, it was as if I felt God say to me, *I appreciate what you've said, son, but faith is not hindsight. Faith is proclaiming the mountain when you're lying facedown in the valley. I want to use you where you are.*

I recited Hebrews 11:1 in my head: "*Now faith is the substance of things hoped for, the evidence of things not seen.*" What happened next would become one of the most important decisions I ever made. I asked my mother, "Mom, can you take my picture?" I wanted photographic evidence of the mighty miracle that God was about to do in my life, which meant that I needed a "before" picture.

Mom ignored me, which was surprising. I didn't have the strength to argue with her, so I let it go. But the next day, I made the same request: "Mom, can you take my picture?" Again, she disregarded my request. The following day, I pushed myself out of bed and stood ungainly in front of our kitchen pantry. This time, I would not be denied. I straightened my bony shoulders and declared, "Mom, I really need for you to take my picture."

"Jordan, why do you insist I do this? I can barely stand to look at you; it breaks my heart. Why do you want me to take your picture now? Can't we wait until you're well?"

For whatever reason, God gave me the strength to say, "Mom, you need to take this picture of me now, at my worst, because the world won't believe what God is going to do."

Mom acquiesced and took a snapshot of me that has now been seen by millions around the world. The photo is repulsive. I look like a Holocaust survivor, and I mean that in all reverence because our family lost relatives in the Nazi death camps. As you can see, I was skin and bones, weighing 111 pounds.

I'd like to tell you that I woke up the next morning, and—"poof"—I was healed, but that didn't happen. Instead, I woke up as sick as ever. Many more days and many

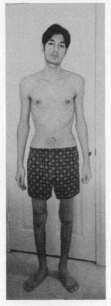

BEFORE

weeks passed by, and my condition remained the same—poor. But my faith that God would heal me never wavered, even when I heard about old friends from high school telling others, "Remember Jordan—the guy who carried his Bible to school? He's sick and dying. Where is his God now?"

God knew exactly what He was doing. I read in 1 Corinthians 1:27 that "God chose the foolish things of the world to shame the wise; God chose the weak things of the world to shame the strong," and He had a plan to use me when I was at my weakest. I also knew that the apostle Paul had written, "I will boast all the more gladly about my weaknesses, so that Christ's power may rest on me" (2 Cor. 12:9).

When God looked upon me, He did not see failure or weakness; He saw a shapeless lump of clay He could mold, and I let Him grab hold of my life.

Going Under the Knife?

Even though I was convinced that God would either heal me or direct me to medical treatment that would cure me, I often lacked hope. More pages on the calendar flew by. After nearly two years of my suffering, doctors urged my parents and me to opt for the surgical removal of virtually all of my large intestine and some of my small intestine. In surgical terms, doctors called it a colostomy. For the rest of my life, I would have to wear bags attached to my abdominal wall to handle my bodily waste.

In day-to-day practical terms, I would be semifunctional, but that was certainly better than living the life of a partial invalid. Feeling that I had run out of options, I consented to going under the knife in the early part of 1996.

About a week before we were to proceed, I overheard my father speaking with a man from San Diego.

"I know why your son is not well," he said.

Dad took a resigned breath. Plenty of well-intentioned friends and acquaintances—and leading experts like Dr. Robert Atkins—had tried to share their insight on why I was not able to lick my ailments. Over a two-year period, I had probably tried five hundred different treatments—gadgets, gizmos, pills, and potions. They ranged from conventional drugs like prednisone to some pretty edgy stuff:

- Taking adrenal cortical extract, or ACE, an extract of bovine adrenal glands
- Being injected with sheep cells from embryos
- Drinking large amounts of cabbage juice
- Injecting myself with a cocktail of assorted vitamins and minerals
- Consuming Chinese and Peruvian herbs, Japanese kampo, olive leaf extract, and shark cartilage
- Taking IVs of an extract of the Venus flytrap

Despite subjecting myself to these unconventional treatments and diets, none of them worked.

The next day I spoke with the man named Bud, and he told me why he believed I was ill and, more important, how I could regain my health.

"Jordan, you're still sick because you're not following the health plan in the Bible."

I had read more than three hundred health books in search for a cure, but I had never thought of the Bible as a health book. God's Word was a spiritual book, not a book on physical health.

But the more I thought about it, the more Bud's idea made sense. I decided to investigate what the Bible said about living a healthy life. Hope welled up in my heart, and that hope caused a slight grin to form. I hadn't smiled in a long time because, if truth be told, I had been miserable for nearly two years. *Maybe God does not want to just heal my body. Maybe He wants to do so with a plan that is totally duplicable, that anyone can follow. Maybe God wants to use my experience to help other believers escape the bondage of sickness and disease.*

I immediately grabbed my concordance and tore it open, looking up every Scripture in the Bible that had to do with health, food, or healing. What I learned is the basis for this book—that God's chosen people, the Israelites (who the Bible calls the world's healthiest people), lived a life totally separate from the rest of the world. A life based on the commandments of the God of Abraham, Isaac, and Jacob.

"Mom, I'm going to get well," I declared, "and God is going to use my illness for good. God isn't going to waste my pain."

A few weeks later, I flew to San Diego to live close to the man who told me about the Bible's health plan. By that time I was using a wheelchair, but my hope was in the Lord. I purchased a dilapidated RV and put myself in God's hands for forty days and offered my body as a living sacrifice.

Forty is a biblical number. The great Flood of Noah lasted forty days. Moses spent forty days on Mount Sinai receiving the Commandments from God. The spies from Exodus were out in the field forty days. Nineveh was allowed forty days to repent. Elijah and Jesus both fasted for forty days, and Jesus spent forty days on earth after His resurrection. Since time immemorial, God has transformed many a life spiritually and physically in forty days. I would devote forty days to the purpose of getting well God's way.

At a park near Mission Bay, I lowered my head and prayed, "Lord, I don't have much to give to You, but whatever I have is Yours. I'm going to take the next forty days to study Your Word, to see what You have to say about living a life that's physically, spiritually, mentally, and emotionally pleasing to You."

I feasted on the Word of God and ate what God said to eat. I learned principles of hygiene and studied everything that God told His people would make them healthy. I offered everything I had to the Lord and became that living sacrifice.

I'm here to tell you that God healed my body in forty days. I was physically reborn and gained twenty-nine pounds during that time. My healing wasn't instantaneous, but it was miraculous nonetheless.

During my illness, if you had asked me the one thing that I wanted from God, what would that have been? Without hesitation, I would have asked to be physically healed. So many times we ask God for something we are

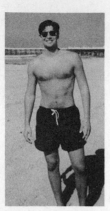

AFTER

desperate to receive, but He wants to give us much more. If you asked me today what is the greatest miracle God worked in my life, I wouldn't tell you that it was my physical healing, although that was a miracle. But I would tell you that the greatest miracle of my life is the passion, vision, and purpose that God birthed in my heart to help transform the health of His people, one life at a time.

AIMING HIGH

I left San Diego with a renewed sense of purpose and began asking the Lord to teach me how to help His people rebuild their bodies, God's temples. I began studying sports medicine, naturopathic medicine, nutrition, and natural therapies. I enrolled at the only naturopathic university in North America that taught from a biblically based curriculum.

I went on to receive doctoral degrees in naturopathic medicine and nutrition in 2001 and 2003, respectively. In my personal life, I met a beautiful young woman named Nicki, whom I married in 1999. After battling a two-and-a-half-year stint of infertility, we became the proud parents of Joshua Michael in May 2004.

Everyone knows someone—a family member, a loved one, a close friend, or a casual acquaintance—who is in poor health or is chronically ill. We may live in the richest country with a health-care system that is the envy of the world, but we are an amazingly unhealthy society. We fill up doctors' waiting rooms with aches and pains and ailments that cost billions of dollars annually to diagnose and treat. We overeat, fail to exercise, and wonder why we weigh more and get less out of life.

In the Battle of the Bulge, we're losing decisively, which carries all sorts of implications for our culture. One of the great political debates in Washington and statehouses today is how to pay for the nation's burgeoning health-care costs. But if fewer people were sick, we'd need less medical attention, which would mean insurance companies would pay on fewer claims, which would translate into lower premiums. Lower health-care costs would mean more of the uninsured could afford medical insurance. The fact is that we wouldn't have a health-care crisis if we didn't have so many unhealthy people in this country.

The latest crisis du jour is America's growing obesity problem. All you have to do is scan the newspaper or a newsmagazine and you'll come across an article about how we've become a fat, sick, and tired people. The statistics certainly bear up to any heavy scrutiny. Today, 65 percent of U.S. adults are classified as overweight by the Centers for Disease Control. Compare that to the early 1980s, when less than half (46 percent) of American adults were considered overweight.[1]

But that's not all. When you take a closer look at our overweight population, one-third of the adult American population is considered *obese*, meaning that they weigh at least fifty pounds over their ideal body weight. Then there are the morbidly obese—those who weigh three hundred, four hundred, or even five hundred pounds. According to a study performed by the *Archives of Internal Medicine,* the ranks of the extremely obese grew from one in two thousand in 1986 to one in four hundred in 2000.[2]

Being overweight predisposes one to all sorts of diseases and causes incredible amounts of stress on the body's organs, like the heart, lungs, and liver. Hips and knees break down from massive weight because they weren't designed to hold up a human being weighing something north of three hundred pounds. The liver, kidneys, and colon work overtime to process the gluttonous amounts of food and drink that pass the taste buds and travel down the gullet.

If Americans continue to become obese in these same heavy percentages, my one-year-old son, Joshua, may be part of the first generation to live *fewer* years than today's life expectancy, which is 72.5 years for men and 78.9 years for women, according to the National Center for Health Statistics. Furthermore, researchers say that if trends continue, one out of three children born after 2000 will develop type 2 diabetes, which leads to adult blindness and kidney failure. An even grimmer statistic is that those who develop type 2 diabetes before the age of fifteen have a shortened life expectancy of approximately fifteen years.[3]

As I mentioned before, I don't believe God's people are one bit healthier than the general population. While I've seen studies suggesting that those who go to church live longer, that doesn't mean we're living healthier. Bill Tanner of Christian Care Medi-Share, a nonprofit ministry in which members "share" one another's medical expenses, said that while believers in Jesus tend not to smoke or drink in the same numbers as everyone else, many in the church have not taken seriously the role that nutrition and exercise play in their lives. "All you have to do is go to any church potluck or listen to a gasping, overweight pastor, and you'll know what I mean," said Tanner.

I can say "amen" to that. Just thinking about the Wednesday night youth group and all the pizza, doughnuts, and ice cream makes my arteries harden. I can also remember a few church potlucks featuring the following main dishes: mounds of fried chicken and smoked barbecue—shredded pork drenched in a molasses-based sauce; the high-carb side dishes: greasy onion rings, funny-looking potato salad, and runny coleslaw; and the over-the-top desserts: three-inch-high lemon meringue pie, cinnamon-dusted peach cobbler, and apple pie topped with whipped cream.

The church has its fair share of sick and hurting people. These days when I speak at churches, I can't help hearing about the substantial number of people seeking prayer for cancer treatments, heart ailments, arthritis, and liver problems. From my vantage point, ill health is the number-one subject of prayer requests for churches and ministries. I've also taken notice of prayer requests for tough cases: children fighting diabetes, thirty-year-olds battling Parkinson's disease, and fifty-something schoolteachers exhibiting the first stages of neurological disorders such as dementia and Alzheimer's disease.

Don't we know that we're setting ourselves up for debilitating disease and/or early death by making poor choices in what we eat and how we live? Of course we do. You and I live in the Information Age, when our knowledge reportedly doubles every four to five years. To put things in a modern-day perspective, a weekday edition of the *New York Times* newspaper offers more information than the average person living in seventeenth-century England would come across in a lifetime. Although more and more information is available than at any other time in human history, I can't say we're any healthier in the twenty-first century. In fact, the research shows that we're becoming *less* healthy.

Information is not the same as knowledge. Knowledge is acquired only when one is able to understand, interpret, and synthesize information productively, toward some valued purpose. This distinction between information and knowledge is crucial. In *The Great Physician's Rx for Health and Wellness*, my goal is not merely to gather and present information, but to help you gain genuine knowledge, understanding, and, more importantly, wisdom.

A LACK OF KNOWLEDGE

When answering the question of why believers are not as healthy as they should be, I am reminded of what God spoke through His prophet Hosea thousands of years ago. In addressing the moral and spiritual decay of the nation of Israel, the Lord said, "My people are destroyed for lack of knowledge" (Hosea 4:6 NKJV). Notice that the Lord said, "My people," meaning believers, Christians, and churchgoers just like you and me. He wasn't talking about pagans or nonbelievers. He said, "My people are destroyed for lack of knowledge"!

I'm convinced that too many people coast through life without realizing that at least 80 percent of diseases are lifestyle-related. We must not be thinking about the significance of what we eat, the quantities we consume, and our sedentary, yet fast-paced, high-stress lifestyles; otherwise we wouldn't be surprised when a Southwest Airlines gate agent politely demands that we purchase a second seat.

Our collective "lack of knowledge" may be wrought from the explosion of too much *conflicting* information about diet and health. With so many voices shouting for attention, it's tough to know whom to believe. Many so-called expert recommendations of what constitutes healthy living are here today and gone tomorrow. Remember how ten years ago everyone was saying that eggs were bad for you? The nutritional logic traveled along these lines:

1. High cholesterol levels are bad for the heart.
2. Eating foods high in cholesterol raises cholesterol levels in the blood.

3. Eggs are high in cholesterol.
4. Therefore, eggs are bad for the heart, so don't eat eggs.

Now health experts are wising up to the benefits of the egg, a nutrient-dense food that packs six grams of protein, a bit of vitamin B-12, vitamin E, lutein, riboflavin, folic acid, calcium, zinc, iron, and essential fatty acids into a mere seventy-five calories. Eggs have the highest-quality protein of any food, except for mother's breast milk. So now the nutritional experts have egg on their faces, saying it's okay to eat them. In moderation, of course. (They have to cover their bases.)

The latest diets and the latest food fads come and go because people aren't looking at a single, constant source of good nutrition and healthy living—the Bible. It all began nearly four thousand years ago when God led the people away from Egypt. "Because I love you"—I'm paraphrasing what God told the Israelites—"I will give you commandments to make you a separate people. I am a jealous God. I want you as My own. I am going to give you ways to eat, ways to live, and ways to keep yourselves clean. Follow My way, and you will become a city on a hill. I will put you on a pedestal, and you will be My trophy."

When Moses led the Hebrews into the desert and across the Red Sea, Psalm 105:37 (NKJV) tells us that there was not one "feeble among His tribes." That's amazing, especially since historians believe that more than two million people were part of the Exodus—and they didn't leave anyone—sick or healthy, young or old—behind! Despite being in Egypt, the Israelites had followed God's health plan in a foreign land where they were enslaved.

You may be reading this and thinking, *It's too hard to follow a healthy lifestyle in today's world.* Try doing it while you're being whipped for not turning straw into brick fast enough! When the time came to gather their belongings and depart, they left Egypt as a vibrant, energetic, and healthy nation.

So there was not *one* feeble among all His tribes. Can you say that about your congregation? What about your place of work? What about your family? What about your life?

You can't argue with the way things turned out for the Israelites after they reached the Promised Land. Scripture tells us that the Israelites were healthier, had more wisdom, and provoked their neighbors to jealousy. Throughout history, the Jewish people have been the most hygienic and healthiest race on the planet—as long as they held true to God's commandments.

Their hygiene has protected them from virulent diseases. When the bubonic plague swept through Europe in the Middle Ages and wiped out more than a quarter of the population, many small pockets of observant Jews escaped the Black Death, and for that they attracted much persecution. Medieval cities were filthy places without modern sewers or garbage collection, and rats (which carried the fleas hosting the plague) lived in intimate contact with humans. The Jews, however, knew that rats were "unclean" animals and stayed clear of them. They followed God's simple hygiene commandments that the rest of the world thought were ridiculous. For instance, in the Middle Ages, people used a slop bucket as the household toilet, and they became so inured to having sewage around that they slept in close proximity to their own human waste.

Compare this form of dirty hygiene to the Jewish practice of burying human waste since the days of Exodus. Nor would Jews of the Middle Ages drink from city wells, because they knew the water was unclean. In order to stay kosher, Jews had to draw water from country springs.

Speaking from a hygienic standpoint, God's chosen people avoided the Black Death like, well, the plague. This shouldn't surprise us because the Jewish people have been keeping themselves separate and clean since they received this promise in Exodus 15:26:

> If you listen carefully to the voice of the LORD your God and do what
> is right in his eyes, if you pay attention to his commands and keep all
> his decrees, I will not bring on you any of the diseases I brought on the
> Egyptians, for I am the LORD, who heals you.

Think about the context of this Scripture. The Egyptians happened to be the most medically, culturally, and technologically advanced people in the world. They invented the calendar and hieroglyphics, a system of writing using characters in the form of pictures. They operated looms to weave cloth for clothing and made paper from papyrus reed plants. They used geometry to reset the boundaries of their fields after the Nile flooded. Two of the seven wonders of the ancient world lay within Egypt—the Lighthouse of Alexandria and the Great Pyramid of Giza. (And the Great Pyramid is the only surviving member of the seven wonders.)

On a medical note, they knew about diseases and attempted to treat them. Of course, the pharaohs and their families eventually succumbed to what ailed them, but we know what diseases caused their deaths because the Egyptians discovered a clever method of preserving bodies to remain lifelike. The process, which we call mummification, involved embalming the bodies and wrapping them in strips of linen.

When modern-day scientists unwrapped and studied these mummies thousands of years later, they determined that Pharaoh and his family suffered from health problems that may sound familiar to you: bone deterioration or osteoporosis, joint degeneration or arthritis, calcification of the arteries or heart disease, and malignancies similar to today's cancers. In other words, the most medically, culturally, and technologically advanced society was populated by men and women with subpar health.

Could it be that believers today—God's called-out people, the ecclesia, the church—are inheriting the health curses of Egypt rather than the health promises of Israel? These days, the United States of America is the world's supreme superpower, but statistically speaking, we can hardly be called a world leader in good health. This is why I believe—and am personally convicted— that we as God's people should offer our bodies as living sacrifices by following His ultimate health plan for us.

Let me conclude by offering four reasons why.

1. *When you offer your body as a living sacrifice by following God's ultimate health plan, you'll enjoy long life and peace.*

Although our time on earth comes with no ironclad guarantees—I learned that lesson as a twenty-year-old—I believe God desires that we live as long as He intended us to live. After all, He owns our bodies not only spiritually, but also physically. It's sad that so many people—good, productive people—die young needlessly and rob God of using their bodies for His glory.

The writer of Proverbs urged, "My son, do not forget my teaching, but keep my commands in your heart, for they will prolong your life many years and bring you prosperity" (3:1–2). I don't know about you, but I'm signing up for that long-term health plan.

We can't escape the fact that God set forth physical principles that govern our planet. Some may say, "If I get sick, I'll just count on God's supernatural healing." Or just before they step into the brightly lit fast-food restaurant, they may say, "I'll pray for God to change those double-deluxe bacon cheeseburgers into something healthy for me." I don't see that happening because God's principles for good health are like His principle of gravity. I wouldn't jump off the top of a ten-story building and pray that God would give me the legs of a cat, which would enable me to make a safe two-point landing without breaking all the bones in my body. Although He could make that happen, I wouldn't test Him, because He created the law of gravity. His law states that what goes up must come down; in other words, people who leap off tall buildings go splat on concrete sidewalks.

To those who may say, "What if I don't follow God's commandments involving health? Can I still get to heaven?" my response is, of course you'll get to heaven. You'll just get there a lot sooner.

2. *When you offer your body as a living sacrifice by following God's ultimate health plan, you'll live an abundant life.*

Jesus said, "I came that they might have life, and might have it abundantly" (John 10:10 NASB). God wants you to have an *abundant* life, a term I equate with *performance*, which is a word usually reserved for athletes and entertainers. In the Lord's eyes, however, all of us perform—stay-at-home moms, busy pastors, high-powered executives, and ambitious students.

Automobiles need a certain type of fuel. How do you find out which one? One sure way would be to open the glove compartment and reach for the owner's manual. The reason you can trust the owner's manual is that the same company that created the car also wrote the manual and knows every aspect of the car and how to maintain it so that it can perform to its full potential. In fact, the same people who wrote the manual conceived the car and knew all about it before actually building it. In a similar fashion, the Author and Perfecter of our lives gave us the Bible, which is His manufacturer's manual for our bodies' physical, spiritual, mental, and emotional well-being.

In the front or back of the owner's manual is "Gas Station Information," which states the recommended fuel for the automobile. That's where you learn whether you get off cheap (87 octane) or have to buy the premium stuff (93 octane). If your car calls for 93 octane but you feed it 87, what happens? You won't get optimal performance. The car won't perform the way the creator intended.

Our bodies come standard-equipped with highly tuned, robust engines requiring 93 octane, yet some of us persist in sticking 87 octane into the fuel tank. Perhaps that's why you're sputtering and not handling the road the way you need to. Some of you are even worse off: you're putting in diesel fuel and really gumming up the works.

A young Israelite named Daniel was asked to put the equivalent of diesel fuel into his 93-octane body at one time. It happened nearly twenty-six hundred years ago when he and three friends—captives of King Nebuchadnezzar—were drafted into the Babylonian army. The chief of the king's palace court said, "I need you guys to get up to speed with our advanced high-tech training, so we're going to serve you food from the king's kitchen— the very best." That would be the equivalent today of an NFL training table during summer camp—tons of great food for the warrior class.

Daniel knew that he and his buddies shouldn't eat from the king's training table because unclean meats would be served. "I have never defiled my body and gone against God's commandments," he said respectfully to the chief official. "Give us a chance to follow God's health plan. Give us ten days, and better yet, if we're not performing better than your army, we'll follow the king's advanced diet and health program."

Ten days later, Daniel and his friends had greater appearance, more energy, steadier countenances, and deeper wisdom. Scripture tells us that they subsisted on only fruits and vegetables, which can be a great short-term diet. I believe the reason Daniel ate only vegetable foods for those ten days was to avoid the king's meats, which were either unclean in and of themselves or were offered to idols. And you know what happened? King Nebuchadnezzar appointed them to his regular staff of advisors, where the king found their advice and wisdom to be "ten times better" (Dan. 1:20 NLT) than others who had his ear.

That's what I call living life abundantly. And guess who got the glory that day? It wasn't Daniel or his friends, but God. Don't you want to be a Daniel and transform your culture? Isn't it time you went against the grain and stood up for what you believe in? You can, by living the abundant life and changing your world to the glory of God. Because of Daniel's obedience to God and his courage to stand up for his beliefs, he not only changed his culture, but we are still reaping the benefits of the revelations that Daniel received from God as recorded in Scripture. It's like what my coauthor, Dr. David Remedios, is fond of saying: "Daniel became lion-proof one bite at a time."

By following the Great Physician's Rx, you, too, can be saved from the lion's den of ill health and disease.

3. *When you offer your body as a living sacrifice by following God's ultimate health plan, you'll honor your family.*

The best way to honor those who matter most to you—your spouse, your children, and your extended family—is by staying here on this earth for them. I'm the proud father of a one-year-old son who runs around the house with the cutest grin on his face. Joshua is so much fun to be around that I can hardly stand to leave him in the morning—and leaving to go out of town is nearly torture. I want to be there for my son—to be a father and a role model to show him God's love, just as I want to be there for my wife, Nicki, as a husband and best friend.

I recently spoke at a large church where I shared this message. At the end of the service, the pastor came onto the stage and told the congregation that what I said really hit home with him. He recounted how his father, a pastor and great man of God, died at the age of fifty-six, leaving behind a devoted wife and five children who would miss out on his love and wisdom. He would never get to hold any of his grandchildren. The pastor then went on to say that he really missed talking to his dad about the Lord and still misses the wisdom that his father imbued upon him.

What about you? Who counts on you to be around? Maybe you're serving

Are Believers Healthier Than Our Neighbors?

You would think that being a Christian, with its constraints on sexual behavior and attitudes regarding vices like smoking and excessive drinking, would set the table for a healthy lifestyle.

That's what you would think.

But Purdue University sociology professor Kenneth Ferraro believes that religious people are more likely to be overweight than the nonreligious.

The culprit?

Overeating, he says, may be the one sin that Christians fail to confront.

Although the Bible frowns upon gluttony—Proverbs 23:21 notes that "drunkards and gluttons become poor"—I think God's people are overweight because they eat the wrong foods, not because they indulge themselves with apple pie à la mode on Sunday afternoons.

Professor Ferraro released his study in 1998 and opined that overweight people find solace and acceptance in churches, which may explain his findings. Baptists were the heaviest, with Jewish, Muslim, and Buddhist adherents the least overweight.[4]

---

in a ministry. Maybe your coworkers, your employees, or your employer counts on you. God has a purpose for your life, and when you're called to serve Him in ministry, every minute is precious. Every year we have more to offer, not less, because we have wisdom and experience on our side. Use that wisdom to establish a health legacy for your future generations. In order to start a health legacy, you may have to take a look at yourself.

On many occasions, a mother will tell me that she has the toughest time getting her children to eat healthy: "All they want is junk, junk, junk—hot dogs, pizza, ice cream, candy, and soda."

As a new parent, I now realize the truth that I've been told for years:

children don't do what we say; they do what we do. Because of this, I often ask the mother, "Mom, what's your diet like?"

"Uhhhh, well, you know, I don't have time to eat well. I'm too busy."

Come on, parents. Start a health legacy by modeling a healthy lifestyle. If you teach your children the principles of good health by setting a good example, your children will reap a lifetime of health. Remember that Proverbs 22:6 (NKJV) tells us, "Train up a child in the way he should go, and when he is old he will not depart from it."

Following God's health plan has become a high priority in my life, but I wasn't given the best set of genes. You know what? I have decided to start a health legacy in my family, and I believe my son, Joshua, and my future generations will reap the rewards. What the devil meant for bad, God is using for good. Wouldn't you like to start a health legacy today and lay the foundation for a healthy future for all your generations?

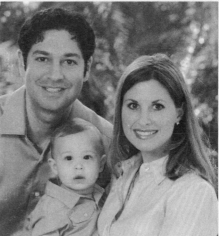

Jordan, Joshua, and Nicki Rubin

4. *When you offer your body as a living sacrifice, you'll honor God.*

Two thousand years ago, Jesus asked His disciples, "Who do the people say I am?" Then He turned to the wild one named Simon, and He asked him, "Who do you say I am?"

Simon Peter didn't flinch. "You are the Christ, the Son of the living God," he replied.

Blessed are you, Simon son of Jonah, for this revelation did not come from man, but by My Father in heaven. And I tell you that you are Peter [—I'm giving you a new name that means "rock" or "foundation"—]

and on this rock I will build my church [or ecclesia, which means "called-out people"] and the gates of Hades will not overcome it, responded Jesus. (See Matt. 16:13–18.)

Peter was called out, and in the same fashion, we are God's called-out people—His church. The fact that we make Sunday church services special is evidenced by the clothes we wear, the manners we keep, and the pleasantries we show to our neighbors and fellow churchgoers. I can still remember being told as a youngster to be "real good in church." Sometimes some of my Sunday school classmates would utter the word, "Don't say that!" Or Mom or Dad would hiss, "Can't you see that we're in church?"

Why do we act this way? Because we must believe that God can see us and hear us better in our church buildings than, say, our living rooms. So we're on our best behavior on Sunday mornings in church, even though we slip a little between Monday and Saturday.

Thank God for the wonderful and beautiful churches we have in this country to worship in. So how would you feel if someone walked up the middle aisle of your church with a bag of rotting garbage over his right shoulder? Shocked, right? Then how would you feel if he dumped its stinking contents all over the place? Blasphemy, right? You'd be furious at that individual for dumping garbage inside your beautiful church.

Yet every day God's people all over the world are poisoning their bodies—God's temples—without giving it a second thought. Paul asked, "Do you not know that you are the temple of God and that the Spirit of God dwells in you? If anyone defiles the temple of God, God will destroy him. For the temple of God is holy, which temple you are" (1 Cor. 3:16–17 NKJV).

Notice that the apostle Paul was writing to the church in Corinth, not to unbelievers. I believe that the promise of this passage is coming to pass, and we are seeing God's children suffering and dying. Your body is God's temple here on earth, and He's given you everything you need to live a long, abundant life that honors your loved ones and the Lord of the universe.

PAYING A GREAT PRICE

I'll never forget my first car, a Honda Prelude. Since I used my allowance and busboy earnings to pay for it, I made sure I took extra care of this beauty. I washed it often and waxed it four times a year. I kept it in the garage at night. I even read the owner's manual!

Why did I baby this bucket of aluminum, plastic, and vinyl? Because I had paid a great price for it—all my savings from years of allowance and after-school jobs. God has paid the greatest price for you. He shed every last drop of life. He gave you His only begotten Son, who died a horrible death on a Roman tree. Because He paid such a great sum for you, He gave you instructions on how to get the most out of life for seventy, eighty, ninety, or one hundred years on earth. He gave you an owner's manual to help you live and to honor Him physically, spiritually, mentally, and emotionally.

Since it's no mistake that you're holding this book in your hands, I believe God is speaking to you about starting your own health legacy, which is why I challenge you to offer your body as a living sacrifice, especially in view of His incredible mercy and goodness toward you.

To lead you on your journey to healthy living, I will spend the next seven chapters handing you seven keys that will unlock your health potential. I believe each and every one of us has a God-given health potential that can be unlocked only with the right keys. I want to challenge you to give God the next seven weeks of your life to incorporate these timeless principles and allow God to transform your health and your life.

Many people have asked me, "Is it ever too late to start God's health plan?" The only way you could start this program too late would be if you started tomorrow. May God bless you as you walk through the straight and narrow gate that leads to good health and longer life.

Beloved, I pray that you may prosper in all things
and be in health, just as your soul prospers.
—3 JOHN 1:2 (NKJV)

What's Behind the Great Physician's Rx?

R𝒙   You can search through the Bible for the phrase "Great Physician," but you won't find that description in any of the sixty-six books of God's Word. Yet ask any churchgoer today who the Great Physician is, and you'll have a quick answer: Jesus Christ, the Son of God.

How did our Lord become known as the Great Physician?

William Hunter, a nineteenth-century Methodist clergyman who served as a pastor in Pennsylvania and Virginia, wrote three collections of hymns during his lifetime, including his best-known effort, "The Great Physician Now Is Near," penned in 1859. The opening stanza goes like this:

The great Physician now is near,
The sympathizing Jesus;
He speaks the drooping heart to cheer;
O hear the voice of Jesus!

Pastor Hunter was probably inspired by the seventy-five references to the healing work of Christ in the New Testament, including Matthew 9:12: "On hearing this, Jesus said, 'It is not the healthy who need a doctor, but the sick.'"

David Stevens, M.D., author of *Jesus, M.D.*, said that the four Gospels record more instances of Jesus' healing than of His preaching or teaching. "That is why down through the centuries, one of the cherished names for Christ has been the Great Physician," Dr. Stevens stated.

The "Great Physician" appellation is entirely appropriate in the context of good health, and I strongly believe the Bible is an authoritative source on what we should eat and not eat, and how we should live. God has written to us a prescription for good health; it's up to us to fill that prescription every day of our lives.

KEY #1

Eat to Live

The LORD alone led him, and there was no foreign god with him. He made him ride in the heights of the earth, that he might eat the produce of the fields; He made him draw honey from the rock, and oil from the flinty rock; curds from the cattle, and milk of the flock, with fat of lambs; and rams of the breed of Bashan, and goats, with the choicest wheat; and you drank wine, the blood of the grapes.

—Deuteronomy 32:12–14 (NKJV)

After our first child, Joshua, was born on Memorial Day weekend in 2004, my wife, Nicki, bore the brunt of the feeding duties. It was up to her to nurse Joshua with the best nutrients that God in His wisdom devised—a mother's breast milk.

Whenever Joshua cried during the night, Nicki rubbed her tired eyes and dutifully got out of bed to feed our infant. I often joined her to show my support and love, and when I say *often,* I mean it. Okay, maybe it wasn't as often as Nicki wanted, but I woke up most of the time. I was just as excited as she was about this new life God had given and entrusted us with.

Sometime before his first birthday, an interesting thing happened: it was becoming apparent to both of us that Nicki was not producing enough milk to satisfy our big, bouncing boy. A nursing mother normally produces between twenty-three and twenty-seven ounces of milk per day, but that wasn't enough for Joshua, who communicated his desire for more milk through wailing tears. We needed to supplement his diet of mother's milk with his first solid foods.

Uppermost in our minds was introducing his little stomach to foods healthy and easily digestible. I decided that his first solid food should be a cooked egg yolk from a soft-boiled or coddled egg. To prepare this nutritional powerhouse, I began by boiling water—yes, I know how to do that—and carefully placing an egg, which is high in omega-3 fatty acids, vitamins A and D, and lutein, into the water. I let the solitary egg boil for three or four minutes, or until the yoke was soft and warm.

When the egg was finished cooking, I rinsed it with cool water. Then I cracked the shell and removed the yolk from the egg white, which I didn't plan to serve to Joshua because egg whites can be highly allergenic to infants.

Like any proud pop, I'm happy to report that Joshua loved his first bites of solid food—and showed us his bright orange cheeks to prove it. A week later, I introduced him to mashed pieces of fresh, organic Florida avocado, which has an abundance of enzymes, healthy fats, vitamin E, and fiber. He was all over that avocado, although he asked me several times where the tortilla chips were. (Just joking.)

I believe more than ever that one of the best things Nicki and I can give Joshua is a healthy start in life as he weans himself from breast milk and begins eating solid foods. We want to raise Joshua to "eat to live"—the first key to unlocking your health potential—not to "live to eat." To help him understand what that means, Nicki and I will be teaching our son these important concepts: eat what God created for food, and eat food in a form that is healthy for the body.

Scripture suggests three boundaries that we can use to identify what God intended for us to eat, according to my friend Rex Russell, M. D., author of *What the Bible Says About Healthy Living*, and they are noted here.

1. When God calls an item food:

God said, "I give you every seed-bearing plant on the face of the whole earth and every tree that has fruit with seed in it. They will be yours for food." (Gen. 1:29)

"You will eat the plants of the field." (Gen. 3:18)

"These are the animals you may eat: the ox, the sheep, the goat, the deer, the gazelle, the roe deer, the wild goat, the ibex, the antelope, and the mountain sheep." (Deut. 14:4–5)

2. When God brings items to His people as a gift:

"Also the food I provided for you—the fine flour, olive oil and honey I gave you to eat." (Ezek. 16:19)

3. If Jesus ate or served an item:

"He took the seven loaves and the fish, and when he had given thanks, he broke them and gave them to the disciples, and they in turn to the people." (Matt. 15:36)[1]

Dr. Russell has made a list of foods that Scripture tells us are designed for health and that may be enjoyed. They were created for food, as opposed to foods that are changed or converted into something that humans think is better. If any of the following foods are altered, they lose many of their health benefits. Here is Dr. Russell's list, followed by where each item is mentioned in Scripture:

- almonds (Gen. 43:11)
- barley (Judg. 7:13)
- beans (Ezek. 4:9)
- bread (1 Sam. 17:17)
- broth (Judg. 6:19)
- cakes (2 Sam. 13:8 [NKJV], and probably not the kind with frosting)
- cheese (Job 10:10)
- cucumbers, onions, leeks, melons, and garlic (Num. 11:5)
- curds of cow's milk (Deut. 32:14)
- figs (Num. 13:23)

- fish (Matt. 7:10)
- fowl (1 Kings 4:23)
- fruit (2 Sam. 16:2)
- game (Gen. 25:28)
- goat's milk (Prov. 27:27)
- grain (Ruth 2:14)
- grapes (Deut. 23:24)
- grasshoppers, locusts, and crickets (Lev. 11:22)
- herbs (Exod. 12:8)
- honey (Isa. 7:15) and wild honey (Ps. 19:10)
- lentils (Gen. 25:34)
- meal (Matt. 13:33 KJV)
- pistachio nuts (Gen. 43:11)
- oil (Prov. 21:17)
- olives (Deut. 28:40)
- pomegranates (Num. 13:23)
- quail (Num. 11:32)
- raisins (2 Sam. 16:1)
- salt (Job 6:6)
- sheep (Deut. 14:4)
- sheep's milk (Deut. 32:14)
- spices (Gen. 43:11)
- veal (Gen. 18:7–8)
- vegetables (Prov. 15:17)
- vinegar (Num. 6:3)[2]

These foods are nutritional gold mines, filled with essentials for building healthy cells in your body. God's dietary guidelines contain no refined or processed carbohydrates, no altered or damaged fats, and no artificial sweeteners. The typical American diet strays far from God's design with its glamorous array of techno-foods replete with empty calories, refined carbohydrates, and woefully inadequate nutrition. A diet based on eating whole and natural foods harvested directly from the Creator's bounty, however, nourishes and satisfies us. That's one more reminder why it's important to (1) eat foods that God created and (2) in a form that is healthy for the body.

You may have read those two statements and wondered how they apply to your life. Perhaps you're thinking, *It can't be this simple.* Well, it is and it isn't. While fresh fruits, farm-grown vegetables, and protein-rich meat are readily available in our land, the genius of man has figured out how to prepare, manufacture, cook, microwave, and market mass-produced foods in ways not always healthy for us. Too many of the so-called foods sold in our nation's supermarkets and too many of the meals prepared in restaurants are not really food because they were not created by God but were largely put together in man-made laboratories.

Like sheep following the next one off a cliff, we are passing through checkout lines with shopping carts filled with processed foods missing many of the nutrients that God intended us to receive. As for eating out, don't get me started on how we've become a country that loves deep-fried, greasy food high in calories, high in fat, high in sugar, and—in most people's minds—high in taste. When you add it all up, the acronym for the "standard American diet" is SAD—and what nearly 300 million Americans eat each and every day *is* sad. For adults, this usually means:

- a breakfast of a Danish or a bowl of sugary cereal drenched in 2 percent milk and a cup of caffeinated coffee stirred with nondairy creamer and artificial sweeteners.
- a midmorning snack in the employee lunchroom—a glazed doughnut or a plain bagel smeared with margarine or cream cheese.
- a lunch consisting of a turkey sandwich (made from processed turkey breast) on white bread, some kind of chips, and a diet soft drink.
- an afternoon snack from the vending machine—a candy bar and another soft drink bubbling with sugar or artificial sweetener.

- a dinner of heated-up frozen pizza (pepperoni or Canadian bacon) and a salad bowl of iceberg lettuce served with a creamy, full-fat ranch dressing.
- a dessert of chocolate chip ice cream, topped with chocolate sauce.

I'm vastly oversimplifying things, of course, but I'm also not taking into account that *one-fourth* of the American adult population frequents a fast-food restaurant *every single day* of the year.[3]

EAT CLOSE TO THE NATURAL SOURCE

Going back to the example of the typical American diet that I just described, which foods were in a form that God created? One could say that God created the coffee beans and the iceberg lettuce, but everything else was mass-produced in some industrial bakery or far-off factory using ingredients that had been stripped clean of nearly all the nutrients and pumped up with additives and preservatives.

The Great Physician's Rx for Health and Wellness calls for eating foods as close to the natural source as possible. This "natural source" was first described in the opening chapter of Genesis when God said, "Let the waters swarm with fish and other life. Let the skies be filled with birds of every kind . . . Let the earth bring forth every kind of animal—livestock, small animals, and wildlife" (1:20, 24 NLT).

After God created all these animals, we learn that when the Lord God made the heavens and earth:

> there were no plants or grain growing on the earth, for the LORD God had not sent any rain. And no one was there to cultivate the soil. But water came up out of the ground and watered all the land. And the LORD God formed a man's body from the dust of the ground and breathed into it the breath of life. And the man became a living person. (Gen. 2:5–7 NLT)

That first man—Adam—was probably hungry before his first coffee break, but there were no vending machines or Jack in the Box drive-thrus in the Garden of Eden. Instead, there was plenty of low-hanging fruit for him to grab and eat, even though Scripture does not reveal what kind of fruit he preferred. Knowing that the fruit was grown in the perfect and pristine Garden of Eden, we have to believe that it tasted great and was brimming with nutrients.

Later on, when Adam and Eve had left their bite marks on fruit from a tree that God had told them *not* to eat from, the days of *la dolce vita* were over. After their banishment from the Garden, the First Couple had to "scratch a living" (Gen. 3:17 NLT) from the fields by the sweat of their brows, but at least they were eating natural grains. (The Bible says that Noah and his family were the first to receive permission to eat meat.)

Adam and Eve and their descendants ate foods in forms healthy for their bodies, which speaks to the second foundational principle of eating. When we eat foods that God created in forms that are healthy for us, our bodies are nourished and able to perform at optimal levels. Foods that God created are what we call "natural."

So much of what passes for food these days is as far from natural as a snowboarder skiing uphill. On supermarket shelves from Portland, Oregon, to Portland, Maine, you'll find that most of the food is man-made—something God did not create. That's because food-manufacturing conglomerates have excelled in the last one hundred years at taking something that God created—wheat, for example—and turning it into something totally unhealthy by stripping out the God-given nutrients and adding chemicals by the truckload. A tube of Pringles, which are cloned crisps of processed potatoes and additives, offers little, if any, real nutritional content. That's because Pringles are not food in a form healthy for the body.

The difference between what our American culture stomachs and what people eat elsewhere was demonstrated in the days after the horrific tsunami struck Southeast Asia. Western aid groups rushed in, and in the Sri Lankan town of Galle, the famished refugees opened cardboard boxes packed in the United States only to discover cans of . . . mixed vegetables in cream sauce. When the Sri Lankan people attempted to eat the canned vegetables, they got sick because their stomachs weren't used to digesting vegetables swimming in a chemical-laden, cream-based liquid. Their bodies preferred their green beans and corn fresh.

The more convenient foods are, the less healthy and farther away from God's design they are. You see it every time you walk into a supermarket. Sure, the grocery chains sell fresh fruits, vegetables, and meats, but few of those foods are organically grown or produced. Instead, supermarkets offer a tremendous variety of convenience foods—ready to eat or ready to be heated up in the microwave. In our time-starved society, the quicker dinner gets on the table, the better.

If that's the way you want to shop, your neighborhood supermarket will entice you to buy from the inventory of several thousand different brands totaling one million items. The canned goods and breakfast cereals and golden apples are stacked perfectly; nothing is out of place. Track lighting illuminates the fresh produce, while an abundance of cheery signs remind shoppers about the "Extra Savings!" The aisles are wide enough for two carts to pass each other, but not too wide: grocers want anything that catches your eye to be at arm's length. At both ends of the aisles, end caps feature specials of the week, like twelve-ounce bags of Lay's Cheddar and Sour Cream Potato Chips for $1.99.

In supermarkets you can find 157 kinds of breakfast cereal, 22 brands or types of peanut butter, and 25 brands of chocolate chip cookies. Despite this great variety, most of these food items are not even *close* to a food that God created in a form that is healthy for the body. Earlier I mentioned one of the staples of most diets around the world—wheat. After the harvest, wheat stalks are trucked to flour mills and rinsed with various chemical bleaches that sound like a vocabulary test from high school biology class: nitrogen oxide, chlorine, chloride, nitrosyl, and benzoyl peroxide. (By the way, benzoyl peroxide is a popular ingredient in over-the-counter acne medications.) The result is that half of the healthy fatty acids are lost in the milling process, as well as the wheat germ and bran, which contain vitamins and fiber. By removing most of the naturally occurring nutrients and adding chemicals and a few isolated and synthetic vitamins and minerals, we've managed to take a healthy food that's been on families' tables for centuries—usually in the form of bread, pasta, or baked goods—and turn it into one of the most highly allergenic, difficult-to-digest substances.

After processing, the "enriched flour"—whoever came up with calling denuded wheat "enriched flour" deserves some sort of marketing award—is packed up and shipped to bakeries, where it becomes the main ingredient in bread and a zillion other food products. (If you read your labels, much of the "wheat bread" found in supermarkets is made from—you guessed it—white enriched flour.)

I'm happy to report that whole wheat bread made from unprocessed whole grain flour, which is how God created wheat to be milled, is becoming more readily available as customers demand it. I wonder sometimes, though, if we should follow the lead of the Swiss government, which places a tax on the sale of white bread to make whole wheat bread cheaper.

Producing foods as cheaply as possible is the mantra of today's agribusiness. Another heavily processed commodity is sugar, which is found in nearly every man-made food, from ketchup to peanut butter to teriyaki sauce. Sugar comes to us from sugarcane, which is then processed 99.9 percent. I'm sure research scientists are working overtime to remove the last one-tenth of 1 percent in sugarcane that's healthy.

Biochemists are also working on ways to preserve foods for longer and longer shelf lives since all foods eventually lose their freshness and rot. In biblical times, people didn't have the option of freezing food or storing it in a refrigerator. They ate food fresh from the field, fresh out of the oven, or fresh from the fire. They also preserved foods for short periods by the process known as fermentation or culturing. They didn't attach a "shelf life" to foods in those days.

In our culture, because of refrigeration, we're able to preserve food longer than it normally should be healthy. I have an Australian friend, a bread maker and fermentation expert, who bakes with only whole grains. He believes that the invention of the refrigerator has been one of the worst things to ever happen to our health. Since we *can* refrigerate foods, we fill our refrigerators and freezers with too many convenience foods that are unhealthy for us instead of buying fresh foods that have to be eaten right away, lest they spoil. In most instances, the more convenient a food is, the more apt it is to be unhealthy and farther away from God's design.

People in biblical times did have a way to preserve foods, which was fermentation. The Israelites discovered that fermenting foods made them healthier and easier to digest, as opposed to today's preservatives, which rely on chemical compounds to keep the food from spoiling. Americans think that every household in the world has a refrigerator, but in various developing countries, as well as significant pockets of Europe, Asia, and South America, refrigeration is reserved for the well-to-do. Everyone else relies on fermentation to preserve foods and beverages as a means of protection from dangerous bacteria.

Fermentation—the culturing or natural processing of foods with the intentional growth of bacteria, yeast, or mold—has a long history. The Chinese have fermented cabbage for centuries. The Romans also learned to ferment cabbage, or what is known today as sauerkraut. Eastern Europeans discovered ways to pickle green tomatoes, peppers, and lettuce. Asians became skilled at preparing elaborate fermented foods such as kimchi, a condiment composed of cabbage, other vegetables, and seasonings. And in nearly every culture, dairy products were used to make lacto-fermented foods such as yogurt, kefir, cheese, cottage cheese, and cultured cream (also known as crème fraîche).

Every sauce and condiment has its beginnings as a fermented food and throughout history has always been healthy. The Chinese are generally credited with inventing ketchup, which started out as a fermented fish brine sauce known as *ke-tsiap*. When sailors brought stone jars of *ke-tsiap* home to England, they added pickled cucumbers (another fermented food) with kidney beans and oysters. Then English settlers in New England added tomatoes in the late 1700s, and before you knew it, McDonald's was handing out ten-gram packets of ketchup by the millions.

Today's ketchup, however, is loaded with vinegar and sugar and corn syrup, which is only one more example of how we have taken these great and wonderful foods and made them extremely poor for our health. Condiments such as ketchup and mustard have ceased to be aids to digestion, as they used to be, and are now used to give food a little more tang.

TURNING A CORNER

As you can probably surmise by now, I'm a proponent of natural foods grown organically, foods that God created for us to eat in a form that's healthy for the body. These principles are core to the Maker's Diet, an eating plan that I introduced in my first book, *Patient, Heal Thyself* (published in 2002), and discussed in great detail in *The Maker's Diet* (released in 2004). The Maker's Diet is based on the Bible, proven through history, and confirmed by science.

Eating foods produced sustainably, which are organically grown or raised, is foundational to the Maker's Diet. What do I mean when I say "produced sustainably"? Regarding fruits and vegetables, this refers to a system of farming that maintains and replenishes soil fertility without the use of toxic and persistent pesticides and fertilizers. Organic agricultural practices cannot ensure that products are completely free of residues, although methods are used to minimize pollution from air, soil, and water. Organic foods are minimally processed without artificial ingredients, preservatives, or irradiation (like from a microwave oven) to maintain the integrity of the food.

Most people, when they think of organic food, picture a head of leafy lettuce or plump red tomatoes fresh from the vine. Organic foods are much more than that: they include cereals, dairy products, and meats, the latter coming from livestock that graze on unsprayed fields of grass and are fed with organic feed, not pumped up with antibiotics or growth hormones. Organic food production costs more than conventional foods since larger and more expensive demands are placed upon the producer.

It's less expensive for commercial farmers to raise crops inorganically because they've adopted methods that rely on dousing their fields with chemical pesticides, herbicides, and fertilizers. These synthetic fertilizers stimulate rapid plant growth, but they bring along unintended circumstances: the fertilizers are made up of nitrogen salts, which return little, if any, vital minerals to the soil. Thus, the nutritive value of foods grown in these soils has declined significantly in the last hundred years. All told, Americans are subsisting on a diet of nutrient-poor foods of both plant and animal origin.

The word is getting out that there's a healthier option, which is why the latest buzzword these days is *organic*. Consumers concerned about taste and quality are becoming more demanding in what they eat, and "Organically Grown" is seen as the new Good Housekeeping seal of approval. Even the nation's largest producer of snack chips, Frito-Lay, has released its first-ever line of snacks made with organic ingredients. Now you can buy Tostitos Organic Blue Corn Tortilla Chips, Lay's Natural Country BBQ Potato Chips, or Natural Cheetos White Cheddar Puffs, all made from organic grains.

Hmm. Many people intuitively know that when they find the magic word *organic* labeled on the package or signage, that means it's something better for them to eat. With thousands of food growers and manufacturers jumping on the organic bandwagon—and trying to claim that their product was organic when maybe it really wasn't—the U.S. Department of Agriculture stepped in and passed new regulations for the organic produce industry in 2001. This USDA organic logo gives consumers more confidence that whatever is labeled "organic" adheres to the stated definition that the food must be free of genetically modified organisms, was produced without pesticides or synthetic fertilizers for plant foods, and must be free from hormones and antibiotics for animal foods.

A Look at Other Diets

The Great Physician's Rx for Health and Wellness relies on our eating natural, organic whole foods, properly prepared, to unlock nutrients to fuel and replenish our bodies. So what does that look like in practice? How do we put it all together?

I talked about the explosion of diet and nutritional information in the introduction. These days, all you have to do is watch an afternoon of TV talk shows, and you'll hear plenty of conflicting nutritional advice from health and wellness authors talking up their latest ideas—and hawking their books.

Listen, I would love to get on those shows so that I can join the debate and share the biblical truths for health, but I'm amazed at what passes for the "gospel truth" about living a healthy life. There is so much conflicting information out there that I don't know how the public—listening with half an ear anyway—keeps it all straight. The right health information comes from the Bible, history, and science—in that order.

Back when I was a 104-pound stick figure in the mid-1990s, low-fat, high-carbohydrate diets popularized by engineer Nathan Pritikin and Dean Ornish, M.D., were making the rounds on afternoon talk shows. The Pritikin diet is an almost vegetarian regimen that encourages the consumption of large amounts of whole grains and vegetables. The Ornish diet is a vegetarian diet high in grains and legumes (like beans and peas). It calls for avoidance of foods containing cholesterol and saturated fat, and the diet severely limits all foods containing fats, including coconuts, nuts, seeds, avocados, chocolate, and olives. In a nutshell, so to speak, the Ornish diet is 10 percent fat, 20 percent protein, and 70 percent carbohydrates, compared to the typical American diet, which is 45 percent fat, 25 percent protein, and 30 percent carbohydrates.

People listened—and voted with their buying choices. That's when we started seeing store shelves stocked with low-fat, reduced-fat, and fat-free versions of everything from peanut butter to ice cream. *Step right up. Get your fat-free blueberry muffins right here. . . .* The problem with fat-free blueberry muffins, besides tasting like sugar-frosted cardboard, is that they have nearly the same amount of calories as the full-fat version.

It turns out that the idea of taking the fat out of foods to reduce the total caloric intake *did not* stop Americans from getting fatter. In fact, we have gotten *heavier* in the last decade, as witnessed by all the newspaper articles about the runaway U.S. "obesity epidemic."

After the low-fat craze came the low-carb vogue, which is where we are today. The evangelists leading the low-carb movement are two cardiologists: Dr. Robert C. Atkins (who died in 2003) and Dr. Arthur Agatston, creators of the Atkins Diet and the South Beach Diet, respectively. Their premise is that reducing the intake of carbohydrates like bread, pasta, and rice will reduce insulin levels and cause your body to burn excess body fat for fuel.

Although low-carb diets offer improvements in insulin and blood sugar, these health plans call for a high consumption of meat products that God calls unclean (as I'll detail shortly), encourage the consumption of artificial sweeteners, and allow only small amounts of nutrient-rich fruits and vegetables. These low-carb diets point adherents toward highly processed snack foods, such as pork rinds, and food bars loaded with chemicals, which do not embrace my second criterion: we are to consume foods in forms healthy for the body.

From my interaction with church folks around the country, I've found that Christians have latched on to the low-carb craze popularized by the Atkins and South Beach diets, and to some extent, the Zone diet by Barry Sears. But there's more than one way to starve yourself, as the old joke goes. Let's take a closer look at other popular diets.

THE VEGETARIAN DIET

Vegetarianism is still popular among Christians, but it depends upon what your definition of *vegetarian* is. Not all vegetarians are created equal, as you will see:

- Lacto vegetarians do not eat any animal flesh, but they do eat dairy products.
- Ovo vegetarians do not eat flesh or milk products, but they do eat eggs.
- Lacto-ovo vegetarians do not eat animal foods, but they do eat eggs and dairy.
- Semi-vegetarians do not eat red meat, but they will eat fish, eggs, and dairy products. Some semi-vegetarians claim they can eat chicken as well, but I don't see how you can call yourself a semi-vegetarian when you eat poultry.
- Vegans do not eat any animal products at all, choosing to rely on plant-based food for their nutrition. Vegans are so extreme that some won't eat anything that comes from a creature—like honey from bees.

My Take

I don't consider lacto-ovo vegetarians to be true vegetarians, although I think it's healthy to eat free-range eggs and organic dairy products whether you choose to eat meat or not. Vegans are probably healthier than strict vegetarians (who eat mostly cooked grains) because they are eating most of their foods raw, which makes them easily digestible and high in many vitamins and minerals. Vegans are still missing crucial nutrients, however.

If you're a vegan or a vegetarian—and you're just about to heave this book against a wall—hear me out a little longer. If you don't see yourself eating meat or any food that comes from an animal source again—I say "again" because the vast majority of us consumed animal foods at one time or another—then you need to optimize your health by consuming plenty of omega-3 fatty acids, which are found in flaxseed and flaxseed oil. You also need to consume healthy, saturated fats found in coconuts and coconut products, and monounsaturated fats from olives, olive oil, macadamia nuts, and avocados. Consume your grains in raw, soaked, or sprouted form, and make sure that your nuts and seeds are soaked so that they don't have too many enzyme inhibitors and are easy to digest. While it's good to eat some foods in a raw form—such as many fruits and vegetables—some foods are easier to digest when cooked, such as broccoli, cauliflower, and many beans and legumes.

At the end of the day, though, I don't believe a vegetarian or vegan diet is the healthy way to go through life. I've studied this issue, and I've been particularly influenced by the teaching of Stephen Byrnes, Ph.D., author of *The Myths of Vegetarianism.*[4] Dr. Byrnes says that many vegetarian health claims cannot be substantiated, while others are simply false and dangerous.

Here are several myths that he knocked down:

Myth #1: The human body is not designed for meat consumption. To the contrary, Dr. Byrnes says. Our physiology indicates that we are omnivores, and an in-depth comparison of the human digestive system reveals that it's closer in anatomy to the carnivorous dog than the herbivorous sheep.

Myth #2: Meat contains numerous harmful toxins. Some claim that animal flesh is loaded with poisons and toxins, such as the germ that causes mad cow disease and salmonella. I agree that commercially raised livestock are filled with hormones, nitrates, and pesticides, which is why I advocate eating range-fed organic and pasture-fed meat. Mad cow disease, or bovine spongiform encephalopathy (BSE), is another concern to keep an eye on, but outbreaks have been far and few between, especially in this country. Eating organic beef is a great way to avoid BSE since there are strict rules prohibiting cows from eating parts of other diseased cows.

Myth #3: Vegetarians live longer and have more energy than meat eaters. Vegetarians like to say that they live ten years longer than the meat-eating population, but again, those claims appear to be anecdotal. Little research has been done on vegetarians' longevity, although one study showed that while vegetarians have lower rates of heart disease, their death rates for all causes of death were higher.[5]

As for the question about vegetarians having more energy, studies have shown that athletes who "carbo-loaded" before a big race or athletic event had less endurance than those who "fat-loaded" with a juicy steak the night before competing.

I think God designed our bodies to eat meat, and it is certainly biblical to eat animal flesh. The Bible recounts meat being eaten by Abraham, Isaac, Jacob, Moses, and David. Jesus ate fish when He performed the miracle feeding of the five thousand, when He sat down with the disciples at the Last Supper, and then at a meal after the Resurrection. Our bodies need properly raised meat for us to perform at our best.

Plant foods are extremely beneficial for us, yet they do not contain all the essential amino acids found in animal proteins. Our bodies need fat-soluble vitamins, particularly vitamins A and D, and while plant foods contain precursors to vitamin A and we can get vitamin D from the sun interacting with our skin, we need to eat meat to get optimal amounts of essential fat-soluble vitamins.

I've heard a lot of vegetarians say, "I can't eat meat because it isn't what it used to be. Today's meat is loaded with chemicals and hormones."

My response is fairly simple: Today's lettuce is pretty toxic as well. Every food group has been subjected to man's abuse of this earth and all the pollution we've heaped upon it. Vegetable foods are no different.

It's all about quality. If you buy organic, if you shop for sustainably produced animal food, then you're purchasing some of the healthiest food you can buy, especially if it's prepared properly. This includes dairy, this includes poultry, and this includes fish and eggs. All of these foods are wonderful sources of concentrated nutrients that do not, contrary to popular belief, contribute to heart disease or introduce toxins into the body.

The Low-Carb Diet

It's the new scarlet letter—the red letter *A* logo that's stamped on foods qualifying them as Atkins products. The Atkins seal of approval means that the food is carbohydrate-friendly to those on the low-carb lifestyle. You also probably noticed that restaurants have scrambled to update their menus with Atkins-friendly choices. While some studies demonstrate that those on the Atkins, South Beach, Zone, or Sugar Busters diet lose weight in the short term, the jury is still out over whether people can maintain their weight loss and their health over the long term.

I've already talked a little about low-carb diets, which limit carbohydrates so that the body can burn fat. The basic science behind the low-carb approach is this: reduce your intake of high-carbohydrate foods, such as white flour and sugar, and increase your intake of high-protein sources, such as meat, fish, and dairy. At first blush, following the Atkins diet looks like you're robbing the bank: you can gorge yourself with steaks, bacon, creams, cheeses, and eggs to your heart's content, but don't you dare reach for a bread roll.

Eating rolls, pasta, and other high-carbohydrate foods causes your body to produce excess insulin in the bloodstream, which leads to weight gain and other health problems. If there is too much insulin in the bloodstream, the body responds by turning the sugar into fat. Hence, if you cut way back on high-carb foods, you'll produce less insulin, which cuts down on fat storage. Strict reduction of carbohydrate intake induces a process known as *ketosis*, in which the body produces something known as ketones and uses fat as the preferred fuel rather than carbohydrates. Many people on low-carb diets notice a more efficient metabolism and a suppression of hunger urges. This is why low-carb diets are also referred to as *ketogenic* diets.

My Take

Low-carb diets are attractive because you lose weight quickly when you're on them, but the weight comes right back on once you resume eating carbohydrates, such as baked potatoes, bread, or fettuccini. Ketogenic diets are extremely high in fat and protein, which is to be expected when you eat so much meat and saturated fat, and that may not necessarily be good for you. Besides, I've long felt that the high consumption of carbohydrates doesn't make you fat: it's the overconsumption of the wrong foods—such as carbohydrates high in calories and low in nutrients—that keeps the pounds resting in the midsection.

My biggest beef with low-carb diets is their reliance on biblically unclean meats and artificial sweeteners, and the lack of emphasis on the quality of foods. In short, popular low-carb diets regularly break both of the eating principles that I believe in: they recommend things that God did not create for food, and they recommend foods in a form not healthy for the body.

NEW-AGE DIETS

In the midst of my two-year health crisis, I grasped at many dietary straws. Some were vegetarian-based; others were based on Eastern philosophy such as macrobiotics. If I was attuned with my "universal consciousness," I could achieve "unity and holistic health" through "visualization" and "letting it be."

I refused to be taken in by the gobbledygook, and so should you. You'll find *The Great Physician's Rx for Health and Wellness* to be biblically based and scientifically sound. It's a plan that is sure to help your body, God's temple, achieve the health that you've always dreamed of.

The Creator's Basic Food Groups

You are what you eat.

We've all heard that fundamental aphorism at one time or another, but have you ever stopped and considered what that simple statement means? Whatever you eat positively or negatively affects the health of the entire body, including the digestive tract, which affects virtually all other bodily systems. If you've ever experienced digestive problems, you know exactly what I mean, because as the gut goes, so goes the body—the immune system, heart, lungs, blood supply, brain, and nervous system. That's why it's important to pay attention to the proteins, fats, and carbohydrates that you eat during the day.

Our diets used to be pretty simple until the 1900s. You ate what was raised on the family farm or, if you lived in the city, what was *harvested* from the family farm—fruits, vegetables, wild grains and seeds, raw, unpasteurized dairy products, and meat from animals that grazed the fields. Wild game was obtainable, and since many people lived near an ocean or a waterway, fresh fish was readily available.

I believe God gave us physiologies that crave these foods in their natural state because our bodies were genetically set for certain nutritional requirements by our Creator. The craving for junk food, however, has been manipulated by restaurants and companies that sweeten meats with various "secret sauces" and cover everything else in melted cheese and bacon. The strategy has worked: I estimate that more than half of the so-called foods available today weren't eaten by our ancestors.

Whatever we eat—good or bad—is a protein, a fat, or a carbohydrate. Let's take a closer look at these macronutrients:

The First Word on Protein

Proteins are the Legos—the essential building blocks—of the body. The English word *protein* is derived from the Greek term *proteios*, which means "of primary importance or that which comes first." All proteins are combinations of twenty-two amino acids, which build body organs, muscles, and nerves, to name a few significant things. Proteins are required for the structure, function, and regulation of the body's cells, tissues, and organs; and each protein has unique functions. Examples are hormones, enzymes, and antibodies. Even when healthy people eat healthy food, however, their bodies cannot produce all twenty-two amino acids—eight amino acids are missing. These eight essential amino acids must come from other sources outside the body. Since the body needs those eight amino acids badly, it just so happens that animal protein—chicken, beef, lamb, dairy, eggs, and so on—is the only complete protein source providing the Big Eight amino acids.

Now, that doesn't mean you have to eat meat. As I noted earlier, lacto-ovo vegetarians must consume lots of high-quality protein sources such as organic eggs and cultured dairy. Strict vegetarians have a much more difficult time meeting their protein needs. Nuts, seeds, legumes, and cereal grains are other decent protein sources for vegetarians, who must be careful to give the body enough protein to produce key essential amino acids like methionine, cysteine, and cystine, which are crucial to the brain and nervous system. Sally Fallon, president of Weston A. Price Foundation and author of *Nourishing Traditions*, warns vegetarians that their diet often leads to deficiencies in many important minerals as well. "This is because a largely vegetarian diet lacks the fat-soluble catalysts [vitamins and vitamin-like factors] needed for mineral absorption," she said.[6]

This is why I'm not a big fan of vegetarianism. Think about it: our ancestors received most of their protein from meat, fish, eggs, and cultured dairy products, yet they rarely experienced heart disease. I know this may sound confusing because a lot has been written about the dangers of meat—especially beef—causing heart disease and colon cancer, but this could not be farther from the truth. Meat—even red meat—does a body good, and Sally Fallon agrees with me. "Current wisdom dictates that Americans should at least reduce their consumption of red meats and the dark meats of birds because these meats contain more saturated fat than fish or white poultry meat," she wrote in *Nourishing Traditions*, "but even this restriction is ill-advised."[7] As long as you're eating clean meat from organically raised cattle, sheep, goats, buffalo, and venison, and not assembly-line cuts of flank steak from hormone-injected cattle eating pesticide-sprayed feed laced with antibiotics, you're going to be eating healthy.

Fish with scales and fins caught from oceans and rivers provide the essential amino acids as well. Supermarkets are stocking these types of foods in greater quantities these days, and of course, you can find them in natural food stores, fish markets, and specialty stores. A complete listing of excellent sources for these proteins is found in the GPRx Resource Guide.

THE SKINNY ON FAT

The low-fat craze from the mid-1990s is responsible for today's conventional wisdom that anything with fat in it is bad for you. A lot of people—especially weight-conscious teenage girls—have been taught to *hate* any food having even a speck of fat. Sure, eating the wrong fats adds pounds to your midsection, clogs your arteries, and puts you at risk for developing cancer, but eating too little fat is just as deadly. Since the Israelites were instructed to eat the fat of the land, so to speak, why didn't the Creator know that saturated fats and cholesterol are the main causes of coronary disease and malignancies?

Actually, and to no surprise, the opposite is true. By giving us these healthy animal fats, God in His infinite wisdom provided us with a concentrated source of energy, and these very fats are the source material for cell membranes and various hormones. Without fats providing satiety, we would be hungry within minutes of finishing a meal. Who would have thought that fats were so important—or good for you?

But you have to eat the right fats—foods loaded with omega-3 polyunsaturated fats and monounsaturated (omega-9) fatty acids, as well as healthy saturated fats. These good fats are found in a wide range of foods, including salmon, lamb, and goat meat, goat's and sheep's milk and cheese, walnuts and olives. It's also better to eat butter—yes, old-school butter—than margarine, which is a man-made, chemically altered fat. The Medical Research Council found that men eating butter ran half the risk of developing heart disease as those eating margarine.[8]

In addition, Greeks, Austrians, and the Swiss are known for their high-fat diets (lots of butter and cheese), but they rank in the top half-dozen countries for longevity. And much has been made about the French, who never met a cream dish they didn't like. A French woman, Mireille Guiliano, topped the book charts with *French Women Don't Get Fat: The Secret of Eating for Pleasure,* a book about how to have your cake and eat it, too.[9]

Fats rich in omega-3 and saturated fats such as medium-chain and short-chain fatty acids play a crucial role in the body's chemistry. Sally Fallon points out that saturated fatty acids constitute at least 50 percent of all cell membranes, play a vital role in the health of our bones, enhance the immune system, protect the liver from alcohol and other toxins, and guard against harmful microorganisms in the digestive tract.

Not all fats are good for you, and I want to make that clear. You want to steer away from hydrogenated fats, which have been associated with a host of maladies, including diabetes, obesity, and cancer. Hydrogenated fats are found in practically every processed food from Triscuits to Wonder Bread, from Twinkies to Skippy peanut butter. Most of the oils used in households today—soybean, safflower, cottonseed, and corn—are partially hydrogenated oils, which, by definition, are liquid fats that have been injected with hydrogen gas at high temperatures under high pressure to make them solid at room temperature.

I urge you to cook with butter or extra-virgin coconut oil, which is a miracle food that few people have ever heard of. Coconut oil was the "go-to" oil of its day until cooking oil manufacturers found a way to produce their products cheaper and push coconut oil off the store shelves. That's too bad because foods cooked in coconut oil taste great. Coconut oil is packed with antioxidants and reduces the body's need for vitamin E. You can tell which oil is better just by comparing how fast real canola oil or safflower oil becomes rancid when sitting at room temperature. Coconut oil shows no signs of rancidity even after a year at room temperature.

THE TRUTH ABOUT CARBOHYDRATES

If everybody loves Raymond, then everyone loves carbohydrates even more. You see it every time you're invited to a dinner party when folks congregate around the chips and crackers. And who can refuse dessert?

Carbohydrates are the starches and sugars produced by plant foods, and like fats, they've been getting a bad rap lately from the purveyors of popular diets like Atkins and South Beach. I'm the first to agree that the American diet is weighted way too heavily on the carbohydrate side, especially when you consider how many foods contain sugar. It's normal in this country to eat sugar-laden foods with every meal: breakfast with its sweet cereals, break time with soda or coffee mixed with sugar, lunch with its cookies, and dinner with its sugary desserts. Here's how much sugar we eat: a United States Department of Agriculture study in 2000 revealed that we eat an average of *thirty-two teaspoons* of sugar each day in our foods.[10]

Sugar comes in so many forms that it's hard to keep track of the names used for it these days. If the food label utilizes descriptions like corn syrup, high fructose corn syrup, sucrose, corn sweeteners, sorghum syrup, fruit juice concentrate, molasses, maple syrup, or honey, you're eating a form of sugar. Some sugar-containing foods are healthier than others, however, and these include honey, maple syrup, dehydrated cane juice, or unrefined sugar.

The other main carbohydrate form is starch, which is found in plant-based foods such as rice, potatoes, corn, and grains. When carbohydrates are eaten, the digestive tract breaks down the long chains of starches into single sugars, mainly glucose, which is a source of immediate energy. If these calories are not expended, however, the body converts them to fat.

The problem with carbohydrates is that we eat too many *refined* carbohydrates. Where kids once ate apples and oranges, now they eat Betty Crocker Fruit Roll-Ups, which are leather-like strips of fruit-flavored candy. Where adults once ate raw almonds or cashews, now they eat Planter's Honey Roasted Peanuts, caked in sugar. Where families once drank fresh-squeezed orange juice, they now serve Sunny Delight in the morning, which is little more than orange soda, minus the bubbles.

The refining process strips grains, vegetables, and fruits of their vital fiber, vitamin, and mineral components. "When we consume refined sugars and starches, particularly alone, without fats or protein, they enter the bloodstream in a rush, causing a sudden increase in blood sugar," says Sally Fallon. "The body's regulation mechanism kicks into high gear, flooding the bloodstream with insulin and other hormones to bring blood sugar levels down to acceptable levels. Repeated onslaughts of sugar will eventually disrupt this finely tuned process." That's why you "crash" when you overdose on sugar; the body cannot cope with the spike in blood sugar levels.

The Great Physician's Rx for eating foods that God created in a form healthy for your body will stop the crash-and-burn cycle. Whenever possible, eat your carbohydrates fresh and unrefined. This includes large amounts of fruits and vegetables, properly prepared grains, and small amounts of honey and other healthy sweeteners.

THE LAND OF MILK

The following list describes today's dairy products: pasteurized, homogenized, vitamin D fortified, and skimmed, which is the removal of fat. Oh, and I need to add antibiotics and hormones to the list because today's dairy products come from cows chewing on feed with added antibiotics and injected with hormones to boost milk production.

A century ago, cows produced four hundred to five hundred pounds of milk annually. Thanks to "modern" farming methods, today's "supercows" regularly produce between twenty thousand and thirty thousand pounds of milk each year. Holy cow![11]

Or "poor cow," I should say. I don't envy their lives: standing in a milking parlor and being hooked up to a milking machine every twelve hours. Due to excessive milking, their four udders are usually excoriated and infected, so the veterinarian administers more antibiotics.

Their milk travels through the milking machine and into pipes that lead to a holding tank, where it is cooled to thirty-eight degrees. A milk truck arrives to transport the milk to a factory, where it is heat-treated to destroy disease-causing bacteria. This process is known as pasteurization, named in honor of Louis Pasteur, the French scientist who invented the process in 1865.

Pasteurization, like antibiotics, kills both good and harmful bacteria. The process also destroys the enzymes in milk, which makes milk harder to digest, and lowers the potency of some vitamins in milk.

I believe it's better to drink raw or unpasteurized milk from a certified clean source. This type of milk is available because of improved sanitation methods in the milk production industry, including the use of stainless steel tanks. Only California and a handful of other states, however, allow raw, unpasteurized milk to be sold. If you happen to live in one of those states, you'll find raw milk to be delicious with a consistency closer to cream.

I also highly recommend eating fermented dairy products such as yogurt, kefir, hard cheeses, cultured cream cheese, cottage cheese, and cultured cream. Those who are lactose-intolerant can often stomach fermented dairy products because they contain little or no residual lactose, which is the type of sugar in milk that many find hard to digest.

Goat's milk is even more digestible because its protein is easier to digest, contains a little less lactose, and is filled with vitamins, enzymes, and protein. Although it does have a more pungent smell and taste than cow's milk, you should be aware that outside the United States, 65 percent of the world's population drink goat's milk—and they find goat's milk to be delicious. Goat cheese is a wonderful food to add to your salads.

The Fiber of Life

Our last entrant in the Great Physician's parade of foods is fiber, or what Grandma called "roughage"—foods that contain fiber help keep you regular. Fiber is the indigestible remnants of plant cells found in vegetables, fruits, whole grains, nuts, seeds, and beans. As they work their way through the digestive tract, they increase the elimination of waste matter in the large intestine and give you an urge to have a bowel movement. Eating fiber can turn the frown right side up for those people walking around with constipation.

Since we're on the subject, the kind of fiber that promotes colon health is found in low-carbohydrate, high-fiber foods such as broccoli, cauliflower, soaked or sprouted seeds, nuts, grains, berries, celery, greens, and fruits. Fruits and vegetables with edible skins, like apples, berries, and tomatoes, are especially high in fiber. These foods are right in the bull's-eye of a healthy diet.

Not enough fiber in the diet, however, means increased transit time for the food to wend its way through the small and large intestines before being expelled through the colon. High-fiber diets cut down on that transit time, so food has less time to putrefy in the colon, and toxins are quickly flushed out of the system.

Another way to classify fiber is by how easily it dissolves in water. Soluble fiber, which is found in oatmeal, nuts and seeds, beans, apples, pears, strawberries, and blueberries, partially dissolves in water. Insoluble fiber, which cannot be broken down by the water, does not dissolve in water and is credited with reducing the risk of colon cancer. Certain weight-loss programs promote foods high in insoluble fiber, such as whole grains, barley, brown rice, cereals, carrots, cucumbers, zucchini, and tomatoes, because these foods satiate hungry appetites without a whole lot of calories.

Americans rarely consume enough fiber each day, eating only around ten grams a day, when we should be eating double or triple that amount. With a reputation for "getting things moving" in the gastrointestinal tract, for preventing type 2 diabetes, for lowering cholesterol, and for carrying on the fight against colon cancer, fiber is a healthy addition to any diet.

The Top Healing Foods

The following is a list of what I call "healing foods" that should become part of your everyday diet. Remember, when you're eating a meal, it is best to consume the proteins, fats, and vegetables first before eating any high-starch carbohydrates like potatoes, rice, grains, and bread. In other words, going out to a nice tablecloth restaurant and filling up on bread and butter *before* the entrée is served is the absolute *wrong* way to eat. Leave the bread and rice or potatoes until the end of the meal, and better yet, if you're satisfied, leave them out altogether.

The foods I'm about to describe are your best choices for ensuring long and abundant life.

1. Fish and Fish Oil

Perhaps you've noticed that warehouse clubs like Costco are selling three-pound packages of Atlantic salmon. While it's great to see more people eating the tender pink meat of this wonderful fish, most of the salmon sold commercially these days is grown on fish farms. From birth until death, the salmon spend several years lazily circling concrete tanks, fattening up on pellets of salmon chow, not streaking through the ocean eating small marine life as they're supposed to. Feedlot salmon do not compare to their cold-water cousins in terms of taste or nutritional value. Since salmon caught in the wild are a richer source of omega-3 fats, protein, potassium, vitamins, and minerals, purchase fresh salmon and other fish from your local fish market or health food store that is labeled "Alaskan" or wild-caught. Wild-caught fish is an absolutely incredible food and should be consumed liberally. If you aren't able to consume enough fish, you should consider adding cod-liver oil to your daily diet.

Cod-liver oil is one of the best sources of omega-3 fatty acids out there. I'll have more to say about this extraordinary nutritional resource in the next chapter, but in study after study, cod-liver oil has been acknowledged to play a leading role in the development of the brain, the rods and cones of the retina of the eye, the male reproductive tissue, lubrication of the joints, and the body's inflammatory response.

2. Cultured Dairy Products from Goats, Cows, and Sheep

Dairy products derived from goat's milk and sheep's milk can be healthier for some individuals than those from cows, although dairy products from organic or grass fed cows can be excellent as well, as long as the dairy is non-homogenized. Goat's milk is less allergenic because it does not contain the same complex proteins found in cow's milk. Goat's milk contains higher amounts of medium-chain fatty acids (MCFAs) than other milks, and contains 7 percent less lactose than cow's milk. It's been said that raw or cultured goat's milk fully digests in a baby's stomach in just twenty minutes, while pasteurized cow's milk takes eight hours. The difference lies in the goat milk's structure: its fat and protein molecules are tiny in size, which allows for rapid absorption in the digestive tract.

I do not recommend drinking 2 percent or skim milk, even though we're told that it's healthier for the body than the full-fat version. The reason I say this is that removing the fat makes the milk less nutritious and less digestible, and can cause allergies.

3. Olive Oil

Long a staple in Mediterranean diets, olive oil is a natural juice that preserves the taste, aroma, vitamins, and properties of the olive fruit. Studies have shown that olive oil, high in monounsaturated fatty acids and antioxidants, protects us from heart disease by controlling LDL (or bad) cholesterol levels while raising HDL (or good) cholesterol levels. Researchers believe that various properties of olive oil, such as flavonoids, squalene, and polyphenols, may protect us from cancer. Flavonoids and polyphenols are antioxidants, which help prevent cell damage from oxygen-containing chemicals called "free radicals." I do not recommend using high-quality extra-virgin olive oil in cooking, however, because certain nutrients in the olive oil break down when subjected to high heat.

4. Small Fruits Such as Figs, Grapes, and Berries

The next time you play Bible Trivia, you'll know the answer to the question "What was the first fruit mentioned in Scripture?"

The answer is the fig, which is mentioned in Genesis 3:7. Whether eaten fresh or dried, figs are a good source of fiber and potassium, a mineral that helps control blood pressure. Many people are potassium-deficient because they do not eat enough fruits and vegetables, and they consume high amounts of sodium found in processed foods. Low intake of potassium-rich foods plus high intake of sodium equals hypertension. Grapes are a wonderful source of fiber and antioxidants. Berries are true nutritional powerhouses. They are low in calories and among the highest antioxidant-containing foods on the planet. Some scientific evidence even suggests blueberries may prevent age-related memory loss.

5. Soups and Stocks

I was rarely sick growing up, but on the few occasions when I caught a cold, Mom served up a heaping helping of "Jewish penicillin," otherwise known as homemade chicken soup. There's something about making zesty soup from scratch with fiber-rich vegetables such as celery, carrots, onion, and zucchini. Now that's *mmm, mmm good.*

Stocks, which are also called broth, are extremely nutritious and swimming with minerals, cartilage, collagen, and electrolytes. Meat, fish, and chicken stocks also contain generous amounts of natural gelatin, an odorless, tasteless substance extracted by boiling bones and animal tissues. Easy to digest, gelatin aids in digestion.

Chicken stock, for example, is made mostly of chicken parts with a low flesh-to-bone ratio. Backs, necks, and breastbones produce the best stock. Stocks and broth are especially beneficial to people with intestinal disease because they are high in nutrients that the gastrointestinal tract can easily absorb.

6. Healthy Saturated Fats

For fifty years, Americans have been told to avoid the fats found in butter and whole milk, even though human beings have been eating butter from grass-fed cows and other animal fats for thousands of years. Instead of these healthy saturated fats, our diets have increased the intake of polyunsaturated and hydrogenated fats, mainly because of the increased consumption of processed oils. Yet the verdict is in: the rate of heart disease has steadily increased, and we have a growing obesity problem in this country.

Whole milk butter produced from cattle grazing in rapidly growing grasses is loaded with vitamins A, D, and E. The reason I say "rapidly growing" is that the quality of the vitamins is directly related to the quality of the cow's foraging. As long as the cows have fresh, fast-growing grass to munch on, the milk will be high in vitamin content.

I've already talked about the value of cooking with extra-virgin coconut oil. Use it anytime you cook foods in a pan or bake something in the oven. Extra-virgin coconut oil has been shown to help balance the thyroid and improve metabolic function, so keep that in mind if you're trying to lose weight.

7. Honey and Pomegranate

Mankind's oldest sweetener—honey—comes from the nectar of flowers and nature's most efficient factory—the beehive. The Bible mentions honey or honeycomb more than forty times, and the Promised Land was described to the Israelites as the land of "milk and honey" (Exod. 13:5 NKJV). After Jesus had risen from the dead, the first food He ate was "broiled fish and some honeycomb" (Luke 24:42 NKJV).

Another first-rate source of antioxidants, honey plays a role in the prevention of cancer as well as heart disease, and wipes out the bacteria that cause diarrhea.[5] It's best eaten the way God had the bees create it: raw and unheated, which preserves the naturally occurring enzymes and bee pollen.

The Bible refers to the pomegranate, which has 613 seeds, as the fruit of royalty. It is renowned for its antioxidant qualities.

8. Soaked and Sprouted Seeds and Grains

Tasty foods rich in antioxidants are sprouted grains, seeds, and nuts, which retain their plant enzymes when they are not cooked. This process greatly helps digestion. When soaked or allowed to germinate, these abundant sources of nutrients transform into nutritional powerhouses that produce vitamin C and various vitamin B's—B2, B5, and B6. Those with wheat intolerances may want to try sprouted wheat bread because the digestive system will be more apt to accept sprouted grains. Soaked and sprouted seeds are great parts of a healthy diet.

9. Cultured and Fermented Vegetables

Often greeted with upturned noses at the dinner table, fermented vegetables such as sauerkraut, pickled carrots, beets, or cucumbers are overlooked, even though they are some of the healthiest foods on the planet. Raw cultured or fermented vegetables supply the body with useful organisms known as probiotics, as well as many vitamins, including vitamin C. If you've never put a fork on any of these foods, I urge you to sample sauerkraut or pickled beets, which are readily available in health food stores.

10. Organ Meats

Here's another esoteric food that doesn't land on too many plates these days, and even leading natural health authorities don't issue a "buy call" on organ meats because of their fear that these meats, such as the liver or the heart, contain too many toxins.

I concur with that fear, but consuming liver from organically raised, grass-fed cattle mitigates those concerns in my mind. By eating the most nutrient-dense parts of the cattle, such as the liver, you consume nature's richest sources of vitamins A, D, B6, and B12; folic acid; iron; and various fatty acids.

11. Fermented Beverages

Few people have heard of fermented beverages such as kefir, grape cooler, natural ginger ale, kombucha, and kvass, but they are worth checking out in well-stocked health food stores. They can even be made at home. These beverages contain lactic acid and supply beneficial probiotics, enzymes, and minerals to the digestive system. Fermented beverages relieve constipation problems, cleanse the colon and gallbladder, aid in the relief of arthritis, and promote overall well-being.

12. Green Vegetables

Right behind organ meats in nutrient density are green vegetables, which say "radiant health" in various hues of blue, purple, red, and yellow. When served farm fresh, green vegetables do not contain additives, preservatives, food colorings, or artificial flavorings.

It's universally recommended that you eat three to five or more servings daily of leafy green vegetables to maintain a healthy body. Greens contain large amounts of beta-carotene and folic acid, which lowers elevated blood levels of homocysteine, a known precursor to coronary heart disease. Folic acid can be destroyed in the cooking process, so green vegetables are best eaten raw, as in a salad, or lightly cooked by steaming.

Most canned vegetables should be "canned" because the manufacturing process destroys vitamins. The only exception is canned tomatoes, whose carotenes remain intact during the canning process. Frozen vegetables are okay, but just okay. You're always going to be better off eating fresh, organic vegetables picked and packaged from the farm.

I know that incorporating the foods I've been describing probably involves a whole new paradigm of eating, but I encourage you to take small steps. You'll be glad you did because you'll feel better and live longer.

The Dirty Dozen

The following twelve so-called foods or food ingredients or components are some of the most popular and least healthy things you can put into your mouth:

1. pork products

2. shellfish and fish without fins and scales (catfish, shark, eel)

3. hydrogenated oils (margarine, shortening, etc.)

4. artificial sweeteners (aspartame, saccharine, sucralose)

5. white flour

6. white sugar

7. soft drinks

8. pasteurized, homogenized milk

9. corn syrup (high fructose corn syrup)

10. hydrolyzed soy protein (imitation meat products)

11. artificial flavors and colors

12. excessive alcohol

ORGANIC IS THE WAY TO GO

The Great Physician's Rx for Health and Wellness is to consume vegetable foods that were grown properly without the use of pesticides, herbicides, and fungicides in healthy soil. If we're talking about food from animals, this means raising the animals the way they're supposed to be treated because the health of the animal is intricately related to the health of the meat, eggs, or milk it provides, which, in turn, is related to our health.

Regarding the consumption of meat in your diet, I strongly urge you to eat meats that are organically raised, or designated as grass-fed or at least free-range. When these animals are fed grasses supplemented with organically grown grains, they lead healthy, happy lives and eat the foods they were meant to eat.

I strongly believe there are meats that you *shouldn't* eat, the meats that God called "unclean" in Leviticus and Deuteronomy. I'm talking about pork, shrimp, and lobster, to name three of the most popular foods in America.

You may be scratching your head and saying, "Are you kidding me? Give up BLT sandwiches and scampi with pasta?" That's exactly what I'm saying, even if you have a fondness for fried catfish, shrimp gumbo, and black-eyed peas seasoned with ham hocks.

God, in His infinite wisdom, didn't beat around the burning bush when He directed Moses to tell the Israelites, "Of all the animals that live on land, these are the ones you may eat: You may eat any animal that has a split hoof completely divided and that chews the cud" (Lev. 11:2–3). Examples of these types of animals are cows, goats, sheep, oxen, deer, buffalo, and other wild game.

Here are some other points that the Lord made in Leviticus:

- The camel, though it chewed the cud, did not have a split hoof, making it unclean to eat.
- Badgers, rabbits, and pigs fit the same description. "You must not eat their meat or touch their carcasses; they are unclean for you," the Lord said in Leviticus 11:8.
- Birds or fowl that ate flesh, like vultures, were unclean, but birds that pecked on insects and grains for food—like quail or doves—were clean.
- Hard-shelled crustaceans such as lobster, crabs, or clams were to be avoided, as well as some smooth-skinned species, such as catfish and eel.
- Fish that could be eaten were ones with fins and scales, like trout, snapper, and grouper.

I recommend that you read Leviticus 11 and Deuteronomy 14 to digest the full flavor of what God said about eating clean versus unclean animals. His categorizations are elaborate and leave nothing to chance, but the main reason why God labeled certain animals, birds, and fish "unclean" is that they are scavengers . . . bottom-feeders . . . mobile trash compactors.

Consider how we look at pigs, for instance. Hog producers call pork America's "other white meat," but they sure don't call them "swine" because that conjures up images of dirty-snout pigs standing knee-deep in muck and their own excrement. Yet there's another reason why God forbade the Hebrew people from putting bacon on top of their cheeseburgers, and it's because He knew something about a pig's physiology, which makes sense, since He created the pig.

Pigs have a simple stomach arrangement: whatever a pig eats goes down the hatch, straight into the stomach, and out the back door in four hours max. As far as their diet goes—well, let's just say that pigs are barnyard animals famous for eating any swill thrown their way. They feast on slop and whatever else they can find under their muddy feet—even the carcasses and body parts of other pigs. To give you a word picture demonstrating how pigs will eat *anything*, I heard a story about a pig farmer who stacked ten pigs in individual wire cages on top of one another. He fed the pig in the penthouse cage a normal diet and let the rest of the pigs eat the droppings from the pig above. Everyone survived just fine.

Now, compare the pig's digestive tract to that of animals the Lord said the Israelites *could* eat: Animals that chewed the cud and had a split hoof included cows, goats, sheep, oxen, deer, buffalo, and so forth. These animals made the Creator's all-star list because they essentially have *three or four* stomachs—the alimentary canal, the stomach, and a secondary cud receptacle—to "wash and rinse" their vegetarian-based diet. Instead of a speedy four hours to digest their food, these "clean" animals take a leisurely twenty-four hours.

Another point is that the Hebrew words used to describe "unclean meats" can be translated as "foul," "polluted," and "putrid," the same terms used to describe human waste. I believe God was quite serious when He directed us to keep unclean meats at arm's length. Don't think that the Lord banned pork from the Israelite diets because they lacked refrigeration in those days, or that storing ham, bacon, or baby back ribs in a cool environment makes them "safe" for modern-day consumption. And don't think that we now have ways to make pigs healthy, because we don't. I know some farmers are now producing organic pork, which sounds like an oxymoron, but God excluded them because they are unclean animals and unfit for human consumption.

Why did He give us these rules? The answer is contained in Leviticus 11:43–44: "Do not defile yourselves by any of these creatures. Do not make yourselves unclean by means of them or be made unclean by them. I am the LORD your God; consecrate yourselves and be holy, because I am holy." Another verse, Deuteronomy 14:2 (NKJV), is also pertinent: "You are a holy people to the LORD your God, and the LORD has chosen you to be a people for Himself, a special treasure above all the peoples who are on the face of the earth." He's saying that He wants us holy, or separate from the world, so He has given us distinctions in what we should and shouldn't eat.

God knew that lobsters, crabs, shrimp, and catfish are bottom-feeders. They troll along the seabed or lakebed, sustaining themselves on, for lack of a better term, fish droppings. The good news is that they purify water; the bad news is that their diet is gulping you-know-what. Whatever they consume goes straight into their system, which explains why scientists measure pollution in the water by checking the flesh of crabs, clams, and lobsters for toxin levels.

PROVOKING CONTROVERSY

I recognize that striking pork and shellfish from your diet is one of the most controversial aspects of the Great Physician's Rx, but I can assure you that it's for the betterment of your health. There's a reason why Jesus did not touch the shrimp cocktails when the hors d'oeuvres were passed around or feast on pork barbecue during His time on earth—those were unclean foods. What was unclean for the Israelites and for Jesus thousands of years ago is still unclean today, and that's why I don't want to go against His commands. The God I serve is the same yesterday, today, and forever, and He never has made and never will make a mistake.

You may say, "Hey, I'm a New Testament believer. I've been saved and redeemed by the blood of the Lamb of God, so I am released from the Old Testament law." I agree, in the sense that I don't believe we are under obligation to practice ceremonial law associated with the Levitical system of sacrifice and atonement. However, while we are released from sacrificing animals to atone for our sins—Jesus took those sins with Him to the cross—I still believe His dietary commandments are relevant and important to us today and should be observed for our own good.

A good example can be found in Matthew 15:16–20 (NLT), when Jesus answered a question posed by Peter:

> "Don't you understand?" Jesus asked him. "Anything you eat passes through the stomach and then goes out of the body. But evil words come from an evil heart and defile the person who says them. For from the heart come evil thoughts, murder, adultery, all other sexual immorality, theft, lying, and slander. These are what defile you. Eating with unwashed hands could never defile you and make you unacceptable to God!"

What Jesus was pointing out was that breaking the traditions of man (otherwise known as the man-made rabbinical fence around the Torah) or instructions will not *defile* a person, but He wasn't saying you wouldn't be *harmed* by what you ate.

Let me explain this another way. Imagine that you were invited to the biggest church potluck ever, one where the buffet table ringed the perimeter of the fellowship hall. Just about every food known has been set out . . . New York strips fresh off the barbeque, sweet corn on the cob, robust salads, and homemade desserts. At the same time, some folks brought their favorite scampi and pasta dishes, while another family went all out and brought a pot of steaming lobster. Some harried couples didn't have time to cook, so they stopped by the supermarket and purchased a case of Twinkies for the dessert table.

You are free to pick and choose what you want to eat from those buffet tables; that's called God's grace. But what would be the healthiest items to put on your plate? I don't think lobster, scampi with pasta, and Twinkies would be wise choices.

There's an important part of Scripture that addresses this issue. In Acts 10, Peter, raised Jewish like the rest of the twelve apostles, had a vision in which the sky opened and a large sheet was lowered—a sheet containing all sorts of animals, reptiles, and birds, "unclean" meat to the Jewish culture:

> Then a voice said to him, "Get up, Peter; kill and eat them."
>
> "Never Lord," Peter declared. "I have never in all my life eaten anything forbidden by our Jewish laws."
>
> The voice spoke again, "If God says something is acceptable, don't say it isn't." The same vision was repeated three times. Then the sheet was pulled up again to heaven. (Acts 10:13–16 NLT).

When people disagree with me, saying it's okay with God if we eat pork and shellfish, they refer to this section of Scripture. What happened there is that God was breaking down the walls that separated Jews from Gentiles, whom the Jews regarded as unclean people. Dr. Rex Russell says he believes the best interpretation of the vision is God was instructing Peter that fellow-shipping with believing Gentiles, whom God had cleansed through Jesus, was not only acceptable but beneficial. There is no record in Scripture or in history that Peter or any of the apostles ever ate flesh from animals that God called "unclean."

Ah, but what about the second half of Romans 14:20? Paul wrote, "All food is clean, but it is wrong for a man to eat anything that causes someone else to stumble." And a few verses earlier, Paul stated, "I am fully convinced that no food is unclean in itself" (Rom. 14:14).

Was Paul really declaring all foods clean? No, because the word for food was never used in Scripture to refer to an "unclean meat." Unclean meats were described in a similar fashion as "waste," but never as food. Also, if you look at the Greek terminology, the word for clean in Romans 14:20 is *katharos*, which means "without blemish or spotless," and it referred to an incident (Mark 7:5–15) when the disciples ate without having first washed their hands—not the type of food they were eating. In Romans 14:14, the word for unclean is *koinos*, which means "common," so Paul was saying that just because meat that was lawful to eat may have been associated with idol worship didn't mean it was no longer fit for human consumption. If we view his words from this angle, Paul wasn't discussing dietary laws at all.

What it boils down to for me is that God has called pork products and shellfish "unclean" for thousands of years, so why would I introduce unclean meats into my body, which is called "God's temple" in 1 Corinthians 3:16?

It's almost a running joke for Nicki and me, but it happens almost every time when we go out to a nice French restaurant in West Palm Beach. After we are seated at a white-linen-covered table with a picturesque view of the ocean, the waiter, who's dressed in coal-black slacks and a starched white shirt, says in a heavy accent, "Madame et monsieur, would you be interested in our special tonight?"

"Sure," I reply, knowing what he'll say next.

"Monsieur, ze special tonight is pork tenderloin, stuffed with crab, ringed with scallops, and drizzled in a lobster sauce."

I nod my head, and Nicki stifles a laugh. In my mind, though, the waiter has just said, "Monsieur, ze special tonight is fresh garbage, ringed with raw sewage and drizzled with solid waste."

So, would I be sinning if I ordered the chef's special that evening?

The answer is no. Eating bacon won't cause you to lose your salvation, nor will you be sinning. Although there are no spiritual consequences to eating unclean meats, I believe there are physical consequences that must be faced. Remember in the Introduction how I talked about the folly of testing God's law of gravity by stepping off a ten-story building? If I stepped off a ledge ten stories above the street, I wouldn't lose my salvation, but I sure would get to heaven sooner because there are physical consequences to falling ten stories without a parachute. In the same manner, eating unclean foods fouls the body and may lead to increases in heart disease and cancer by introducing toxins into the bloodstream. God declared those meats unclean because He understands the ramifications of eating them.

I've eaten pork—knowingly—on only one occasion in my life: the time I tried some bacon when I was seventeen years old. The more I've been sharing the message of good health, the better I understand that my actions have great ramifications beyond myself. In terms of eating junk food, I haven't strayed much off the reservation, although I will confess a weakness for Cherry Vanilla Häagen-Dazs ice cream about once a year.

As I encourage people around the world to live a healthy life, I know that my health is not my own. I'm very aware that everyone is looking for fakes because we live in an age of hypocrisy and cynicism, a time when you have to parse political statements to glean the truth from the kernels of double-talk. Recently I traveled to the National Nutritional Foods Association Southeast trade show, where I had been asked to be the keynote speaker for an evening session. You should have seen the dinner that some key Maker's Diet partners and I provided: wild salmon, grass-fed organic beef, organic potatoes, quinoa (an ancient grain), sprouted whole grain bread, and organic green salad. My mouth waters just describing it, and the four hundred natural food store owners and managers in attendance dug in with gusto.

Afterward, a store owner told me, "I really want to thank you for dinner tonight. I've been coming to these conventions for twenty years, and this is the healthiest meal I've ever had. Do you know what we were served by the sponsors of the breakfast event this morning?"

"No," I replied.

"We had scrambled eggs, ham, bacon, English muffins, margarine, sugary cereal, and jams—at a health food show!"

I was amazed, although maybe I shouldn't have been. So few people in any industry or marketplace will stand up for what they truly believe. Their actions are dictated by political correctness and an unwillingness to go against the flow. One time after church, an acquaintance walked up to me and said, "If we're supposed to eat healthy, why does the world tell us to eat junk food? Why is all the advertising on TV for foods that are bad for you?"

"Look at what you're asking," I replied. "God's truths are always hated by the world; you see it in the types of shows on TV, music on the radio, and images in magazines and on billboards. The envelope is always pushed. Remember, when Jesus was on this earth, men despised Him. He went against the grain."

Christians are just as blind in the area of health as the rest of the world. We make every excuse in the world. We love our Krispy Kremes, we love our McDonald's burgers, and we love our holiday hams.

But you know what? I believe that every time we eat what we shouldn't, the adversary smiles because he knows, at that moment, we've become less effective for the kingdom.

I believe with all my heart that *The Great Physician's Rx for Health and Wellness* will allow us to unlock our health potential, fulfilling God's purpose for our lives.

LIFESTYLE CHANGES

As you "eat to live," I would like to turn your attention to several eating strategies that you should try to incorporate into your life. Some of these ideas will be reintroducing old habits that you last practiced in grammar school; other ideas will sound new to you.

1. *Chew Food as Slowly as You Can*

We should all heed this advice, including me; I have wolfed down more than a few meals on the go. But I've become a much better "chewer"; in fact, if you were to eat out with me sometime, you'd be surprised at how long I take to chew my food. It has taken some effort on my part to reprogram the way I eat, yet I know that a conscious effort to chew food slowly ensures that plenty of digestive juices are added to the food as it begins to wind through the digestive tract.

Chewing foods properly allows enzymes in your saliva to turn the food into a near liquid form before swallowing. The act of working your jaw also sends a neurological message to your stomach and pancreas to increase acid and digestive enzyme production because food's on the way.

People who eat quickly and gulp their food like ravenous wolves can develop heartburn and cause food to back up in the stomach. Chewing slowly allows you to savor the smell and taste of the food, which is why eating is enjoyable, right?

I recommend that you chew each mouthful of food twenty-five to fifty times. I know that seems like a pretty arduous task, but chewing your food thoroughly—especially foods high in carbohydrates—can enhance the digestive process and reduce post-meal bloating. Chewing slowly and thoroughly can also help maintain a healthy weight as you allow your brain to register the amount of food you are consuming. Put simply, people who chew more consciously eat less.

In addition, don't chew on a piece of gum between meals. Slapping a stick of chewing gum in your mouth and chewing away starts those valuable digestive juices flowing—but then nothing gets sent down the hatch! Since gum is full of sugars, artificial sweeteners, and chemicals anyway, it's better not to chew gum at all.

And that old adage your mom drummed into you from the time you could sit at the dinner table—"Don't talk with food in your mouth!"—still rings true. Chewing food while regaling your guests about your gallbladder operation interferes with optimal digestion and may lead to another condition—persona non grata.

2. Practice Fasting Once a Week

We read in Isaiah 58:6, 8: "Is not this the kind of fasting I have chosen: . . . to set the oppressed free and break every yoke? . . . Then your light will break forth like the dawn, and your healing will quickly appear." I'm a firm believer in the value of giving the body's digestive system time off from the round-the-clock digestive cycle that so many people put their bodies under these days. Your liver—the hardest-working organ God gave you—will thank you.

Many people aren't aware that this wondrous organ performs five hundred different functions for the body.[12] Among them is filtering blood to remove toxins and germs such as viruses, bacteria, and yeast. The liver also processes fats, proteins, and carbohydrates, and breaks down any chemicals, hormones, or metabolic waste circulating through your bloodstream.

Don Colbert, M.D., author of *Fasting Made Easy*, compared the liver to a swimming pool filter, saying that a pool filter would have to clean half of the pool's water *every minute* to keep up with what your liver does every minute you draw breath.[13] When working efficiently, the liver filters out 99 percent of the germs and toxins in your blood before sending the cleansed blood back into circulation.

To work efficiently, your liver could use some downtime, and fasting provides that. Taking a sustained break from eating will improve your physical health in ways you can't understand, but there's a spiritual side to fasting that must be addressed as well. Something about denying your growling stomach leads to greater self-control and opens one up, I believe, to hearing what God wants to say to you. The Bible is full of references to fasting—seventy-four in all—and tells how spiritual giants such as David, Daniel, and Paul experienced periods of fasting before launching themselves into doing God's work.

From my reading of Scripture, I spotted three types of fasts:

1. *The Esther Fast.* For three days, you don't eat or drink a thing—a total fast. This was described in the fourth chapter of Esther, when Esther was deciding whether to risk her life by approaching King Xerxes after he decreed that all Jews must be annihilated on a single day. Before approaching the king to beg him to change his mind, Esther asked the Jewish people not to eat or drink for three days. Afterward, God worked a tremendous miracle to save His chosen people.

Elsewhere in Scripture, we learn that Paul, after being blinded on his way to Damascus, "was three days without sight, and neither ate nor drank" (Acts 9:9 NKJV).

I don't recommend a strict Esther fast these days because of our overall poor health and number of toxins swirling around in our bloodstreams. Abstaining from food is one thing, but we need water and other liquids to help expel toxins from the bloodstream as they are being released during a fast.

2. *The Daniel Fast.* I spoke of the Daniel fast in the introduction, when Daniel and his buddies refrained from eating the typical Babylonian diet (with its rich foods and/or unclean meats) and subsisted on vegetables for ten days. What I find worthy of notice is that the Bible says that Daniel and friends outperformed their Babylonian counterparts and "looked healthier and better nourished than the young men who had been eating the food assigned by the king" (Dan. 1:15 NLT). Daniel and his three friends continued on this diet for three years.

The Daniel fast, which was a vegetable diet, can be applied today in two ways: (1) eating only raw vegetables, fruits, nuts, seeds, and juices; or (2) avoiding solid foods and drinking only raw vegetable and fruit juices to cleanse the digestive system. I view the Daniel fast as an excellent way to break free from food addictions (like sitting down with a half-gallon of cookie dough ice cream every night) and start over again.

A twenty-one-day fast is also mentioned in the Bible. The tenth chapter of Daniel describes how he ate "no choice food; no meat or wine touched [his] lips" (Dan. 10:3) for three weeks. Extended fasts should be performed only under the strict supervision of a licensed physician.

3. *The Forty-Day Desert Fast.* Scripture tells us that Moses and Jesus endured forty-day total fasts *without drinking liquids.* That sounds like a miracle to me because the body's internal organs would be seriously damaged if you attempted that today—if you survived. It's generally accepted that the body cannot go more than three days without hydration. The tragic Terry Schiavo situation in the spring of 2005 proved that it is possible to go longer than three days without water, but that was an unusual situation. Although I've heard of other people completing forty-day water-only fasts, these extended fasts should be undertaken only under medical supervision.

I think it's better—and more realistic—to concentrate on completing a one-day partial fast once a week. I've found that Thursdays or Fridays work best for me because the week is winding down and the weekend is coming up. For instance, I won't eat breakfast and lunch so that when I break my fast and eat dinner that night, my body has gone between eighteen and twenty hours without food or sustenance since I last ate dinner Wednesday or Thursday night.

Fasting is a form of discipline that isn't easy for someone who's never done it. If you've never voluntarily fasted for a day, I urge you to try it—preferably toward the end of the week. The benefits are immediate: you'll feel great, lose weight, look younger, save money, save time, and become closer to the Lord. Fasting is a means of denying the flesh because the stomach *and* the brain work overtime in reminding you, "Hey! I'm hungry!" That's why they call it the "fasting headache."

When you fast and pray (two words that seem to go hand in hand in

Scripture), you are pursuing God in your life and opening yourself to experiencing a renewed sense of well-being and dependence upon the Lord.

Here are some dos and don'ts regarding fasting:

- Remind yourself that it's going to be difficult, especially the first time or two you fast. There will come a point, though, when your hunger will subside and your energy will increase.
- Drink only water or raw juices. Drinking pasteurized orange juice or a smoothie isn't really fasting. But you should drink water or raw juices as if you're running the Boston Marathon. Water and fresh juices do not require the digestive system to work hard and thus give your body the time off it needs to rest and repair. The idea is to flush toxins from your body. Water and fresh juices can also satiate the hunger pains some, but don't drink ice-cold beverages. It's better to drink room-temperature water or fresh juices at room temperature so as not to shock the stomach.
- Before you set out to fast, make a list of prayer requests that you would like God to answer. Every time you experience hunger pangs, ask the Lord to do a work in that area of your life or a loved one's life.
- Schedule a quiet time with the Lord. Keep a Bible handy. It's amazing what God will show you as you give up sustenance for Him. Use a journal to write down what you feel God is saying to you. Many people feel that during times of fasting, they hear God's voice more clearly than at any other time.
- Maintain a normal schedule. Staying busy helps the hours pass quickly, and light exercise such as functional fitness (which I'll describe in Key #4), walking, or deep breathing can be beneficial as well.
- Break your fast with vegetable juices, fruits, and raw cultured dairy products. This is not the time to cook thick, juicy steaks on the barbecue or eat baked potatoes topped with shredded cheese and sour cream. Remember: your stomach has contracted somewhat during the fasting period, so "gentle" foods are the way to go. I often break a fast with a large green salad and some fresh vegetable juice, followed by a

healthy meal of chicken soup or salmon and steamed veggies with fruit. For dessert, I treat myself to a smoothie.

I'LL DRINK TO THAT

Since fasting restricts you to drinking water and fresh juices, this is a good spot to talk about the importance of staying hydrated when you're *not* fasting.

Water—which, in its pure form, is odorless and colorless—is the perfect fluid replacement. Only God could come up with a calorie-free and sugar-free substance that regulates body temperature, carries nutrients and oxygen to the cells, cushions joints, protects organs and tissues, removes toxins, and maintains strength and endurance. Water makes up 92 percent of your blood plasma and 50 percent of everything else in the body.

The problem is that people don't drink enough water, or the liquids they do gulp down aren't healthy for them—coffee, sodas, and Mocha Frappuccinos. People who think it's nothing to chug a thirty-two-ounce Big Gulp filled with Pepsi cringe at sipping regular old . . . water. Yet replenishing the body with water throughout the day is vital because fluids in urine eliminate waste products, and fluids elsewhere in the body dissipate excess heat and cool the body.

Since the most oft-quoted advice in health books is to "drink eight glasses of water each day," I already know what you're thinking: *If I drink that much water, I'll be running to the toilet every twenty minutes!*

Yes, you do go to the bathroom more often when you're well hydrated, but is that so bad? The body needs plenty of water, and if it doesn't receive enough, we settle for far less than vibrant health. "Every twenty-four hours, the body recycles the equivalent of forty thousand glasses of water to maintain its normal physiological functions," says F. Batmanghelidj, M.D., author of *You're Not Sick, You're Thirsty!* "If you think you are different and your body does not need eight to ten glasses of water each day, you are making a major mistake."[14]

Sip water throughout the day. I set a forty-eight-ounce bottle of water on my office desk as a reminder to keep putting fluids into my system. My record for drinking water is one and one-quarter gallons of water in a day during a fast, but I won't reveal how many trips I made to the bathroom. I also drink water before each meal and before, during, and after exercise, knowing that I need extra fluid to offset perspiration. I've learned through personal experience that if I fail to drink enough fluids before or during my exercise periods, my body goes into the tank. Sooner or later, I'll hit the wall.

One thing I don't drink while I exercise is the sugar-and-salt cocktail known as Gatorade, which commands 80 to 90 percent of the sports drink market in America. I'll be up front about this: my feelings about Gatorade aren't derived from the fact that this sports drink was invented at my rival school, the University of Florida, and named after the Gator football team. I'd be saying the same thing if this stuff was called "Seminolade."

My gripe with Gatorade is that it's a combination of nonpurified water; sucrose, glucose, and fructose (which are nothing more than sugars); and artificial colors with some potassium and sodium (the electrolytes) thrown into the mix. In other words, Gatorade is artificially colored and flavored sugar water with a salty aftertaste. Contrary to their claims, I believe Gatorade and other power drinks do more harm than good. It would be better during workouts to consume natural mineral or spring water, or fresh vegetable or diluted fruit juices.

I'm also not a big fan of fitness waters like Propel, which was created by the makers of Gatorade. Propel is basic H_2O in various flavors—lemon, orange, and berry—with four B vitamins and two antioxidants (vitamins C and E) added in. In case you're wondering how a manufacturer can pour additives into water and still call it water, the International Bottled Water Association (yes, there is one) decided that if the additives don't add up to more than 1 percent by weight of the final product, then it can be sold as water. I'm still shaking my head over seeing a product with four grams of sugar in each bottle on the same shelf as bottled water, but that's America for you. When it comes to something as basic as water, you should accept no imitations. I hate to see such a wonderfully healthy resource perverted, so to speak, to satisfy our taste buds.

Water is an overlooked resource by those seeking to lose weight. Many times dieters, I've found, confuse hunger and thirst. They think they're hungry when actually they're dehydrated. Drinking fluids will not only hydrate the body for all the good reasons I've just described, but it will put a damper on those hunger pains coming from the pit of the stomach.

If you're trying to lose weight, drink an eight-ounce glass of water the next time you feel hungry. Drinking a glass a half hour before lunch or dinner will act like a governor on an engine, taking the edge off your hunger pangs and preventing you from raiding the fridge or pillaging the pantry.

What about our favorite hot beverages?

Regarding tea and coffee, is our obsession with hot drinks making us sicker? Although many health experts disagree whether consuming caffeinated beverages such as coffee and tea is healthy, history tells a different story. Coffee and tea have been consumed for thousands of years by some of the world's healthiest people. While I'm not a huge fan of coffee or a coffee drinker myself, I will say that fresh ground organic coffee flavored with organic cream and honey is fine when consumed in moderation (one cup per day). Teas and herbal infusions (beverages made from herbs and spices other than the actual tea plant, which are often mistakenly called teas) are another story altogether.

Infusions of herbs and spices such as teas have been a part of nearly every culture at every time of history. In fact, consuming organic teas and herbal infusions several times per day can be one of the best things we can do for our health. Green and white tea, for example, provide the body with antioxidants such as polyphenols, which help reduce cellular damage and oxidative stress. There have been many studies identifying anti-cancer compounds in tea as well as compounds that help increase metabolism. Teas and herbal infusions can provide energy, enhance the immune system, improve our digestion, and even help us wind down after a long day.

You'll find that I recommend a cup of hot tea and honey with breakfast, dinner, and snacks. I also recommend consuming fresh-made iced tea, as tea can be consumed hot or steeped and iced. Please note that drinking tea cannot be considered a substitute for drinking water. While tea provides many great health benefits, nothing can replace pure water for hydration. You can safely and healthfully consume two-to-four cups per day of tea and herbal infusions, but you still need at least six cups of pure water.

As far as caffeine is concerned, I believe teas' benefits are better delivered in teas containing caffeine. Since tea leaves naturally contain caffeine, the Creator obviously intended for us to consume tea in its most natural form. One word of caution: if caffeine tends to keep you up at night, you should avoid consuming caffeinated teas after 6 p.m. For an evening treat, try consuming a caffeine-free herbal infusion containing relaxing herbs and spices to help you wind down and decompress.

My favorite tea blends contain combinations of tea (green, black, or white) with biblical herbs and spices such as grape, pomegranate, hyssop, olive, and fig leaves. Even though I have never thought of myself as the tea-drinking type, Nicki and I enjoy these biblical tea blends each and every day. (See the GPRx Resource Guide, page 339, to find my favorite tea and herbal blends.)

Nutrition in a Bar

What about energy bars?

In an effort to eat healthy and lose weight, many Americans have turned to consuming energy bars as a convenient meal replacement or an in-between snack. This may sound like a good idea, but in reality, many energy bars are no healthier than a Snickers candy bar. In fact, many energy bars contain harmful ingredients such as artificial sweeteners, chemicals, preservatives, and synthetic nutrients.

If you find it difficult to sit down to a home-cooked healthy breakfast every morning, or if you find yourself frequenting the vending machines during your snack breaks, you can eat healthy whole food bars as a meal replacement, healthy snack, or afternoon pick-me-up. In my quest for consuming and providing for others the healthiest and most convenient functional foods available, I have developed whole food bars containing recommended amounts of protein, omega-3 fats, fiber, and probiotics. Whole food bars are great for people of all ages and are great for children as a quick breakfast, a healthy snack for lunch, or a treat when they get home from school. These whole food bars contain the highest-quality protein, carbohydrates, fats, and fiber, as well as vitamins, minerals, probiotics, and enzymes.

The healthiest and most functional food bars today contain compounds known as beta glucans from soluble oat fiber, which provide the following benefits:

- helps lower serum cholesterol and triglycerides
- promotes maintenance of healthy blood sugar levels
- supports healthy immune function
- promotes digestive health
- promotes maintenance of healthy body weight

In addition to all of the wonderful health benefits, whole food nutrition bars taste great. (For information on healthy whole food bars that I recommend, see the GPRx Resource Guide, pages 329–30.)

NUTRITION IN A SHAKE

Ten years ago, most people gagged at the thought of drinking a smoothie, probably because they pictured themselves swallowing a foul mixture of brewer's yeast, avocado, and wheat germ.

That perception is rapidly changing, thanks to juice bars like Jamba Juice, which are sprouting up like spring mushrooms in malls and airport concourses across the country. In fact, some in the fast-food business are predicting smoothies will be the next big craze. That's why you're seeing stores like Planet Smoothie, Tropical Smoothie, Smoothie Island, Smoothie America, Smoothieville, and Smoothie King whipping up sweet confections of frozen fruit, juice, frozen yogurt, and ice across the fruited plain. Smoothies, punched up with vitamins, mineral supplements, and protein powders, are being called the power drink of the future.

Smoothies were surely created shortly after the invention of the blender. No one can recall when the word *smoothie* was coined, but I can remember drinking Orange Julius concoctions, a distant relative to the modern-day smoothie, when I was a kid. Smoothies are certainly better for you than drinking a Pepsi or chocolate milk, but I would shy away from smoothies made with frozen yogurt, which are not much healthier than ice cream. As long as you stick with the smoothie recipes in appendix A of this book, you should be okay, and you should view commercially made smoothies like energy bars: some are good for you, while others are nothing more than vitamin-enriched liquid candy.

Going hand in hand with the Jamba Juices of the world are homemade smoothies, which almost always include a dollop of protein powder mixed in with fresh fruit and juice. Protein powder is much more mainstream than it was even five years ago, and now it's sold in laundry-sized tubs at Wal-Mart and nationwide pharmacy chains like Longs Drugs.

Health-conscious families, especially those into exercise and athletics, are firing up blenders every morning. Now, I'm all for making a smoothie for breakfast, especially if you include some green food in the mixture. But I want to include a cautionary message, and it's that commercially made protein powder—such as soy, milk, or whey protein—is not as healthy as it may seem. It is extremely difficult without modern-day technology to extract the protein from the whey of cow's milk or from the soybean. Bottom line: most protein powders are highly processed and derived from cows that have been injected with hormones, have been fed antibiotic-rich grain, and have never seen the light of day. Most soy protein powders are produced from genetically modified soybeans.

Many whey- or soy-based protein powders also contain artificial sweeteners, flavorings, and additives. Some labels say the product contains dextrin, high fructose corn syrup, sucralose, aspartame, or acesulfame-K, which are sugars or artifical sweeteners. Since sugars are not healthy and artificial flavors and sweeteners are chemicals, I would not consider these protein powders to be ideal substances.

While some protein powders are better than others, superior protein powders are whey protein powders made from grass-fed, free-range cows, fermented soy protein, and my personal favorite, protein powder made from goat's milk, which is easily digestible, contains enough fat for the nutrients to be absorbed, and is a food that God created in a form healthy for the body. (For recommended sources of protein powders, see the GPRx Resource Guide, page 337.)

You'll also find a number of great smoothie recipes in appendix A, but if you're having difficulty making time to even prepare a smoothie, I recommend consuming a powdered smoothie mix that only requires mixing in water. When consuming a powdered smoothie mix, I recommend using one that is organic, high in antioxidants, fiber, and probiotics and that contains compounds known as beta glucans from soluble oat fiber. Smoothie mixes with the recommended daily amount of beta glucans from soluble oat fiber have been shown in research to reduce the absorption of excess dietary fat, slow the absorption of carbohydrates (sugars and starches), increase the feelings of fullness (satiety), and provide needed dietary fiber. For information on my favorite whole food smoothie mix, see the GPRx Resource Guide, page 329.

With the help of functional whole food bars and smoothies, eating healthy has never been as convenient. Although I've done my best to establish that there are no reasons to veer off of my health plan, just in case you do so, there are ways to minimize the damage.

THE URGE TO CHEAT

Maybe you can't stop yourself from reaching for the cookie jar before dinner or indulging in a midnight snack. Maybe you're trying to be good by staying away from sandwiches, pastas, rice, and potatoes because you have problems with your blood sugar.

The *glycemic index* refers to how foods affect blood sugar levels and is a valuable measure of how quickly the carbohydrates in foods are broken down into simple sugars. Foods with a high glycemic index are the usual suspects: bread and rolls made from white enriched flour, starchy potatoes, and sugary sweets, to name a few. If you eat a typical lunch of a turkey-and-cheese sandwich and Lay's potato chips, followed by a Famous Amos chocolate chip cookie, you'll see your blood-sugar level rise dramatically because high-carbohydrate intake causes the body to produce insulin in the bloodstream. When blood sugars are high, cells burn sugar instead of fat, which is how fat accumulates in the body.

Controlling this blood sugar/insulin response is the essence of low-carb diets, as I described earlier in this chapter. Of course, you're going to be better off eating foods with a lower glycemic index most of the time: fruits, vegetables, salads, and whole grain products. This fits hand in glove with the essence of *The Great Physician's Rx for Health and Wellness*, which helps you lose weight while reprogramming the body to eat foods that God created—and stop the cravings for junk food.

Cravings are very difficult to deal with, especially for those addicted to their favorite carbs: French fries, doughnuts, and pasta. The mind practically goes to war with the body, demanding, "I want my carbs, and I want them now!"

The husband-and-wife team of Richard and Rachael Heller, Ph.D.'s and professors who have retired from the Mount Sinai School of Medicine in New York, say that their years of research and thousands of case studies have led them to this piece of advice: if you're going to cheat, do it all in a one-hour time frame.

Why sixty minutes, which they are very strict about? The Hellers say that when the body has been deprived of insulin-releasing foods high in carbohydrates for two consecutive meals, the body starts making adjustments: it releases less insulin because it's not expecting the next meal to be heavy in carbohydrates. When that happens, "less insulin is released; less fat is stored; and more fat is used up. The lowered level of insulin also allows the brain chemical serotonin to act as it should—as an appetite regulator. You will probably eat far less than you would if you had been eating three consecutive carbohydrate-rich meals," the Hellers write in *The Carbohydrate Addict's Diet*.[15]

If, however, you cheat—fall off the wagon, stuff yourself, pig out—then the body responds by releasing a second phase of insulin, which produces more fat cells. This second insulin phase usually kicks in between seventy-five and ninety minutes after you begin eating. If you stop cheating *before* sixty minutes are up, however, the second phase of insulin release manages to stay low.

So, if you're hanging out at a Super Bowl party or a lazy Sunday-after-church barbecue, the *last* thing you want to be doing is grazing on chips and dip and deviled eggs and potato salad and cheeseburgers and s'mores all afternoon and into the evening. Continuous eating for five hours can send your insulin readings shooting to the moon. So the next time you're cheating, check your watch. By limiting the "damage" to one hour, you limit the overproduction of insulin, which ultimately leads to weight gain.

There's another approach you can take the next time you feel the urge to overeat or eat poorly. I once ate dinner with Nick Yphantides, M.D., and author of *My Big Fat Greek Diet* (Thomas Nelson Publishers, 2004). I thought I had a remarkable story until I heard what happened to Dr. Nick, a family physician from San Diego. Apparently Dr. Nick had ballooned to 467 pounds when he reached his mid-thirties. Here was a guy as fat as the Goodyear blimp counseling his patients on the pros and cons of the Atkins diet versus the South Beach Diet. Tired of saying, "Do as I say, not as I do," Dr. Nick embarked on a one-year mission to get healthy. He took a leave of absence from his practice and traveled around the country going to major-league baseball games while drinking protein shakes. He lost 270 pounds, or as he put it to me, "the equivalent of two American women, who weigh, on the average, 135 pounds."

During his morbidly obese days, Dr. Nick said he got used to blithely eating way past the discomfort level, which meant that he was not paying attention to his body's signals *Hey! Stop eating!* It was like he was running red lights at intersections.

Dr. Nick trained his body to brake for yellow lights. He did this by asking himself three questions as he ate:

1. Is my body saying that I've had enough?
2. Is my stomach satisfied?
3. Am I full yet?

If he could say yes to any of these three questions, it was time to put his fork down.

In working with obese people wanting to eat healthy and the right amount, I counsel them to put the fork down before the plate is clean or seconds have been served and ask themselves if they're full. Some people would do well to try this when their plate is half empty.

If you're overeating, then please know that you don't have to clean your plate. I know—your mom said, "You need to clean your plate because kids are starving in Africa." I heard the same line at home, but if you don't finish your food, you'll end up being healthier and live longer—and perhaps you'll be able to participate in a short-term missions trip to Africa someday.

So look for the yellow light and don't feel you have to clean your plate.

LOOKING AHEAD

You've heard how Nicki and I are being oh-so-careful to start Joshua on the right foods as his life begins. We want him to be an effective member of God's kingdom, someone who'll grow up without being slowed down by any of the health problems that plague many adults (such as allergies, diabetes, digestive problems, or obesity).

We want the best for our son, but there's a difference between *wanting* something and then *making* the necessary sacrifices to achieve it. My wife and I understand that feeding Joshua a healthy organic diet involves more shopping and more food preparation, but at his age, we remind ourselves that his stomach and digestive tract are a blank slate. Feeding him the right foods right out of the starting gate will point him down a path toward growing up into a vigorous young man who will serve the Lord and glorify God with his physical health. In that way, he'll eat to live, not live to eat.

EAT: WHAT FOODS ARE EXTRAORDINARY, AVERAGE, OR TROUBLE?

In the following lists, each category includes foods in descending order based on their health-giving qualities. Foods at the beginning of the list are healthier than those at the end.

Extraordinary

Extraordinary foods are those that God created for us to eat and are in a form healthy for the body. If you are struggling with poor health, it is best to consume foods from the extraordinary category more than 75 percent of the time. These extraordinary foods impart health benefits and can bring about regeneration of body, mind, and spirit. For recommendations of sources and brands of the healthiest foods, see the GPRx Resource Guide.

Meat *(Grass-fed organic is best.)*
    meat bone soup or stock
    liver and heart (must be organic)
    lamb
    buffalo
    elk
    venison
    beef
    goat
    veal
    jerky (with no chemicals, nitrates, or nitrites)
    beef or buffalo sausage (with no pork casing)
    beef or buffalo hot dogs (with no pork casing)

Fish *(Wild- or ocean-caught is best, and the fish must have fins and scales.)*
    fish soup or stock   trout
    salmon   tilapia
    halibut   orange roughy
    tuna   sea bass
    cod   snapper
    scrod   sardines (canned in water
    grouper   or olive oil only)
    haddock   herring
    mahimahi   sole
    pompano   whitefish
    wahoo

Poultry *(Pastured and organic is best.)*
    poultry bone soup or stock
    chicken

Cornish game hen

guinea fowl

turkey

duck

chicken or turkey bacon (with no pork casing)

chicken or turkey sausage (with no pork casing)

chicken or turkey hot dogs (with no pork casing)

Lunch Meat (Organic, free-range, and hormone-free is best.)

turkey

chicken

roast beef

Eggs (High omega-3/DHA or organic is best.)

chicken eggs (whole with yolk)

duck eggs (whole with yolk)

fish roe or caviar (must be fresh, not preserved)

Dairy (Organic is best.)

kefir made from raw goat's milk

kefir made from raw cow's milk

raw goat's milk hard cheeses

raw cow's milk hard cheeses

goat's milk plain whole yogurt

organic cow's milk yogurt or kefir

raw cream

Fats and Oils (Organic is best.)

oil, coconut, extra-virgin (best for cooking)

oil, olive, extra-virgin (not for cooking)

oil, butter (ghee)

butter, goat's milk, raw (not for cooking)

butter, goat's milk

butter, cow's milk, raw, grass-fed (not for cooking)

butter, cow's milk

avocado

coconut milk/cream (canned)

oil, unrefined flaxseed (not for cooking)

oil, unrefined hemp seed (not for cooking)

oil, expeller-pressed sesame

oil, expeller-pressed peanut

Vegetables *(Organic fresh or frozen is best.)*

raw fermented veggies (no vinegar)

squash (winter or summer)

broccoli

artichokes (French, not Jerusalem)

asparagus

beets

cauliflower

brussels sprouts

cabbage

carrots

celery

cucumbers

eggplant

pumpkins

garlic

onions

leafy greens (kale, collard, broccoli rabe, mustard greens)

salad greens (radicchio, escarole, endive)

okra

lettuce (leafs of all kinds)

spinach

mushrooms

peas

peppers

string beans

tomatoes

sprouts (broccoli, sunflower, pea shoots, radish, etc.)

sweet potatoes

sea vegetables (kelp, dulse, nori, kombu, and hijiki)

white potatoes

corn

Fruits (Organic fresh or frozen is best.)

blueberries	pineapples
strawberries	bananas
blackberries	mangoes
raspberries	papayas
lemons	dried fruits (no sugar or sulfites)
limes	raisins
apples	figs
apricots	dates
grapes	prunes
melons	peaches
oranges	grapefruit

Grains and Starchy Carbohydrates (Organic is best, and whole grains and flours are best if soaked for six to twelve hours before cooking.)

sprouted bread (see the GPRx Resource Guide, page 328)

fermented whole grain sourdough bread (see the GPRx Resource Guide, page 328)

sprouted whole grain cereal (see the GPRx Resource Guide, pages 328–29)

quinoa

amaranth

buckwheat
millet

Sweeteners
unheated raw honey
date sugar

Beans and Legumes (Best if soaked for twelve hours.)

miso
lentils
tempeh
natto
black beans
kidney beans
navy beans
white beans

pinto beans
red beans
split peas
garbanzo beans
lima beans
broad beans
black-eyed peas
soybeans (edamame)

Nuts and Seeds (Organic, raw, and/or soaked is best.)
almonds (raw or dry roasted)
pumpkin seeds (raw or dry roasted)
hemp seeds (raw)
flaxseeds (raw and ground)
sunflower seeds (raw or dry roasted)
almond butter (raw or roasted)
tahini (raw or roasted)
pumpkin seed butter (raw or roasted)
hemp seed butter (raw)
sunflower butter (raw or roasted)
walnuts (raw or dry roasted)
macadamia nuts (raw or dry roasted)
pecans (raw or dry roasted)

hazelnuts (raw)
Brazil nuts (raw)

Condiments, Spices, and Seasonings (Organic is best.)

salsa (fresh or canned)
tomato sauce (no added sugar)
guacamole (fresh)
soy sauce (wheat free, tamari)
apple cider vinegar
herbs and spices (no added stabilizers)
Herbamare seasoning
Celtic sea salt
Real salt
sea salt
mustard
ketchup (no sugar; see the GPRx Resource Guide, page 342)
salad dressings (no canola oil)
marinades (no canola oil)
omega-3 mayonnaise
umeboshi paste
flavoring extracts such as vanilla or almond (alcohol-based, no sugar)

Snacks

healthy whole food bars (see the GPRx Resource Guide, pages 329–30)
goat's milk protein powder
flaxseed crackers
Healthy Macaroons (see the GPRx Resource Guide, page 339)
Healthy Trail Mix (see appendix A, page 273, for recipe)
organic cocoa powder
organic chocolate spreads (see the GPRx Resource Guide, page 343)
carob powder

Beverages
   purified, nonchlorinated water
   natural sparkling water, no carbonation added (e.g., Perrier)
   unsweetened or honey-sweetened herbal teas (green tea, black tea, white
      tea, red tea, oolong tea, mate, and herbal infusions)
   raw vegetable or fruit juices
   lacto-fermented beverages
   coconut water

Average

Foods in the average category should make up less than 50 percent of your daily diet. If you are struggling with your health, it is best to limit consumption of average foods to less than 25 percent of your daily diet. It may be wise in the early going to avoid these foods until symptoms are under control.

Dairy (Organic is best.)
cheese (cow, goat, or sheep)	low-fat yogurt
cow's milk cottage cheese	fat-free yogurt
cow's milk plain sour cream	almond milk
cream cheese	oat milk
heavy cream	rice milk
cultured whole soy yogurt	soy milk
Amazake	

Fats and Oils
   sunflower oil
   soy oil
   safflower oil

Vegetables (Organic is best.)
   canned vegetables

Nuts, Seeds, Beans, and Legumes *(Organic is best.)*
  tofu
  peanuts (dry roasted)
  peanut butter (roasted)
  cashews (raw or dry roasted)
  cashew butter (raw or roasted, in small quantities)
  soynut butter (in small quantities)

Condiments, Spices, and Seasonings *(Organic chemical- and preservative-free is best.)*

ketchup	marinade
mayonnaise	pickled ginger
salad dressing	wasabi

Fruits
  canned fruit in its own juices

Grains and Starchy Carbohydrates *(Whole grains and whole grain flours are healthiest if soaked for twelve hours before consuming.)*

brown rice	white potatoes
oats	whole-grain pasta (wheat, kamut, or spelt)
kamut	wheat
spelt	rye
barley	whole-grain dried cereal
corn	

Sweeteners

honey	agave nectar
Stevia	xylitol
organic dehydrated cane juice	barley malt
maple syrup	brown rice syrup

Beverages (Organic is best.)
    pasteurized vegetable juices
    pasteurized fruit juices (not from concentrate)
    beer and wine in moderation (organic and/or unpasteurized)
    fresh ground coffee (organic is best, but limit to one cup per day)

Snacks
    Zesty Popcorn (see appendix A, page 321, for recipe)
    baked corn or rice chips
    milk or whey protein powder from cow's milk
    rice protein
    soy protein (nongenetically modified)

Trouble

Foods in the trouble category do not promote good health and should be consumed with extreme caution. If you are generally healthy, you should limit trouble foods to once or twice per week—if you must consume them at all. If you are struggling with health problems, you should avoid these foods completely until symptoms disappear for at least six months. Only then can you eat these foods with extreme caution.

Meat

pork	ostrich
ham	emu
bacon	imitation meat products (soy)
sausage (pork)	veggie burgers
rabbit	

Fish and Seafood
    fried or breaded fish
    Avoid all shellfish, including:

crabs	catfish

oysters
clams
mussels
lobsters
shrimp

eel
squid (calamari)
shark
scallops

Poultry
fried or breaded chicken

Lunch Meat
ham
corned beef
soy lunch meat

Eggs
imitation eggs (e.g., Egg Beaters)

Dairy
soy cheese
rice cheese
homogenized milk
low-fat or skim milk
commercial ice cream with sugar

processed cheese food
American cheese (singles)
yogurt with sugar or artificial sweeteners
any dairy product with added stabiliaers,
preservatives, sugars, or artificial sweeteners

Fats and Oils
lard
margarine
shortening
canola oil

corn oil
cottonseed oil
any partially hydrogenated oil

Nuts and Seeds
nuts roasted in oil

honey-roasted nuts

Condiments, Spices, and Seasonings
    all spices that contain added sugar or preservatives

Fruits
    canned fruits in syrup

Beverages
    commercial beer and wine   fruit juices or drinks with artificial flavors
    sodas   fruit juices or drinks made from concentrate
    chlorinated tap water

Grains and Starchy Carbohydrates
    bread or crackers made with white or unbleached flour
    pastas made with white or unbleached flour
    white or unbleached flour
    dried cereal with sugar
    white rice
    instant oatmeal
    pastries
    baked goods

Sweeteners
    sugar
    corn syrup
    high fructose corn syrup
    all artificial sweeteners, including:
        aspartame   sorbital
        sucralose   maltitol
        acesulfame K

Miscellaneous

snack foods with sugar, partially hydrogenated oils, artificial sweeteners, or unbleached flour

---

Examples of Clean Meats in the Eyes of God

Meat

beef	antelope
elk	buffalo
lamb	venison
goat	sheep

Fish

cod	haddock
mackerel	salmon
tuna	

Fowl

chicken	turkey
quail	pheasant
goose	grouse
duck	guinea fowl

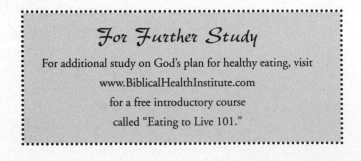

For Further Study

For additional study on God's plan for healthy eating, visit

www.BiblicalHealthInstitute.com

for a free introductory course

called "Eating to Live 101."

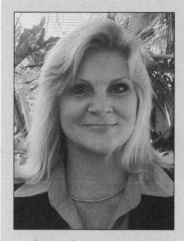

FUEL FOR FAMILY LIFE
by Julie Helm

To say that our family is active is an understatement. Ours has been a pastor's family for nearly twenty-five years, and we currently serve at a rapidly growing, fast-paced mega-church. In the midst of our busy work schedules—and basically doing life together—my husband, Steve, and I are also raising three lively, energetic children (now young adults) serving in their own respective ministries.

Our high-energy lives have sometimes necessitated "fast" options, and we have fallen into the fast-food trappings that many on-the-go families fall into. Fortunately, our drive-thru dinners have been sporadic. After spending most of the day away from each other, it's nice to hang out with *only* the family so that we can reconnect and hear about how our days went. There's nothing better than sharing a home-cooked meal with your favorite people in the world!

Steve and I have always tried to be health-conscious, but we both became more interested in nutrition when our children arrived. I fed them only breast milk for the first year of their lives, and when they were ready for solid foods, I used a baby-food grinder to feed them fresh vegetables and produce from our own garden. We provided the best nutrition possible because we know that our children were the most valuable contributions we would ever make during our lifetime. We wanted them to thrive, and they did—minimal colds, ear infections, and flu bugs compared to other kids.

Our emphasis on healthy eating began to splinter during the teen years, when our extracurricular and sports schedules meant that we were not home as much. That's when we started relying more on fast foods and convenience foods. We knew that we weren't eating the best foods for us, but we learned from it. As a result, we decided that we needed to be as intentional as possible to *never* compromise on nutrition again.

Our family realized that if we were going to faithfully make the trip through life as healthily and effectively as possible, we would have to make some deliberate changes to adopt healthier eating habits for the rest of our lives. Now that Steve and I are in our forties and our children are rapidly entering adulthood, we value the benefits of healthy eating more than ever before.

For our household these days, eating a healthy diet is not only enjoyable, but it also serves as a way to get the most out of our lives—for us personally, for our children, and for our professions. A healthy diet enables us to fulfill our responsibilities to the best of our abilities—and literally fuels our family life!

R͓ THE GREAT PHYSICIAN'S Rx FOR EATING

- *Eat only foods God created.*

- *Eat foods in a form that is healthy for the body.*

- *Chew each mouthful of food twenty-five to fifty times.*

- *At mealtime consume protein, fat, and veggies before starchy carbohydrates or sweet desserts.*

- *Drink six to eight or more glasses of pure water per day, and drink eight ounces of water whenever you feel hungry.*

- *When the plate is half-eaten, take a deep breath and ask yourself if you're still hungry.*

- *Consume one-to-three cups of hot tea blends each day to provide antioxidant protection and maintain a healthy weight.*

- *Consume at least one snack per day (whole food bar or smoothie) containing beta glucans from soluble oat fiber. This promotes good digestion, helps lower elevated cholesterol and triglycerides, maintains healthy blood sugar levels, supports immune system function, and maintains healthy body weight.*

- *Partially fast one day per week.*

THE GREAT PHYSICIAN'S Rx FOR WEEK #1

If you're ready to take the Great Physician's prescription for health and wellness to heart, then I've prepared a 49-day health plan that will revolutionize how you eat and live. This seven-week plan is designed to improve your health, help you lose weight, and lay a strong foundation for a lifetime of superb health for you and your family.

In week one, I'm letting you ease into the Great Physician's health plan by allowing you to eat what you normally eat for several meals, but it won't be long before you're on a whole new track. Yes, this menu plan will involve some change in your shopping habits and what foods that you stock your refrigerator and pantry with, but you're going to notice a big difference in the way you feel.

One note before we begin: You'll find only the first week of the 49-day plan in this chapter. Subsequent weeks will be found in each of the remaining six Keys.

Day 1

Breakfast
    eat what you consider to be your "normal" breakfast

Lunch
    normal lunch

Dinner
    grilled chicken
    green salad with red peppers, red onions, cucumbers, and carrots
    baked sweet potato with butter

Snacks
    normal snacks

Day 2

Breakfast
    normal breakfast

Lunch
    normal lunch

Dinner
    Cilantro-Lime Sea Bass (see appendix A, page 302, for recipe)
    green salad with red peppers, red onions, cucumbers, and carrots
    Garlic Mashed Potatoes (see appendix A, page 302, for recipe)

Snacks
    healthy whole food bar (see the GPRx Resource Guide, pages 329–330, for recommended products)
    piece of fruit

Day 3

Breakfast
    normal breakfast

Lunch
    Oriental Red Meat Salad (see appendix A, page 266, for recipe)
    apple

Dinner
Herb-Baked Salmon with Creamed-Style Spinach
green salad with red peppers, cucumbers, red onions, and carrots
Easy Spanish Rice (see appendix A, page 302, for recipe)

Snacks
cottage cheese, honey, and blueberries
Mango-Berry Smoothie Mix blended in eight-to-twelve ounces of water (see the GPRx Resource Guide, page 329, for recommended products).

Day 4

Breakfast
soft-boiled eggs
sprouted toast with butter (see the GPRx Resource Guide, page 328, for recommended products)
grapefruit

Lunch
Turkey and Goat Cheese Wrap
carrot and celery sticks

Dinner
Chicken Piccata (see appendix A, page 280, for recipe)
Garlicky Green Beans (see appendix A, page 283, for recipe)
Millet Corn Casserole (see appendix A, page 280, for recipe)

Snacks
vanilla protein whole food bar (see the GPRx Resource Guide, pages 329–330, for recommended products)
yogurt, honey, and fruit

Day 5 (Partial Fast Day)

Breakfast
none (partial fast day)

Lunch
none (partial fast day)

Dinner
Soy Ginger Salmon (see appendix A, page 281, for recipe)

green salad with carrots, cucumbers, red peppers, and red onions
cultured veggies

Snacks
none (partial fast day)

Day 6

Upon Waking
twelve-to-sixteen ounces of water

Breakfast
Mexican Omelet (see appendix A, page 266, for recipe)
avocado
salsa
hot tea with honey (see the GPRx Resource Guide, page 339, for recommended
herbal tea blends)
Lunch
Before eating, drink eight ounces of water.
During lunch, drink eight ounces of water or hot or iced fresh-brewed tea with
honey.
Chicken Salad on lettuce or on sprouted or whole grain sourdough toast (see
appendix A, page 303, for recipe)
apple

Dinner
Before eating, drink eight ounces of water.
During dinner, drink hot or iced fresh-brewed tea with honey.
Filet of Grass-Fed Beef (see appendix A, page 296, for recipe)
grilled asparagus with butter
green salad with red peppers, red onions, cucumbers, and carrots

Snacks
raspberries, raw almonds, and raw milk cheese
antioxidant fruit whole food bar (see the GPRx Resource Guide, pages 329–330,
for recommended products)
Drink eight-to-twelve ounces of water or hot or iced fresh-brewed tea with honey.

Before Bed
Drink eight-to-twelve ounces of water or hot tea with honey.

Day 7

Upon Waking

twelve-to-sixteen ounces of water

Breakfast

Easy Fried Eggs (see appendix A, page 306, for recipe)
Blueberry Pecan Pancakes (see appendix A, page 267, for recipe)
hot tea with honey

Lunch

Before eating, drink eight ounces of water.
During lunch, drink eight ounces of water or hot or iced fresh-brewed tea with honey.
Oriental Chicken Salad (see appendix A, page 303, for recipe)
grapes

Dinner

Before eating, drink eight ounces of water.
During dinner, drink hot or iced fresh-brewed tea with honey.
Tropical Chicken and Vegetable Kabobs (see appendix A, page 289, for recipe)
steamed vegetable medley
brown rice

Snacks

Tropical Smoothie Mix blended in eight-to-twelve ounces of water (see the GPRx Resource Guide, pages 329–330, for recommended products)
crackers (whole grain or flaxseed) and cheese
Drink eight-to-twelve ounces of water or hot or iced fresh-brewed tea with honey.

Before Bed

Drink eight-to-twelve ounces of water or hot tea with honey.

KEY #2

Supplement Your Diet with Whole Food Nutritionals,
Living Nutrients, and Superfoods

Their fruit will be for food, and their leaves for medicine.
—Ezekiel 47:12 (NKJV)

I travel a great deal, so everywhere I go, I take a silver case containing a variety of nutritional supplements with me. Whenever I sit down for a meal, whether it's breakfast at home with my family, lunch with colleagues, or a business dinner with associates, I discreetly reach for my silver case and pop it open. I pick out a few whole food living multivitamins and a couple of digestive enzyme caplets. Without further ado, I reach for a glass of water and then it's down the hatch . . . one after another.

In the morning and evening, I gulp down a "green food" supplement, a powdered probiotic formula and a whole food fiber combination. I call this my "cleansing drink." Once a day, usually with dinner, I consume one spoonful of one of my absolute favorite supplements—Icelandic cod-liver oil. (I hope I'm not making you too hungry!)

I ingest supplements three times a day not because I fail to eat healthy, although I sometimes find myself in settings where I'm served meals that aren't the highest quality, if you catch my drift. Ninety percent of the time I enjoy meals that incorporate organic fruits, vegetables, free-range or wild meats, and healthy oils while eschewing white rolls, fried foods, and sugary desserts. At the same time, I realize that the nutrients in today's foods have been depleted by nutrient-barren soils. That's why I cover my bases by taking nutritional supplements, which offer a concentrated source of nutrients that today's animal and plant foods don't always provide.

Back in biblical times, foods coming from the fields contained many more enzymes, minerals, and microorganisms than what's sold in supermarkets today. For the past half century or so, we've been sterilizing our soil with pesticides and herbicides, which means our food—even what is organically grown—doesn't pack the same nutritional punch as it did for our forefathers. That's why I urge you to supplement your diet with whole food nutritionals, living nutrients, and superfoods, which is the second key that will unlock your health potential.

From the outset, though, please know that I'm not one who believes good health can be found in a bottle of pills. After years of study in naturopathic medicine and nutrition, I understand better than most that dietary supplements are just what they say they are—supplements, not a substitute for an inadequate diet.

My friend and colleague Joseph Mercola, an osteopathic physician and founder of www.mercola.com, agrees with me. "There's no question that supplements can compensate for some of the damage that we do to ourselves," he said. "However, my experience is that many, if not most, people use the supplements to justify their poor choice of foods. That makes about as much sense as building a boat with rotten wood and using the best screws in the world to fasten everything together. The boat may hold together, but it will still leak. The boards in the boat are like macronutrients in the body—the protein, carbohydrates, and fats we consume. If we make poor choices here, it really doesn't matter what types of screws we use."[1]

The leaky boat is a great word picture, and I concur with Dr. Mercola that the indiscriminate use of supplements will not compensate for an inferior diet, poor hygiene, lack of exercise, or a life full of stress. Having made this disclaimer, though, let me boldly proclaim that the judicious use of the high-quality whole food nutritional supplements and superfoods can ensure an adequate supply of essential nutrients and beneficial compounds that will help you take long and measured steps toward optimal health. To make this happen, you need to take nutritional supplements that

1. meet a need or a deficiency of the body; and

2. are in a form that the body can utilize.

Since we're talking about supplementing your diet, we'll begin with the starting point for most people—multivitamins.

MULTIVITAMINS

Every major health agency from the American Medical Association to the American Heart Association, the American Lung Association, and the American Dietetic Association—you can see that I'm not even out of the A's yet—recommends that you take a multivitamin daily to ensure good health. Americans have apparently heeded that advice; according to the Council for Responsible Nutrition, a trade association for the dietary supplement industry, 70 percent of Americans take vitamins—usually a multivitamin—at least occasionally.[2]

While that figure might be high (researchers at the Harvard School of Public Health arrived at a more modest estimate of 30 percent),[3] it's my estimation that probably half of Americans rely on vitamin and mineral supplements to ward off illness and fill in the holes of a less-than-perfect diet. These days, multivitamins are mainstream, heavily advertised on TV, touted in national magazines, and part of "starting the day off right." The trouble is that not all multivitamins are created equally.

Let's start with the manufacturing process. Multivitamins—and all supplements, for that matter—are produced in one of five ways, according to the *Encyclopedia of Natural Healing*:[4]

1. *Natural.* The nutrients are derived from vegetable, mineral, or animal sources with little or no processing. Examples would be cod-liver oil, bee pollen, yeast, garlic, kelp, and minerals in their natural form.

2. *Natural source.* Although nutrients come from vegetable, mineral, or animal sources, the product undergoes processing. Examples would be

extracting vitamins A and D from fish liver oil; vitamin E from soy oil; lecithin from soybeans; and digestive enzymes, protein powders, and amino acids from various natural sources.

3. *Nature-identical or bio-identical.* These are laboratory-manufactured nutrients identical in molecular structure and activity in the human body to natural nutrients. These nutrients are manufactured because the cost or difficulty of extracting the same nutrients from all-natural sources would be prohibitively expensive. Examples of nature-identical nutrients include certain B vitamins.

4. *Synthetic.* These laboratory-manufactured nutrients aren't identical, molecularly speaking, to the natural nutrient. For instance, when you find inexpensive vitamin E or vitamin C on the shelf, you can rest assured that it was produced synthetically.

5. *Whole food or food-grown.* It's possible to produce nutritional supplements with raw materials, for example, by adding vitamins and minerals to a living probiotic culture. This form of supplement is the most costly to produce and is highly bioavailable, meaning it's highly usable and available to the body. This is the form of vitamin and mineral supplement that I recommend and use daily. If you are currently using a multivitamin/mineral supplement, I challenge you to switch to a whole food multivitamin for thirty days and feel the difference real food can make.

Multivitamins come packaged in different varieties: tablets and capsules are the most common; powders and liquids are less widespread. I prefer caplets and capsules as a good delivery system to ensure the nutrients get where they need to go. When it comes to capsules, you should look for kosher beef gelatin or vegetarian capsules, rather than the commonly used pork gelatin capsules. You can imagine my feelings about using a multivitamin encased in pork gelatin.

Multivitamins, by simple definition, are a grouping of vitamins and minerals compacted into a single pill or capsule. The idea that we should supplement our diets dates back to the Great Depression era, which, incidentally, coincides with the rapid changes in the manufacture and production of food in this country. Health-minded individuals and companies back in the 1930s introduced wheat and barley grass as our first multivitamins. They said if you mixed some wheat and barley grass (which are abundant in easily absorbable nutrients) into your favorite juice or milk, then you would be "fortifying" your body with nature's best. These cereal grasses, as they are known, were very popular until chemical scientists came along after World War II and discovered ways to synthetically replicate various nutrients in the laboratory.

My research into multivitamins reveals that companies producing synthetically made nutrients dominate much of the commercial supplement market. Vitamin companies—even some well-known and well-trusted names in the natural health field—have succumbed to market forces that are pushing them to sell products for less than the other guy. Their biochemists in white lab coats peer through their microscopes and figure out ways to synthetically create— although I prefer the verb *imitate*—complex structures such as vitamin E, vitamin C, and beta-carotene. They do this by synthesizing compounds that may *look* the same as the nutrients God created in foods. While these isolated nutrients are representative of man's genius inside the laboratory, they are also nutritional folly because they skip the entire process of nature.

There's no doubt that synthetic versions have dropped the price of vitamin supplements to a level that makes them popular and affordable: one can buy ninety vitamin C tablets from a mail-order company for seventy-nine cents or five hundred tablets of one-thousand-milligram vitamin C at a warehouse club for less then ten bucks. Yet the human body was not designed to consume these artificial and unnatural products, especially in the massive amounts that some health professionals advocate. For instance, if you feel a cold coming on and take ten one-thousand-milligram vitamin C tablets in the course of a day, that would be the equivalent of eating 150 oranges. Talk about a colon cleanse! I think it's unnatural—and nearly impossible—to eat 150 oranges in one day, and I don't think God designed us to process ten thousand milligrams of synthetic vitamin C when the flu bug is going around either. That's another reason why you should not take a multivitamin containing synthetic nutrients.

How can you tell if your multivitamin is filled with synthetic nutrients? The place to start is with the fine print on the label affixed to the back of the bottle or plastic container. If, for example, a bottle of chewable vitamin C tablets lists ingredients such as ascorbic acid, natural or artificial orange flavor, sucralose, or yellow 6 lake, then the product is made from synthetic materials. Another tip-off is the letters *dl* in front of the name of the ingredient.

For instance, if you pick up a bottle of vitamin E and see the main ingredient named dl-alpha tocopheryl, that means you're holding a synthetic version. An ingredient named d-alpha tocopheryl (*d* instead of *dl*) would mean that this is natural vitamin E and better for you. In addition, if the label lists many chemical names for various vitamins, such as pyridoxine hydrochloride, thiamin mono-nitrate, or cholecalciferol, you are holding a synthetic multivitamin.

I know that keeping track of all this information is tricky, and perhaps you're ready to throw your hands in the air. Don't, because if your multivitamin label says it "contains no filler ingredients, no artificial ingredients, and no preservatives" and it is a "whole food multivitamin/mineral product," then you're standing on solid ground. But the best way to determine whether your multi is natural or synthetic is to call the company, do your own research, or visit the GPRx Resource Guide at the back of this book for recommended whole food multivitamin brands.

Labels are clearinghouses of other worthwhile information as well, such as how many tablets you should take per serving and when to ingest them. Labels also relay the U.S. recommended daily allowance (RDA) for each nutrient. But don't be too impressed with large amounts of vitamins and minerals far exceeding the RDAs, as the source is very likely synthetic or at the very least isolated and purified, which means that the nutrient is likely missing key co-factors required for its proper function. Another consumer tip is that some companies add insignificant ingredients to make their product's RDA break-down look more impressive.

The natural-versus-synthetic question is central to good health because synthetic vitamins are 50 percent to 70 percent less biologically active than natural vitamins. The dirty little secret in this industry is that our bodies usually do not absorb more than 50 percent of the vitamins and minerals we ingest because of the way our digestive system works. So, if you're taking a multivitamin that is, say, 50 percent less productive for you, and the body absorbs just half of that, you're receiving only 25 percent of the advertised potency. That's a lot of money you're paying to have glow-in-the-dark urine.

So why take multivitamins at all? People say that they want to feel better about themselves and look healthier and younger. Others seek to gain energy that can be applied to their busy, stressful lives. In addition, many people take multivitamins to prevent diseases such as cancer, heart disease, and diabetes. I find nothing wrong with these motives.

When I looked at published research done in the last fifty years or so, however, I discovered something interesting: no doctor, no medical group, no drug manufacturer, and no supplement company has been able to conclusively document that taking multivitamins improves human performance, boosts energy, or reduces the risk for disease. Very few studies could prove that people feel better or experience less disease after taking a multivitamin product!

My inability to find documentation outlining the benefits of vitamins intrigued me, so I began looking into the different forms of vitamins and minerals that were available on the market. I was interested in what these vitamins did, how they worked, and, most important, how humans obtained their nutrients from nature. I needed to see the entire picture.

After prolonged study, I ascertained something so basic that I nearly slapped my forehead. What I learned is that we get our nutrients from eating plants—or from eating the flesh of animals that eat plants. Everything starts with plant life, and plants get their nutrients through biological transmutation. What's that? Biological transmutation is a process in which soil organisms take inorganic nutrients and convert them into organic substances that can be consumed by animals, then by humans, or by humans directly. Put another way, the microorganisms found in soil and on plants secrete various acids and enzymes to break down the inorganic substances and convert them into organic substances that the plants can use.

That's why, at the end of the day, you should search for a multivitamin that is made with organisms found in *dirt*. Yes, you read me correctly, although I do not mean literal dirt, as you will see, but the microorganisms found in pristine, healthy soil.

Back when I was in San Diego seeking a cure for my digestive ailments, I received a package in the mail from my father. I opened it to find a plastic bag containing a black-colored powder. A note said, "I know I promised not to send you anything more to try, but I really think you should add this to your diet. Love, Dad."

I thought I had already tested every known supplement known to man, including thirty different probiotics, which I'll talk about later. None of these supplements did anything special for me, although I could wistfully remember a couple of products that made me violently ill or touched off another round of diarrhea. No wonder I didn't click my heels in happiness when Dad forwarded a package with a friendly appeal to sample the dirtlike substance.

The next time we talked on the phone, he remained confident that this black powder was just the nature-based elixir I needed. "It may look like dirt, but it isn't," he promised. "That plastic bag contains healthy organisms and minerals from the soil."

An article accompanying the package explained that since nutrients had been hijacked from our soil-depleted farmlands, we needed to step up and do something about it. Not only were nutrients and trace minerals AWOL, but "living organisms" in our foods had been wiped out by three things: the pesticide treatment of cropland, pasteurization of dairy products, and modern man's disdain for microorganisms.

As I peered into Dad's plastic bag of black powder, I thought, *What do I have to lose?* Over the next week, I mixed some of this black powder in water and drank the dark-colored cocktail. I also sought out foods containing these beneficial microorganisms. These included raw goat's or cow's milk in the form of fermented kefir, sprouts, organic fruits and vegetables, raw sauerkraut, and carrot and other vegetable juices. These "live" foods retained their beneficial enzymes and microorganisms.

The reason I tell you this is that after my health improved and I resumed a normal life, I continued to seek out supplements made with soil-based organisms and other probiotic microorganisms which are known in the natural health industry as "whole food" or "living" multivitamins. I was convinced that nutrients produced by probiotic fermentation—a process in which beneficial bacteria and yeasts are created into beneficial compounds that enhance digestive and immune system health—are a missing link to good health. These probiotics contained many different compounds, such as organic acids, antioxidants, and key nutrients that were essential to human health. Beneficial microorganisms found in the soil and on plants also played a key role in biological transmutation, which is scientific jargon for evidence of nonradioactive, low-energy transmutation of light elements in plants, animals, and minerals.

I also studied the work of Dr. Weston Price, a Cleveland dentist who lived from 1870 to 1948. As he filled more and more cavities of patients sitting in his dental chair, he wondered, "Could it be our processed foods?" Dr. Price left his practice and traveled around the world studying indigenous people whose teeth and gums were untouched by processed foods. He came into contact with fourteen primitive cultures who not only displayed row after row of healthy teeth, but these smiling men, women, and children also lived healthy lives virtually free of physical disease. When Dr. Price wrote his findings, he was convinced that the standard American diet—SAD—was sending us down the road to perdition. Clearly a man ahead of his time, Dr. Price posited that restoring nutrient-dense foods into our diets would do us a world of good.

When I examined Dr. Price's writings, I paid close attention to the type and form of the nutrients contained in foods—meats, dairy, fruits, vegetables, botanicals, sea vegetables, and mushrooms—that the world's healthiest people consumed. That gave me a baseline to search for a "living" multivitamin that was the sum of nature's richest sources of these key nutrients. Although I couldn't go back to the lifestyle of our ancestors, I could certainly ingest nutrients in the forms they did and get at least part of the way there. My goal was to find a multivitamin that was as close to food as possible, which complies with the second criterion of eating—eat food in a form that is healthy for the body.

That's why I highly recommend that you take living multivitamins in whole food form, also known as homeostatic nutrients, which are vitamins and minerals that have been fermented with probiotic microorganisms and their enzymes. (You'll find a list of such products in the GPRx Resource

Guide.) Basically the nutrient complexes that make up the multivitamins have been put through a fermentation process (similar to the digestive process of the body) that takes the isolated nutrients and recombines them in a form found in food so the body can recognize it and utilize it better.

These multivitamins also contain a broad array of antioxidants from fruits, vegetables, herbs, and spices. Antioxidants are compounds that preserve and protect other compounds in the body from free radical damage. Without going into a long explanation, free radicals are something you don't *want* to run rampant within your molecular system. Free radicals are oxygen molecules with a single electron, but these unstable molecules are known to attack the immune system's cells. Antioxidants neutralize free radicals, which is a good thing.

The most well-known antioxidants are vitamins E and C and beta-carotene. Through scientific research, we've learned that vitamin E is a fat-soluble vitamin present in nuts, seeds, whole grains, apricots, vegetables, and eggs laid by healthy chickens. Vitamin C, chemically known as ascorbic acid, is a water-soluble vitamin present in green peppers, cabbage, spinach, broccoli, kale, cantaloupe, kiwi, strawberries, and citrus fruits and their juices. Beta-carotene is a precursor to vitamin A (which means the body converts beta-carotene to vitamin A) and is present in butter from grass-fed cows, spinach, carrots, cereal grasses such as wheat and barley, squash, broccoli, yams, tomatoes, cantaloupes, and peaches.

Take another look at those foods I just described. Do you think the average person is eating enough of those foods to receive the antioxidants he or she needs? Does a typical American diet of a Danish and coffee for breakfast, hamburger and fries for lunch, and spaghetti and meatballs with garlic bread for dinner fit this bill?

I don't think so, which is why I think everyone needs to take a living multivitamin daily—even folks who eat as healthy as I do. We all need a boost that only a living multivitamin can deliver.

COD-LIVER OIL

Another supplement that I universally recommend is the underappreciated cod-liver oil.

You may be thinking, *You mean that horrible-tasting stuff they gave to me when I was in labor for hours and the baby wouldn't come out?*

No, that would be *castor* oil. Cod-liver oil, on the other hand, contains four nutrients that hardly any of us get enough of. These four nutrients are eicosapentaenoic acid (EPA), docosahexaenoic acid (DHA), vitamin A, and vitamin D.

EPA and DHA are long-chain polyunsaturated fats known as omega-3 fatty acids, which are found in cold-water fish and eggs from chickens that run around and eat worms. Omega-3 is also present in flaxseed oil, hemp seed oil, and pumpkin seed oil, although it occurs as alpha linolenic acid, which must be converted by the body into EPA and DHA.

But EPA and DHA are best found in cold-water fish, especially the golden oils extracted from the filleted livers of Icelandic cod. This rich source of valuable nutrients began showing up in the fishing communities of Norway, Scotland, and Iceland in the middle of the nineteenth century as people discovered the health benefits of cod-liver oil. They endured harsh winters with long periods of darkness in some of the most remote places in the world, so whenever someone came off a fishing boat sneezing up a storm, he couldn't run down to Wal-Mart for some Sudafed or NyQuil.

Instead, they turned to cod-liver oil because they had learned over the years that its medicinal properties were a natural, effective remedy for many of the infections that ailed them. By the 1890s, cod-liver oil was commonly used to treat rickets in malnourished children, and adults relied upon it when they complained of rheumatism or arthritis. People in the old days believed cod-liver oil "lubricated the joints."

Cod-liver oil became popular in this country at the turn of the twentieth century, and I'm sure your parents or grandparents haven't forgotten the time when they held their noses while their parents administered a teaspoon of the fishy-smelling liquid. For a long time, however, cod-liver oil had a reputation as a vile substance. Apprehensive mothers often resorted to a "spoonful of sugar to make the medicine go down," as Mary Poppins used to sing. When improvements in the extraction and preparation of cod-liver oil occurred, progress was made in how it smelled and tasted. These days, cod-liver oil comes in lemon, mint, and other flavors that mask the fishy odor and taste. I'll admit that cod-liver oil is an acquired taste, but after a week or two, you'll get used to swallowing a spoonful.

I added cod-liver oil to my daily diet nearly ten years ago during my recovery from illness, and now I'm to the point where I can drink the stuff right out of the bottle. That's nothing, though, compared to the Hotel Borg in Reykjavik, Iceland, where they serve cod-liver oil in cordial glasses during breakfast!

These days, Icelandic schools have made cod-liver oil a lunchtime staple because of the lack of sunshine in the winter and their recognition that the vitamin D in cod-liver oil builds strong bones and keeps rickets at bay. If schoolkids in Reykjavik can handle cod-liver oil, you can too. I recommend that you place this enduring, time-proven nutritional gem on your list of supplements, and begin taking between one teaspoon and one tablespoon a day. Cod-liver oil helps prevent bone deterioration in adults, improves cardio-vascular function, and contributes to long life. Life insurance data and genetic research have shown that Iceland is now ahead of Japan for longevity, and the Icelandic people are medical marvels, displaying less heart disease and high blood pressure than most people in other cultures of the world.

Your children should be taking cod-liver oil, too, because the fatty acids in cod-liver oil are important for the development of the brain and nervous system. Cod-liver oil helps with concentration. David Horrobin, a medical and biochemical researcher, once told me, "If you want to prevent learning disabilities in your children, feed them cod-liver oil." The omega-3 fatty acids present in cod-liver oil are not only wonderful for your immune system, but for your skin health as well. The high levels of vitamin D are especially helpful if you're very careful about the amount of sunlight you expose yourself to.

Cod-liver oil contains more vitamin A per unit weight than any other common foods—almost three times more than beef liver, the next richest source. Most people are deficient in vitamin A because they don't regularly eat beef liver or butter produced from cows fed only grass from irrigated fields year-round. Vitamin A is not found in carrots or greens, despite what you may have heard; that is beta-carotene, which can be converted into vitamin A by a healthy liver.

Vitamin A is extremely important to the health and integrity of the mucosal linings of the body, such as the gastrointestinal tract and the lungs. When you have a virus or flu, however, your body gets depleted of vitamin A, which is another reason to sip on a teaspoon of cod-liver oil each evening.

Cod-liver oil is the Rodney Dangerfield of nutrition—it doesn't get a lot of respect. Sure, it may be as old as the hills and not real fancy, but study after study shows that people who use cod-liver oil are less likely to develop multiple sclerosis, arthritis, or coronary heart disease. And check this: a study of Norwegian women showed that women who consumed cod-liver oil during pregnancy gave birth to smarter children.[5] That's why cod-liver oil is one of the best-selling supplements in Europe, and it should be the same on this side of the Atlantic Ocean.

Green Superfoods

The average American consumes less than the recommended three-to-five servings a day of "greens," and the most beneficial are the deep green, leafy vegetables. In fact, Americans eat *way less* than they should when it comes to consuming their green veggies. The United States Department of Agriculture estimates that more than 90 percent of the population fails to eat five to nine servings of fruits and vegetables daily, which are some of the most beneficial foods that God created on this planet.

This amazes me in our land of plenty. Here we are, living in a blessed nation where fruits and vegetables are readily available at markets and roadside stands, and people don't avail themselves of these natural foods that are so good for us. Thanks to modern transportation and shipping methods, we can shop for fresh fruits and vegetables year-round: Fuji apples from Chile, ruby red strawberries from New Zealand, Hass avocados from Mexico, and fresh lettuce and tomatoes from our nation's breadbasket every month of the year. Do we eat enough of them? No.

I wonder what those Icelandic fishing families of yesteryear, who would have jumped for joy at the chance to eat a harvest salad in the dead of winter, would think of us now—a culture too apathetic to stock our refrigerators with fresh fruits and vegetables. It just goes to show you the wisdom of Solomon, who wrote: "Some people are so lazy that they won't even lift a finger to feed themselves" (Prov. 19:24 NLT). The ancient king must have known that our culture would squander one of the most powerful weapons against potent diseases. Fruits and vegetables, when consumed at optimal amounts, have been shown in countless studies to protect us against the ravages of heart disease, high blood pressure, cancer, diabetes, and almost every killer disease common to modern men and women.

Besides not eating enough leafy green vegetables, we don't eat enough grass. Yes, I said grass, and I'm not talking about the type you smoke. I'm referring to barley grass, wheat grass, oat grass, and alfalfa grass, which are commonly known as cereal grasses. Barley grass has been a part of a healthy diet since biblical times, mainly because barley was the first green plant to sprout up through the earth after a long winter. The Egyptians, Israelites, Greeks, and Romans made young barley sprouts a dietary staple. I mentioned earlier in the chapter that wheat and barley grasses were promoted in the 1930s as one of the first multivitamins.

Cereal grasses contain a broad array of enzymes, vitamins, minerals, proteins, and chlorophyll, which is the green pigment found in plants. Chlorophyll makes life on earth possible because the oxygen we breathe comes from the chlorophyll-rich green plants. Our human blood is identical to chlorophyll with one exception: the main element in blood is iron, while the main element in chlorophyll is magnesium. Nothing matches the nutritive density found in barley or other grasses such as wheat, rye, corn, rice, oats, sorghum, millet, and spelt.

In the 1930s and 1940s, America's leading scientists, led by agricultural biochemist George Kohler, embarked on grass research at the University of Wisconsin. They compared the growth of guinea pigs fed one of four foods: dried grass powder, lettuce, cabbage, and spinach. The guinea pigs fed dried grass powder thrived and gained normal weight, while those that ate lettuce, cabbage, or spinach lost or barely sustained their weight.[6]

Charles Schnabel, another agricultural biochemist, carried out similar experiments with chickens. Those fed cereal grass increased winter egg production by 94 percent and produced stronger, healthier chicks. Credit was given to the blood-building ability of grasses like wheat grass and barley, thanks to the presence of chlorophyll, which the body transforms into hemoglobin, thereby increasing the red blood cell count and the blood's capacity to deliver oxygen and other nutrients to the cells of the body.[7]

As I learned of the importance of whole food nutrition, I saw the value of taking a "green food" supplement that was a certified organic blend of barley, wheat, oat, and alfalfa grass juices combined with other vegetables, tart fruits, microalgae such as spirulina and chlorella, and sprouted grains and seeds. Once I began blending a couple of scoops of green food into a glass of water or veggie juice, I could tell that I was drinking one of the most nutrient-dense foods on this green earth. That's why I call powdered green foods "superfoods." And while the taste didn't thrill me at first, after regular use, my body actually began to crave it. For those who can't stomach the thought of drinking their greens, you've got no more excuses, because high-quality green foods are now available in caplets.

A combination green superfood product is a "must have" for your daily regimen. (A list of recommended green superfoods supplements can be found in the GPRx Resource Guide, pages 346–347.) A nutritious green superfood powder combines the dietary benefits of whole food living nutrients and often contains whole food fiber sources, and green food powders mix well with water or your favorite fruit or vegetable juice. If you're looking for nutrition on the go before you leave the house for work in the morning, a glass of green superfood powder mixed in water or juice provides convenient nutrition. Green foods also do wonders for keeping you regular.

Final thoughts about green superfood blends: the nutritional content in a high-quality green food powder often has greater amounts of various nutrients, such as vitamin A, riboflavin, folic acid, magnesium, and calcium than single servings of fresh, raw garden vegetables like broccoli, cabbage, carrots, cauliflower, cucumber, lettuce, spinach, and tomatoes. How is this done?

The answer is in juicing, low-temperature drying, and fermentation—

nature's way of preparing foods for easy assimilation into the human body. The fermentation of foods is accomplished by beneficial microorganisms, producing enzymes and organic acids that break down foods into their most usable compounds. You should seek out green food manufacturers that use a fermentation process to make their product. Some companies—like those that produce multivitamins—use fillers since it's an expensive process to transform thirty pounds of wheat and barley grass juices, for example, into a pound of green food powder. If you see ingredients like apple fiber, lecithin, chicory, or inulin on the ingredient label, that's a strong sign that the green food has been diluted by filler ingredients, making it not nearly as beneficial for you.

As the old Joni Mitchell song from the Sixties goes, we need to "get back to the garden."

Eat your green foods.

WHOLE FOOD FIBER

I grew up in south Florida, where the Miami Dolphins are a big deal for pro football fans, which pretty much includes everyone in my part of the state.

Whenever the Dolphins make the playoffs—which hasn't been too often in recent years—a sportswriter with one of the Miami papers goes into the files and rehashes one of the greatest playoff games in NFL history. I'm talking about the January 1982 clash between the Dolphins and the San Diego Chargers, which *Sports Illustrated* named the second-greatest game in NFL history.

Listen, I was a first grader when the Dolphins and the Chargers played that game in the Orange Bowl, which was decided in overtime when Charger kicker Rolf Benirschke nailed a chip-shot 29-yard field goal to win the game.

Rolf was the first NFL player—and probably the first professional athlete—to play with ostomy appliances. Several seasons before that playoff game, he almost died from an inflammatory bowel disease similar to the one that nearly claimed my life. After collapsing on a team flight following a game in New England, Rolf submitted to emergency surgery that removed most of his large intestine—the same surgical procedure that Dr. Wenger feared was in my future. In Rolf's case, his colostomy meant wearing a pair of "pouches" that were attached to the side of his stomach to capture the fecal waste.

I had breakfast with Rolf on a recent trip to San Diego, and I couldn't help thinking that his surgery could have been my fate as well. It's estimated that two million Americans suffer from inflammatory bowel disease (IBD), and thirty thousand new cases are diagnosed in the United States each year.[8] That's more than eighty people a day. IBD generally comes in two forms: Crohn's disease, which is what I had; and ulcerative colitis, which is what Rolf suffered from. Both are chronic digestive disorders of intestines.

If you've never experienced symptoms of IBD, then you have something to thank the Lord for. IBD is an unpredictable illness: some patients recover after a single attack or are in remission for years, while others require frequent hospitalizations and eventual surgery. Around one hundred thousand people a year submit to this life-changing procedure. (Note: a change in bowel habits and pain can be early signs of serious illness. A medical checkup is recommended.)

The reason I'm telling this story about Rolf is to point out the importance of digestive health. If irregularity—or persistent diarrhea or abdominal pain—is a large issue in your life, then a whole food fiber supplement can counteract the refined foods that glut the stomach and cause teeth-grinding pain. If you've been taking laxatives, antacids, or anti-hemorrhoidal or anti-diarrhea medicines, then you're a candidate for a whole food fiber supplement that supplies your body with a highly usable, vegetarian source of dietary fiber.

When searching for a fiber product that's right for you, choose a brand that is made from organic seeds, grains, and legumes that are fermented or sprouted for ease of digestion. One of the best ways to consume whole food fiber is to take it first thing in the morning and just before bed. Just mix it with your green superfood powder, and you've given your body more nutrition than most people get in a week. (For a list of recommended whole food fiber products, see the GPRx Resource Guide, pages 346–347.)

PROBIOTICS

Most people, when they see their family physician for a sinus problem or a nasty bronchitis infection, walk out of the doctor's office holding a prescription for antibiotics. Medically speaking, antibiotics are a variety of natural or synthetic substances that inhibit the growth of—or destroy—microorganisms. Since their discovery in the 1930s, antibiotics have made it possible to cure bacteria-related diseases such as pneumonia, tuberculosis, and meningitis. So if antibiotics are supposed to be good for us, what about probiotics? Does that mean they're bad for us?

Just the opposite, I can assure you. By definition, probiotics are living, direct-fed microbials (DFMs) that promote the growth of beneficial bacteria in the intestines. In fact, I would argue that the lack of probiotics in our diet can be associated with a whole array of intestinal problems like the aforementioned Crohn's disease, gastritis, and ulcerative colitis, along with high cholesterol levels, allergies, skin conditions, frequent colds, and the flu. Our society has developed into an antibiotic culture so intent on destroying bacteria that we've eradicated much of the beneficial bacteria in our bodies and the environment, thanks to the development of antibiotic drugs, the introduction of chlorinated water, the onset of air pollution, and the continued reliance on a poor diet.

After I recovered from my intestinal disorders with the help of beneficial microorganisms from food and supplements, you can bet your bottom dollar that my interest was piqued in this category of human nutrition with so much promise called probiotics. For instance, I learned that the normal human gastrointestinal tract contains hundreds of different species of harmless bacteria, otherwise known as intestinal flora. When the normal balance of these bacteria is disturbed by illness or antibiotic treatment, an imbalance occurs, and the result is often constipation or diarrhea.

Man, did I have terrible bouts of the runs when I was sick. Most days, I had to run to the toilet twenty to thirty times. When I intentionally introduced the right whole food probiotics containing organisms from healthy soil and plants into my system, I experienced profound benefits. Probiotics, I learned, work by colonizing the intestinal tract and crowding out disease-causing bacteria, viruses, and yeasts.

Since it has become my life mission to share what I've learned about how we should eat and stay healthy, I believe it's important to reintroduce beneficial bacteria to our digestive tracts so that we can stave off IBD and other digestive ailments.

Probiotics are available in two formats: food and dietary supplements. Unfortunately we've been sterilizing our soil for the last fifty to one hundred years with pesticides and herbicides, destroying good and bad bacteria. An easy place to find foods containing probiotic bacteria is your grocery store's dairy case, where you can reach for probiotic-rich yogurt, kefir, or raw sauerkraut.

Dietary supplements are a great way to reintroduce beneficial microorganisms into your digestive tract, which can improve bowel and immune system function, increase nutrient absorption, and detoxify the body and its organs. I think the best probiotics are the ones that contain soil-based organisms (SBOs), which are room-temperature stable and do not require refrigeration as most common probiotic supplements do.

In the old days, before farmers called in crop dusters to spray their fields with pesticides, our soils teemed with microorganisms, many of which were beneficial to our digestive tracts and immune systems. I've seen clinical studies showing that people with Crohn's disease, irritable bowel syndrome, constipation, *Candida,* asthma, and other allergies demonstrated dramatic changes in health once they added probiotics to their supplement plan.

Digestive Enzymes

I mentioned that I stock digestive enzymes in my silver supplement case, and I always make sure I take a couple before I dig into a restaurant meal. Let me explain why: when we eat raw foods, such as salad and fruit, we consume the enzymes they contain. When we eat cooked or processed meals, like in a restaurant, however, the body's pancreas must produce the enzymes necessary to digest them. The constant demand for enzymes strains the pancreas, which must kick in more enzymes to keep up with the demand. Without the proper levels of enzymes from foods—either raw or fermented—or from taking supplements, you are susceptible to excessive gas and bloating, diarrhea, constipation, heartburn, and low energy.

Digestive enzymes are complex proteins involved in the digestive process. They are the body's day laborers, the ones responsible for synthesizing, delivering, and eliminating the unbelievable number of ingredients and chemicals that your body uses during the waking hours. When the body produces enzymes, their job is to stimulate chemical changes in the foods passing through the gut. The pancreas, which takes a lead role in producing digestive enzymes for the body, has to keep up by producing pancreatic enzymes. Those with pancreatic problems such as cystic fibrosis usually require some form of digestive enzyme, but junk-food diets, fast chewing, and eating on the run contribute to the body's inability to produce adequate enzyme production and the subsequent malabsorption of food. These problems get worse as we age, not better.

A leading biochemist, Dr. Edward Howell, cited numerous animal studies in his book *Enzyme Nutrition*[9], showing that animals fed diets deficient in enzymes experienced enlargement of the pancreas because the organ was working overtime to produce digestive enzymes. It wasn't long before their health was severely affected. One could eat more raw food in its natural, unprocessed state, but that isn't always possible, as I can attest when I travel or have a heavy social schedule. The last thing you want to eat when you have these types of digestive problems is fried foods because items like fried chicken and French fries must be cooked in oil at higher temperatures than the boiling point, which damages fats and destroys all enzymes.

So, if you're having trouble finding a way to eat enough raw, fresh, live foods like bananas, avocados, seeds, nuts, grapes, and other natural foods, then take plant-based digestive enzymes to ease the digestion of the food. Digestive enzymes are available at your local natural food store, and you can find recommended brands in the GPRx Resource Guide, pages 347–348.

Final Thoughts

There is no doubt in my mind that the right amount of high-quality whole food nutritional supplements can make a big difference in all of our lives. However, keep in mind that the term *supplement* means "in addition to," so I want to encourage you to base your health plan on eating healthy, organic food and using supplements such as a whole food multivitamin, Icelandic cod-liver oil, green superfoods, whole food fiber, enzymes, probiotics, and high-quality protein powders to aid in your quest for a long and healthy life.

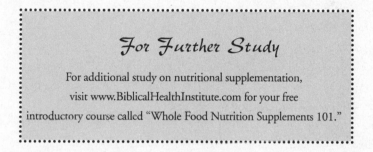

For Further Study

For additional study on nutritional supplementation,
visit www.BiblicalHealthInstitute.com for your free
introductory course called "Whole Food Nutrition Supplements 101."

A PICKY EATER BECOMES EVEN MORE PICKY
by John Norton

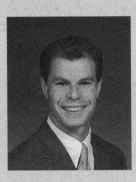

If you had been my friend in college, you would have told others, "Yep, that John sure is a picky eater." That's because I ate corn flakes for breakfast, lunch, and dinner. If I broke things up with a turkey sandwich, you could bet your bottom dollar that I wouldn't eat the crust. Fruits and vegetables? They weren't part of my laissez-faire attitude toward nutrition.

I took a lot of ribbing from my college roommates. Even as bad as their diets were, they were light-years ahead of me when it came to eating right. One day, after enduring another round of teasing, I decided to eat a cob of fresh corn. That wasn't too bad. Then I became more adventurous, sampling green beans and even turkey tetrazzini. You could say that I was expanding my taste buds.

It's a good thing I did; otherwise, I don't think Ruthie would have accepted my marriage proposal. Slowly but surely through the early years of marriage, I added more fruits and vegetables to my diet. I even began eating the skin of the potato!

I noticed the jump in energy when I ate healthy; my performance as a husband, father, and employee improved when I ate foods in their purest and most natural state. I felt better, had more energy, and gained in all areas of performance. That's when I became a believer in eating organic whole foods containing no harmful chemicals such as pesticides, hormones, and antibiotics. I found out through personal experience that the body absorbed whole organic foods immediately, while processed foods containing synthetic chemicals were harder for the body to digest.

This discovery revolutionized my diet, but for my body to be in peak performance, I needed extra help. This is where the area of supplements became a factor. I heard a great word picture about supplements: just as snow can be condensed into a snowball, all the nutrients of whole foods can be condensed into whole food supplements.

I had always thought that supplements were more like meal replacements so that one could reduce calories. That's not the way they work at all. The supplements that my wife and I take are not meant to replace foods or meals. Instead, they simply add to the nutrients that we are already getting from our diet, thereby making sure that we have everything we need for our bodies to perform at the highest levels.

My family and I have incorporated whole food nutrition supplements such as a whole food, living multivitamin, Icelandic cod-liver oil, green superfoods, whole food fiber, enzymes, and probiotics into our diets. We enjoy healthy smoothies fortified with goat's milk protein powder, and we have even convinced our two-year-old to consume some supplements. I know that whole food supplements will never take the place of a healthy diet, but I can tell you firsthand that they have become a great insurance policy for me and my family.

THE GREAT PHYSICIAN'S Rx FOR NUTRITIONAL SUPPLEMENTATION

- *Take a whole food living multivitamin with each meal.*

- *Consume one-to-three teaspoons or three-to-nine capsules of high omega-3 cod-liver oil per day with dinner.*

- *Drink a cleansing drink containing a combination of green superfoods and whole food fiber.*

- *If you want improved digestion, take a probiotic and enzyme blend with each meal.*

- *To ensure optimal protein intake, incorporate an easily digestible protein powder into your daily diet.*

THE GREAT PHYSICIAN'S Rx FOR WEEK #2

Day 8

Upon Waking
   twelve-to-sixteen ounces of water

Breakfast
   hot tea with honey (see the GPRx Resource Guide, page 339, for recommended herbal tea blends)
   Berry Smoothie (see appendix A, page 304, for recipe)
   Supplements: take one or two whole food multivitamin caplets (see the GPRx Resource Guide, page 345, for recommended brands).

Lunch
   Before eating, drink eight ounces of water.
   During lunch, drink eight ounces of water or hot or iced fresh-brewed tea with honey.
   turkey and avocado sandwich on toasted sprouted or whole-grain sourdough bread
   carrot and celery sticks
   Supplements: take one or two whole food multivitamin caplets.

Dinner
   Before eating, drink eight ounces of water.
   During dinner, drink hot or iced fresh-brewed tea with honey.
   Lemon Garlic Chicken (see appendix A, page 305, for recipe)
   pan-roasted, red bliss potatoes
   steamed asparagus
   Supplements: take one or two whole food multivitamin caplets.

Snacks
   Drink eight-to-twelve ounces of water or hot or iced fresh-brewed tea with honey.
   antioxidant fruit whole food bar (with beta glucans from soluble oat fiber; see the

GPRx Resource Guide, pages 329–330, for recommended products)
   sliced apples with nut or seed butter (almond, sesame, etc.)

Before Bed
   Drink eight-to-twelve ounces of water or hot tea with honey.

Day 9

Upon Waking
   Supplements: take one serving of a fiber/green superfood powder (mixed in) or five caplets of a super green formula (swallowed with) twelve-to-sixteen ounces of water or raw vegetable juice. (See the GPRx Resource Guide, pages 346–347, for recommended products.)

Breakfast
   hot tea with honey
   sprouted cereal with four ounces of plain yogurt, goat's milk, or almond milk (see the GPRx Resource Guide, pages 328, 330–331, 335, for recommended products)
   half a cup of berries
   Supplements: take one or two whole food multivitamin caplets.

Lunch
   Before eating, drink eight ounces of water.
   During lunch, drink eight ounces of water or hot or iced fresh-brewed tea with honey.
   Red Meat Chili (see appendix A, page 305, for recipe)
   flaxseed crackers, whole grain crackers, or baked corn chips
   carrot and celery sticks
   Supplements: take one or two whole food multivitamin caplets.

Dinner
   Before eating, drink eight ounces of water.
   During dinner, drink hot or iced fresh-brewed tea with honey.
   Roasted Pastured Chicken (see appendix A, page 320, for recipe)
   Hobo Potatoes (see appendix A, page 306, for recipe)
   steamed broccoli and cauliflower
   Supplements: take one or two whole food multivitamin caplets.

Snacks
   Drink eight-to-twelve ounces of water or hot or iced fresh-brewed tea with honey.
   Chocolate protein whole food bar (with beta glucans from soluble oat fiber)
   Banana Bread with butter (see appendix A, page 312, for recipe)

Before Bed

Drink eight-to-twelve ounces of water or hot tea with honey.

Supplements: take one serving of a fiber/green superfood powder (mixed in) or five caplets of a super green formula (swallowed with) twelve-to-sixteen ounces of water or raw vegetable juice.

Day 10

Upon Waking

Supplements: take one serving of a fiber/green superfood powder (mixed in) or five caplets of a super green formula (swallowed with) twelve-to-sixteen ounces of water or raw vegetable juice. (See the GPRx Resource Guide, pages 346–347, for recommended products.)

Breakfast

hot tea with honey
fried eggs
Easy Oatmeal (see appendix A, page 306, for recipe)
Supplements: take one or two whole food multivitamin caplets.

Lunch

Before eating, drink eight ounces of water.
During lunch, drink eight ounces of water or hot or iced fresh-brewed tea with honey.
sliced turkey and cheese sandwich on toasted sprouted or whole grain sourdough bread
apple
Supplements: take one or two whole food multivitamin caplets.

Dinner

Before eating, drink eight ounces of water.
During dinner, drink hot or iced fresh-brewed tea with honey.
Beef & Chicken Fajitas (see appendix A, page 268, for recipe)
green salad with red peppers, red onions, cucumbers, and carrots
Supplements: take one or two whole food multivitamin caplets.

Snacks

Drink eight to twelve ounces of water, or hot or iced fresh-brewed tea with honey.
flaxseed crackers, baked corn chips, avocado, and salsa
antioxidant fruit whole food bar (see the GPRx Resource Guide, pages 329–330, for recommended products)

Before Bed

Drink eight-to-twelve ounces of water or hot tea with honey.

Supplements: take one serving of a fiber/green superfood powder (mixed in) or five caplets of a super green formula (swallowed with) twelve-to-sixteen ounces of water or raw vegetable juice.

Day 11

Upon Waking

Supplements: take one serving of a fiber/green superfood powder (mixed in) or five caplets of a super green formula (swallowed with) twelve-to-sixteen ounces of water or raw vegetable juice. (See the GPRx Resource Guide, pages 346–347, for recommended products.)

Breakfast

hot tea with honey

cottage cheese with berries and honey

sprouted English muffins with butter (see the GPRx Resource Guide, page 328, for recommended products)

Supplements: take one or two whole food multivitamin caplets.

Lunch

Before eating, drink eight ounces of water.

During lunch, drink eight ounces of water or hot or iced fresh-brewed tea with honey.

Warm Chicken Supreme Salad (see appendix A, page 282, for recipe)

Supplements: take one or two whole food multivitamin caplets.

Dinner

Before eating, drink eight ounces of water.

During dinner, drink hot or iced fresh-brewed tea with honey.

Goat Cheese Stuffed Free-Range Chicken Breast (see appendix A, page 298, for recipe)

baked sweet potato with butter

green beans

Supplements: take one or two whole food multivitamin caplets and one-to-three teaspoons or three-to-nine capsules of high omega-3 cod-liver oil (see the GPRx Resource Guide, pages 345–346, for recommended brands).

Snacks

Drink eight to twelve ounces of water or hot or iced fresh-brewed tea with honey.

apple-cinnamon fiber whole food bar (see the GPRx Resource Guide, pages 329–330, for recommended products)

piece of fruit

Crispy Almonds (see appendix A, page 270, for recipe)

Before Bed

Drink eight-to-twelve ounces of water or hot tea with honey.

Supplements: take one serving of a fiber/green superfood powder (mixed in) or five caplets of a super green formula (swallowed with) twelve-to-sixteen ounces of water or raw vegetable juice.

Day 12 (Partial Fast Day)

Upon Waking

Supplements: take one serving of a fiber/green superfood powder (mixed in) or five caplets of a super green formula (swallowed with) twelve-to-sixteen ounces of water or raw vegetable juice. (See the GPRx Resource Guide, pages 346–347, for recommended products.)

Breakfast

none (partial fast day)

hot tea with honey or raw vegetable or fruit juice

Lunch

none (partial fast day)

sixteen ounces of water or raw vegetable or fruit juice

Dinner

Before eating, drink eight ounces of water.

During dinner, drink hot or iced fresh-brewed tea with honey.

Marinated Baked Salmon with Capers (see appendix A, page 290, for recipe)

cultured vegetables

steamed green beans

green salad

Supplements: take one or two whole food multivitamin caplets, one-to-three teaspons or three-to-nine capsules of high omega-3 cod-liver oil, and one or two capsules of a probiotic/enzyme blend (see the GPRx Resource Guide, pages 345–348, for recommended brands).

Snacks

none (partial fast day)

Drink eight-to-sixteen ounces of water or raw vegetable or fruit juice.

Before Bed

Drink eight-to-twelve ounces of water or hot tea with honey.

Supplements: take one serving of a fiber/green superfood powder (mixed in) or five caplets of a super green formula (swallowed with) twelve-to-sixteen ounces of water or raw vegetable juice.

Day 13

Upon Waking

Supplements: take one serving of a fiber/green superfood powder (mixed in) or five caplets of a super green formula (swallowed with) twelve-to-sixteen ounces of water or raw vegetable juice. (See the GPRx Resource Guide, pages 346–347, for recommended products.)

Breakfast

hot tea with honey
Mushroom Swiss Omelet (see appendix A, page 267, for recipe)
avocado
grapefruit
Supplements: take one or two whole food multivitamin caplets and one or two capsules of a probiotic enzyme blend.

Lunch

Before eating, drink eight ounces of water.
During lunch, drink eight ounces of water or hot or iced fresh-brewed tea with honey.
Chicken Soup
Supplements: take one or two whole food multivitamin caplets and one or two capsules of a probiotic/enzyme blend.

Dinner

Before eating, drink eight ounces of water.
During dinner, drink hot or iced fresh-brewed tea with honey.
Spaghetti with Meat Sauce (see appendix A, page 307, for recipe)
garlic cheese bread
steamed broccoli
Supplements: take one or two whole food multivitamin caplets and one-to-three teaspoons or three-to-nine capsules of high omega-3 cod-liver oil and one or two capsules of a probiotic enzyme blend.

Snacks

Drink eight-to-twelve ounces of water or hot or iced fresh-brewed tea with honey.
Creamy High Enzyme Dessert (see appendix A, page 307, for recipe)
Pepitas (see appendix A, page 269, for recipe)
Berry Smoothie mix blended in eight-to-twelve ounces of water (see the GPRx Resource Guide, page 329, for recommended products)

Before Bed

Drink eight-to-twelve ounces of water or hot tea with honey.

Supplements: take one serving of a fiber/green superfood powder (mixed in) or five caplets of a super green formula (swallowed with) twelve-to-sixteen ounces of water or raw vegetable juice.

Day 14

Upon Waking
Supplements: take one serving of a fiber/green superfood powder (mixed in) or five caplets of a super green formula (swallowed with) twelve-to-sixteen ounces of water or raw vegetable juice. (See the GPRx Resource Guide, pages 346–347, for recommended products.)

Breakfast
hot tea with honey

Berry Smoothie (see appendix A, page 304, for recipe) with two tablespoons of protein powder (see the GPRx Resource Guide, page 337, for recommended brands)

Supplements: one or two whole food multivitamin caplets and one or two capsules of a probiotic/enzyme blend.

Lunch
Before eating, drink eight ounces of water.

During lunch, drink eight ounces of water or hot or iced fesh-brewed tea with honey.

Roast Beef with Marinated Cabbage and Provolone Cheese Wrap (see appendix A, page 289, for recipe)

apple

Supplements: take one or two whole food multivatamin caplets and one or two capsules of a probiotic/enzyme blend.

Dinner
Before eating, drink eight ounces of water.

During dinner, drink hot or iced fresh-brewed tea with honey.

Sweet and Sour Chicken (see appendix A, page 308, for recipe)

Mexican Quinoa (see appendix A, page 308, for recipe)

green salad

Supplements: take one or two whole food multivitamin caplets and one-to-three teaspoons or three-to-nine capsules of high omega-3 cod-liver oil and one or two capsules of a probiotic/enzyme blend.

Snacks
Drink eight-to-twelve ounces of water or hot or iced fresh-brewed tea with honey.

raspberry super green whole food bar (see the GPRx Resource Guide, pages 329–330, for recommended products)

Before Bed

Drink eight-to-twelve ounces of water or hot tea with honey.

Supplements: take one serving of a fiber/green superfood powder (mixed in) or five caplets of a super green formula (swallowed with) twelve-to-sixteen ounces of water or raw vegetable juice.

Key #3

Practice Advanced Hygiene

The clean person shall sprinkle [hyssop and water upon] the unclean on the third day and on the seventh day; and on the seventh day he shall purify himself, wash his clothes, and bathe in water; and at evening he shall be clean.
—Numbers 19:19 (NKJV)

One time I was hastily changing planes in Dallas when I ducked into a Terminal B public restroom before my next flight. After using the facilities, I was dutifully washing my hands when I heard the toilet flush in the stall behind me. I glanced into the mirror and observed a burly man in a business suit zip his fly and quickly exit the premises.

Witnessing that brazen behavior surprised me, although I shouldn't have been shocked because such ill-mannered conduct is commonplace these days. It's absolutely brutal how many millions of people each day fail to wash their hands after they go to the bathroom. They blithely leave the restroom and spread their germs on an unsuspecting public.

In 2003, the Dallas-Fort Worth International Airport was part of a survey sponsored by the American Society of Microbiology (ASM) in which representatives of Wirthlin Worldwide observed 7,541 people in public restrooms at airports in New York, Chicago, San Francisco, Miami, and Toronto. Thirty-one percent of the males did not wash their hands in Dallas, which was better than JFK (37 percent) and O'Hare (38 percent) in New York and Chicago, respectively. Canadian guys were the cleanest of the bunch: 95 percent washed their hands after going to the bathroom. Lumped together, however, 26 percent of males zipped up and bypassed the washbasin.[1]

How did women rate? My wife, Nicki, predicted that women would be cleaner than men, but even she was shocked by the survey results: 22 percent of women failed to clean up at JFK, 15 percent at O'Hare, but at San Francisco International, 41 percent of women, for reasons unfathomable to Nicki or me, left the bathroom stalls without washing their hands and headed straight for the gates. Women were most hygienic north of the border, where 97 percent washed up at Toronto International. In total, 17 percent of women declined to wash their hands after going to the bathroom, which is rather astounding.

Now here's the really interesting part: when the Wirthlin organization conducted a follow-up survey by telephone and *asked* people if they washed their hands after going to the bathroom, 95 percent responded yes. That's human nature speaking loud and clear. Who wouldn't answer in the affirmative if asked whether they wash their hands after taking care of business? I know I would be too embarrassed to tell a pollster otherwise.

It's a shame that so many men and women neglect the most fundamental rule of good hygiene because the hands are one of the five main areas where germs enter the body—the other four being the eyes, ears, nose, and mouth. Since germs prefer to hitchhike rather than fly through the air, tiny microbes find the hands and the soft tissue underneath the fingernails to be staging areas for their assault on the body's immune system. Once germs establish a beach-head on your fingertips, it's a matter of time before you rub your eyes, scratch your nose, stroke your ears, or touch your mouth. Your body's immune system is under attack as the germs, like soldiers assaulting the beaches of Normandy, invade the portals to your body.

Something can be done to repel this raid on your immune system, and that's the practice of advanced hygiene, which is the third key that will unlock your health potential.

BACK IN MOSES' TIME

Practicing advanced hygiene is as essential to optimal health as diet and exercise. I'm talking about a system that has its roots in a plan that God laid out for the

Israelites four thousand years ago in which He instructed them to avoid certain situations where they were likely to encounter germs. Sections of Leviticus, Deuteronomy, and Numbers outline laws that protected the Israelites from communicable diseases. They were told to avoid touching dead bodies, keep corpses away from where they lived, properly dispose of their solid waste, and clean their hands, utensils, and clothing in running water instead of stagnant water in a bowl. In addition, women were given guidelines to follow during menstruation, and the adults were presented with rules for sexual conduct, which condemned same-sex activity, promiscuity, and sexual contact between humans and animals.

Prior to receiving these laws, the Israelites had lived side by side for four centuries with the Egyptian people, who, as I mentioned in the Introduction, were the world's most advanced people at the time. They even had their own medical book called the *Ebers Papyrus*, and their doctors' little black bags contained "medicines" like mouse tails, cat hair, pig eyes, dog toes, breast milk, eel eyes, and goose guts.

Egyptian practitioners' ideas about treating medical ailments ranged from pouring worm's blood on splinters to packing donkey dung on open wounds. These two practices would have been anathema to the Israelites. After Moses communicated God's laws for hygiene, the Hebrew people were forbidden from consuming the blood of animals or coming into contact with the solid waste of animals and humans.

The Israelites may not have known it at the time, but God's laws of hygiene were for their own good. God promised good health to His chosen people if they followed His principles:

If you listen carefully to the voice of the LORD your God and do what is right in his eyes, if you pay attention to his commands and keep all his decrees, I will not bring on you any of the diseases I brought on the Egyptians, for I am the LORD, who heals you. (Exod. 15:26)

Let me show you in one small way how God knew what He was talking about by recounting a modern-day story from my friend, Rex Russell, M.D.

When Dr. Russell was an intern at the University of Kentucky in the late 1960s, he was handed his first surgical case: circumcising a newborn male. A circumcision was about as routine and easy a procedure as a novice doctor could get.

Snip, snip, and in a matter of minutes, Dr. Russell had removed the foreskin of the infant's tiny penis. He carefully bandaged the boy, who displayed a healthy set of lungs for the apprentice doctor and the nurse. Four hours later, however, the three-day-old boy had not stopped crying out in pain. When Dr. Russell removed the bloody bandage and inspected his handiwork, he could see that the infant was still bleeding. His blood was failing to clot.

Medical protocol called for administering vitamin K, a fat-soluble vitamin used as a clotting agent. The infant's bleeding persisted for several days, however, which prompted worries of hemophilia in the young doctor and his supervisors. Finally, four days later, the bleeding stopped, and Dr. Russell and the boy's parents could start breathing again.

Years later, Dr. Russell recalled this case when he was reading in Genesis about how God made a covenant with Abraham and his descendants that He would be their God and give them the land of Canaan as an "everlasting possession."

Abraham's side of the bargain was that every male among his people had to be circumcised, and in those days before anesthetics, I probably wouldn't have looked forward to literally going under the knife, as an adult, on that part of my anatomy either. But Dr. Russell said that Genesis 17:12 leaped out at him, which stated, "For the generations to come every male among you who is eight days old must be circumcised."

Wait a minute—that boy he circumcised in Kentucky was only three days old! Then Dr. Russell remembered reading in a recent medical journal that an infant's ability to clot blood was lowest between the second and fifth days of life. Reason? The body's natural supply of blood-clotting vitamin K didn't build up until after five to seven days of breast-feeding. No wonder God was so specific to instruct Abraham and his descendants to count *eight days* before circumcising their newborn males.

When Dr. Russell stopped and thought about the role of circumcision, he wondered why did God make such a big deal about it anyway? Dr. Russell said that the foreskin provides a warm, moist area for harmful bacteria to grow, so God's command for males to be circumcised stemmed from His loving concern for proper hygiene. "The ongoing value of literal circumcision is shown by medical research," Dr. Russell wrote in *What the Bible Says About Healthy Living*. "It proves that circumcised males have a lower incidence of infections and carcinoma of the penis. Also, the female partners of uncircumcised males have more infections, which in turn result in a higher incidence of cancer of the cervix."

Two more medical physicians, Dr. S. I. McMillen and Dr. David Stern, point out that the health laws of the Bible have a foundation in medical fact. "For centuries epidemics had killed thousands of Egyptians and Hebrews," they wrote in their book, *None of These Diseases: The Bible's Health Secrets for the 21st Century*. "Ancient treatments rarely helped. Often the 'cure' was worse than the diseases. Yet in Exodus 15:26, God made a fantastic promise— freedom from diseases. God then gave Moses many health rules, filling a whole section of the Bible. Moses recorded hundreds of health regulations"—there are more than six hundred in Leviticus alone—"but not a single current medical misconception."[2]

God's principles of hygiene protected the Israelites from germs and disease centuries before mankind had any idea what they were facing. Today, we know a lot more scientifically about why germs do the things that they do and how they enter our bodies. While germs don't necessarily instigate disease, they do cause the body's resistance to weaken by stressing the immune system. When that happens, you're suddenly vulnerable to illness, but there are steps that you can take to defeat the invaders.

Give Them a Hand

You would think that washing your hands after you go to the bathroom would be so elementary that we could dispense with this area in one sentence: *Using a toilet? Then wash your hands, pal.* Unfortunately, if numerous observational surveys of public restrooms are correct (and I believe they are), we still have some learnin' to do.

I don't know what the gals think, but some guys don't believe there's a hygienic reason to wash up afterward. Their mind-set is like that displayed in the old joke about the two men standing side by side at a urinal: one is from Harvard and the other is from Yale. They finish relieving themselves and zip up. The Harvard man walks to the washbasin while the Yale man makes for the exit.

"Wait a minute," the Harvard man interjects. "At Harvard, they teach us to wash our hands after we urinate."

To which the Yale man replies, "And at Yale, they teach us not to pee on our hands."

I'm sure that some guys think just like the man from Yale, but they are so mistaken. Listen, if you're one of those folks who doesn't think it's necessary to wash up after urinating, let me point out that hand washing is the number one way to prevent the spread of infection-causing agents, according to the U.S. Centers for Disease Control and Prevention. Germs aren't necessarily just flung at us by coughs and sneezes—they're *handed* to us during routine physical contact.

The Centers for Disease Control also found that one in four adults do not wash up after changing a baby's diaper, which creates a high risk of infectious diarrhea. Fewer than half of American adults wash after walking their dogs on "poop patrol." Less than one in five wash after handling paper money and coins, a major carrier of disease germs. Homemakers don't wash or clean up as they should after handling raw chicken and other meats during food preparation.

To protect others, as well as yourself, it's vital to keep your hands sanitary and clean. You begin by incorporating the three elements of hand washing: soap, running water, and friction, although I would add a fourth—motivation. There's no excuse on God's green earth why anyone should neglect washing his hands after going to the bathroom, handling meat, or touching doors and other property in public places. A few seconds at the sink can save you hours or even days of discomfort or a trip to the doctor's office.

When it comes to steering clear of germs, I exercise common sense and practice advanced hygiene. For instance, I've done dozens of book signings in the last year, and at these appearances, I usually shake hands with a couple of hundred people. While I'm happy to greet new people in this manner, the moment the book signing is over, I return to my hotel room and wash my hands thoroughly by digging them into a semisoft soap to remove germs from underneath my fingernails. Then I lather the soap over my cuticles for fifteen seconds and rinse with running water as warm as I can stand.

From the hands and fingernails, germs can enter the body through the nasal passageway or the corner of the eyes—the tear ducts—when we touch those areas. All of us rub our faces so often that we don't even know we're doing it half the time, but when skin-on-skin or skin-on-membrane contact is made, we transfer a garden variety of bacteria, allergens, environmental toxins, and viruses from one part of the body to another. In medical terms, it's called auto- or self-inoculation of the conjunctival (the eyes) or nasal mucosa (the nose) with a contaminated finger.

Hand-to-face contact happens dozens, if not hundreds, of times a day. The next time you're sitting in a meeting, straining to stay awake, take a look around. How often does Betty in accounting touch her nose? What about Jeremy from IT? How often is he rubbing his eyes and mouth? And what about those times you pass somebody on the freeway and you notice the driver doing some "nasal maintenance"?

The areas underneath the fingernails, around the membranes of the eyes, and the membranes in the front part of the nasal passageway are key areas to keep clean. I follow a five-step advanced hygiene system at home and on the road that was first developed back in the 1980s. The system is based on research done by Australian scientist Kenneth Seaton, Ph.D., who discovered that ear, nose, and throat problems—which represent 80 percent of visits to doctors' offices—were linked to the fact that humans inoculate their noses, eyes, mouths, and skin with dirty fingernails throughout the day.

Dr. Seaton coined the phrase "Germs don't fly; they hitchhike." He believed that germs were much more likely to be spread by hand-to-hand contact as opposed to airborne exposure. To test his theory, he commenced a research study where ten healthy people were put into a room with ten other people suffering from an active virus. They spent eight hours together. There was only one caveat—no physical contact. At the end of the day, the ten healthy people were tested. How many do you think became infected? The answer was only two.

Dr. Seaton repeated his study with ten healthy people put into a room with ten sick people, but this time they were allowed physical contact. After eight hours, you can deduce what happened: all ten healthy people were infected after exposure through physical contact. I guess you could say that germs fly 20 percent of the time and stick out their thumbs for a ride 100 percent of the time.

If we are to stave off colds, allergies, or the flu, particular attention must be paid to five areas of the body—the hands, eyes, ears, nose, and mouth. After shaking hundreds of hands at a book signing or trade show, I'm well aware that scrubbing my hands isn't enough because 90 percent of the germs hide *underneath* my fingernails, no matter how short I keep them trimmed. To reach those germs hibernating under and around my fingernails, I use a special semisoft hand soap. The creamy-type soap, which comes in a white tub and is rich in essential oils, is *not* directly antibacterial, however. I believe that antibacterial medicines and soaps end up disrupting the delicate balance of microflora necessary for healthy skin.

Each morning and evening, I dip both hands into the tub and plunge my fingernails into the cream. Then I work the special cream around the tips of my fingers, cuticles, and fingernails for fifteen to thirty seconds. When I'm finished, I lather my hands for fifteen seconds before rinsing them under running water. After my hands are clean, I take another swab of special soap into my hands and wash my face.

A Primer on Washing Your Hands

I'm taking nothing for granted here, so if you've been one of those who could use a brushup on this most basic form of hygiene, here are some tips:

1. Wet your hands with warm water. It doesn't have to be anywhere near scalding hot.

2. Apply plenty of soap to the palms of both hands. The best soap to use is a semisoft soap that you can dig your fingernails into (see the GPRx Resource Guide, page 349, for my favorite advanced hygiene products).

3. Rub your hands vigorously together and scrub all the surfaces. Pay attention to the skin between the fingers, and work the soap into the fingernails.

4. Rub and scrub for fifteen to thirty seconds, or about the time it takes to slowly sing "Happy Birthday to Me."

5. Rinse well and dry your hands on a paper towel or clean cloth towel. If you're in a public restroom, it's a good idea to turn off the running water with the towel in your hand. An even *better* idea is to use that same towel to open the door since the door handle is the first place that nonwashers touch after they've gone to the bathroom.

6. Keep waterless sanitizers in your purse or wallet in case soap and water are not available in the public restroom. These towelettes, although not ideal, are better than nothing.

Since I'm aware that the most susceptible entry ports for germs are the tear ducts and nasal passageways, I employ the second step of advanced hygiene, which is called a facial dip. I begin by filling my washbasin or a clean, large bowl with warm but not hot water, and then I add regular table salt and two eyedroppers of a mineral-based facial solution into the cloudy water.

Whether it's morning or evening, I bend over and dunk my face into the water, opening my eyes several times to allow the cleansing water to flush out the membranes around my eyes. Immediately after, I dive in once again, keeping my eyes closed and my mouth out of the water while I blow bubbles through my nose. I call it snorkeling in the sink.

Then I quickly suck a small amount of water into my nose, which does a Roto-Rooter action by scouring out germs that may have been transferred to my nose. If one of my nostrils is partially blocked, I close the open nostril while underwater and slowly inhale to draw the diluted facial solution into the blocked nostril. That maneuver usually unplugs the nostril. Whenever I feel that I'm coming down with a cold or flu, I do the facial wash four to six times that day, and when I wake up the next morning, I'm as good as new.

After my sink snorkeling, I towel off and blow my nose into a tissue. Of course, I do not share the used water in my washbasin with Nicki since that would defeat the purpose of advanced hygiene.

My two final steps of advanced hygiene are applying very diluted drops of hydrogen peroxide and minerals into my ears for thirty to sixty seconds to cleanse the ear canal, followed by brushing my teeth with an essential oil tooth solution to cleanse my mouth of unhealthy germs. Sometimes I use a saline or xylitol-based nasal inhaler to top off my hygiene experience.

I've been following this advanced hygiene protocol ever since I learned about it ten years ago when I was very sick. Since then, I've been virtually illness-free from the usual respiratory illnesses and sinus infections that afflict millions of Americans each day. Practicing advanced hygiene adds three or four minutes to getting ready for work in the morning or going to bed in the evening, but I think that's a small price to pay for not having to deal with the sniffles, a head cold, or worse.

For a listing of my favorite advanced hygiene products, please see the GPRx Resource Guide, page 349.

DAY IN AND DAY OUT

Germs are everywhere, and we're reminded about that every time there's a global outbreak or major flu scare. The SARS (severe acute respiratory syndrome) scare virtually shut down travel to and from Asia in 2003, and there are well-founded fears that we could be headed toward another smallpox outbreak. A couple of years ago, the Norwalk virus shuttered the cruise ship industry while a battery of cruise ships was steam-cleaned from top to bottom. It turned out that the Norwalk virus was transmitted person to person through fecal-oral contact, health authorities said. Translation: the disease was spread by cruise ship workers going to the bathroom and failing to wash their hands properly (if at all). Then their germs contaminated food they handled, like a salad, or the public areas they touched, like a stair railing.

This hit home for me when I recently debarked from a cruise where I was a speaker. The porter carrying our bags remarked, "You're lucky you weren't on the boat that left the day after yours. The whole ship caught a bug, and the passengers and crew all got very sick."

True stories like these cause concern and reflection. For instance, did you know that shopping carts are repositories of bacteria, reportedly carrying 1.4 million bacteria per square inch, which is one thousand times more than on a toilet seat?[3] That's why Publix and Albertson's supermarkets in my home state of Florida place containers of free disinfectant wipes at store entrances so that customers can wipe down their cart handles before fulfilling their shopping duties.

Chuck Gerba, a University of Arizona environmental-microbiology professor, has spent twenty-five years researching the spreading of germs in schools, offices, and public places. "Dr. Germ," as his colleagues call him, says that 80 percent of infections, from cold and flu viruses to food-borne diseases, are spread through contact with hands and surfaces. Since bacteria, viruses, and other germs can survive up to three days on some surfaces, grocery-cart handles can be one of the *worst* places to pick up hitchhiking germs. It doesn't take much imagination to picture a sneezing, coughing mother with a runny-nosed baby gripping the handles of your grocery cart ten minutes before you arrived.

When to Wash Your Hands

- After you go to the bathroom
- Before and after you insert and remove contact lenses
- Before and after food preparation

- Before you eat
- After you sneeze, cough, or blow your nose
- After cleaning up after your pet
- After handling money
- After changing a diaper
- After blowing a child's nose
- After handling garbage
- After cleaning your toilets
- After shaking hands with a bunch of people
- After shopping at the supermarket
- After attending an event at a public theater
- Before and after sexual intercourse

I know: this is sounding like the scenario for a B-grade horror movie—*Attack of the Killer Germs.* I don't want anyone to become paranoid about this because we come into contact with billions of germs every day. Life's too short to pass through like Howard Hughes, the eccentric billionaire who washed his hands until he bled and wouldn't leave a seemingly spotless bathroom until someone else entered and opened the door for him. Hughes became such a germ-a-phobe that he spent the last years of his life living like a circus-freak hermit with long hair and even longer fingernails.

Germs break down your immune system and make you more susceptible to health problems. I believe you can minimize germ infestations when you take key steps to guard yourself against attack, like washing your hands and nails with a good-quality soap and dipping your head into a facial solution, which cleanses your eyes and nasal passageways.

During the cold and flu season, however, many people are afraid they are a ticking time bomb: one false step, and they will blow up like a grenade, sending them to their sickbeds. Actually germs don't quite work that way. They overload the immune system through contact of the fingers with the eyes and nose, and this overload is similar to water filling a balloon in the backyard. If you keep filling the balloon with water, eventually the balloon will expand and expand to the point where one more drop of water will cause the balloon to burst. Our bodies react in a similar manner: the immune system becomes so overloaded that the body reaches a point where it can't take on more germs.

Now, does one water drop cause a balloon to break? No, of course not. It is the accumulation of hundreds of thousands of drops, if not millions, that causes the balloon to explode. It's the same for the germs that attack our bodies.

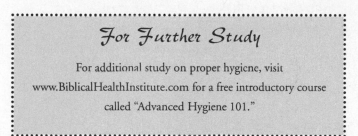

For Further Study

For additional study on proper hygiene, visit www.BiblicalHealthInstitute.com for a free introductory course called "Advanced Hygiene 101."

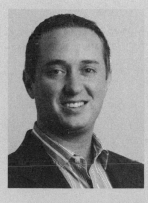

WHY CLEANLINESS IS NEXT TO GODLINESS
by Jason Dewberry

I had this dirty little habit growing up—biting my fingernails. I bit my nails as a youngster because I thought that was the best way to get rid of the dirt beneath my nails. (Yeah, right!)

I'll never forget the scolding I got from my mom, but I thought I was doing something good for my body. "Come on, Mom," I retorted. "Stop bothering me about it. I'm teaching my body to fight germs."

That's the way my eight-year-old mind worked. As I grew up, I became more and more fascinated with hygiene and cleanliness, but not in an obsessive way. I enjoyed learning more about how the introduction of environmental bacteria, viruses, fungi, and other external agents to the body, especially early in life, helped the body develop a potent immune system.

Then my friend Jordan Rubin asked me one day to be a guinea pig for an advanced hygiene system that he was using. Concepts such as "germs don't fly; they hitchhike" and "put less stress on the immune system" struck a chord with me. The application of both the philosophy and the easy-to-use five-step system turned me into a true believer.

I've been following this advanced hygiene protocol for nearly two years, and I can count the number of days that I've been sick on one hand—and I haven't been sick enough to miss work. For someone who flies in airplanes with recirculated air as much as I do, this has been an amazing development.

My wife, Sherry, has adopted advanced hygiene as well, and for as long as she could remember, she battled allergies and headaches. No matter what medication, supplements, or diet program she was on, a runny nose, watery eyes, itchy scalp, night sweats, and congestion were her constant companions. "It's always something," she often said.

The daily cleansing of her nasal passages, as well as other germ-entry points, balanced her body's immune system and significantly reduced her allergic symptoms and headaches. Relief feels like a great gift to her.

Advanced hygiene has also made a difference in our marriage. For years, poor Sherry had to listen to my deep nasal breathing as I slept. "I can't sleep when you snore like that!" she griped. Sherry insisted that I had a form of sleep apnea.

I didn't blame her for feeling that way, but I couldn't control my breathing or snoring, of course. After several months of cleansing my nasal passages by dipping my face into a sink of water with salt and an iodine-based mineral solution, my nocturnal breathing, as I like to call it, became much less frequent, for which Sherry was eternally grateful.

Now I cannot travel without my advanced hygiene system, nor can I wake in the morning or go to bed without performing the hand washing, the facial and nasal rinse, the ear drops, and the tooth and gum solution. Three minutes in the morning and three minutes late at night have made a huge difference in how I feel each day.

Mom, in case you're reading this book, I no longer feel compelled to bite my fingernails. I've found a much better method to keep the germs away.

℞ THE GREAT PHYSICIAN'S Rx FOR ADVANCED HYGIENE

- *Wash your hands regularly, paying special attention to removing germs from underneath your fingernails.*

- *Cleanse your nasal passageways and the mucous membranes of the eyes daily by performing a facial dip.*

- *Cleanse the ear canals at least twice per week.*

- *Use an essential oil-based tooth solution daily to remove germs from the mouth.*

THE GREAT PHYSICIAN'S Rx FOR WEEK #3

Day 15

Upon Waking

Advanced hygiene: for hands and nails, jab fingers into semisoft soap four or five times, and lather hands with soap for fifteen seconds, rubbing soap over cuticles and rinsing under water as warm as you can stand. Take another swab of semisoft soap into your hands, and wash your face. (See the GPRx Resource Guide, page 349, for recommended advanced hygiene products.)

Supplements: take one serving of a fiber/green superfood powder (mixed in) or five caplets of a super green formula (swallowed with) twelve-to-sixteen ounces of water or raw vegetable juice. (See the GPRx Resource Guide, pages 346–347, for recommended products.)

Breakfast

hot tea with honey (see the GPRx Resource Guide, page 339, for recommended herbal tea blends)

Mochachino Smoothie with two tablespoons of protein powder (see appendix A, page 309, for recipe)

Supplements: take one or two whole food multivitamin caplets (see the GPRx Resource Guide, page 345, for recommended products) and one or two capsules of a probiotic/enzyme blend (see the GPRx Resource Guide, pages 347–348, for recommended products.)

Lunch

Before eating, drink eight ounces of water.

During lunch, drink eight ounces of water or hot or iced fresh-brewed tea with honey.

Mushroom, Spinach, and Swiss Wrap (see appendix A, page 290, for recipe)

apple

Supplements: Take one or two whole food multivitamin caplets and one or two capsules of a probiotic/enzyme blend.

Dinner

Before eating, drink eight ounces of water.

During dinner, drink hot or iced fresh-brewed tea with honey.

Spinach and Goat Cheese Meat Lasagna (see appendix A, page 309, for recipe)

Supplements: take one or two whole food multivitamin caplets, one-to-three teaspoons or three-to-nine capsules of high omega-3 cod-liver oil (see the GPRx Resource Guide, pages 345–346, for recommended products), and one or two caplets of a probiotic/enzyme blend.

Snacks

Drink eight-to-twelve ounces of water or hot or iced fresh-brewed tea with honey.

vanilla protein whole food bar (see the GPRx Resource Guide, pages 329–330, for recommended products)

macaroons (see the GPRx Resource Guide, page 339, for recommended brands)

Crispy Pecans (see appendix A, page 270, for recipe)

Before Bed

Drink eight-to-twelve ounces of water or hot tea with honey.

Supplements: take one serving of a fiber/green superfood powder (mixed in) or five caplets of a super green formula (swallowed with) twelve-to-sixteen ounces of water or raw vegetable juice.

Advanced hygiene: for hands and nails, jab fingers into semisoft soap four or five times, and lather hands with soap for fifteen seconds, rubbing soap over cuticles and rinsing under water as warm as you can stand. Take another swab of semisoft soap into your hands, and wash your face.

Day 16

Upon Waking

Advanced hygiene: for hands and nails, jab fingers into semisoft soap four or five times, and lather hands with soap for fifteen seconds, rubbing soap over cuticles and rinsing under water as warm as you can stand. Take another swab of semisoft soap into your hands, and wash your face.

Next, fill basin or sink with water as warm as you can stand, and add one-to-three tablespoons of table salt and one-to-three eyedroppers of iodine-based mineral solution. Swirl water. Dunk face into water and open eyes, blinking repeatedly under water. (See the GPRx Resource Guide, page 349, for recommended advanced hygiene products.)

Supplements: take one serving of a fiber/green superfood powder (mixed in) or five caplets of a super green formula (swallowed with) twelve to sixteen ounces of water or raw vegetable juice. (See the GPRx Resource Guide, pages 346–347, for recommended products.)

Breakfast

Dirty Eggs (see appendix A, page 310, for recipe)
turkey bacon
orange
hot tea with honey
Supplements: take one or two whole food multivitamin caplets and one or two capsules of a probiotic/enzyme blend.

Lunch

Before eating, drink eight ounces of water.

During lunch, drink eight ounces of water or hot or iced fresh-brewed tea with honey.

Oriental Salmon Salad (see appendix A, page 303, for recipe)
carrot sticks
Supplements: take one or two whole food multivitamin caplets and one or two capsules of a probiotic/enzyme blend.

Dinner

Before eating, drink eight ounces of water.

During dinner, drink hot or iced fresh-brewed tea with honey.

EZ Pizza (see appendix A, page 310, for recipe)

green salad with red peppers, red onions, cucumbers, and carrots

Supplements: take one or two whole food multivitamin caplets, one-to-three teaspoons or three-to-nine capsules of high omega-3 cod-liver oil, and one or two capsules of a probiotic/enzyme blend.

Snacks

Drink eight-to-twelve ounces of water, or hot or iced fresh-brewed tea with honey.

Quick Sprouted Apple Crisp (see appendix A, page 310, for recipe)

Tropical Smoothie Mix blended in eight-to-twelve ounces of water (see the GPRx Resource Guide, page 329, for recommended products)

Before Bed

Drink eight-to-twelve ounces of water or hot tea with honey.

Supplements: take one serving of a fiber/green superfood powder (mixed in) or five caplets of a super green formula (swallowed with) twelve-to-sixteen ounces of water or raw vegetable juice.

Advanced hygiene: for hands and nails, jab fingers into semisoft soap four or five times, and lather hands with soap for fifteen seconds, rubbing soap over cuticles and rinsing under water as warm as you can stand. Take another swab of semisoft soap into your hands, and wash your face.

Next, fill basin or sink with water as warm as you can stand, and add one-to-three tablespoons of table salt and one-to-three eyedroppers of iodine-based mineral solution. Swirl water. Dunk face into water and open eyes, blinking repeatedly under water.

Day 17

Upon Waking

Advanced hygiene: for hands and nails, jab fingers into semisoft soap four or five times, and lather hands with soap for fifteen seconds, rubbing soap over cuticles and rinsing under water as warm as you can stand. Take another swab of semisoft soap into your hands, and wash your face.

Next, fill basin or sink with water as warm as you can stand, and add one-to-three tablespoons of table salt and one-to-three eyedroppers of iodine-based mineral solution. Swirl water. Dunk face into water and open eyes, blinking repeatedly underwater.

Supplements: take one serving of a fiber/green superfood powder (mixed in) or five caplets of a super green formula (swallowed with) twelve-to-sixteen ounces of water or raw vegetable juice. (See the GPRx Resource Guide, pages 346–347, for recommended products.)

Breakfast

sprouted dried cereal with yogurt, kefir, goat's milk, or almond milk

banana
hot tea with honey
Supplements: take one or two whole food multivitamin caplets and one or two capsules of a probiotic/enzyme blend.

Lunch

Before eating, drink eight ounces of water.
During lunch, drink eight ounces of water or hot or iced fresh-brewed tea with honey.
Beef Vegetable Soup
flaxseed or whole grain crackers
Supplements: take one or two whole food multivitamin caplets and one or two capsules of a probiotic/enzyme blend.

Dinner

Before eating, drink eight ounces of water.
During dinner, drink hot or iced fresh-brewed tea with honey.
Steak au Poivre (see appendix A, page 311, for recipe)
Sweet Onion Pudding (see appendix A, page 311, for recipe)
Braised Leeks (see appendix A, page 269, for recipe)
Supplements: Take one or two whole food multivitamin caplets, one-to-three teaspoons or three-to-nine capsules of high omega-3 cod-liver oil, and one or two capsules of a probiotic/enzyme blend.

Snacks

apple with almond butter
antioxidant fruit whole food bar (see the GPRx Resource Guide, pages 329–330, for recommended products)
Drink eight-to-twelve ounces of water or hot or iced fresh-brewed tea with honey.

Before Bed

Drink eight-to-twelve ounces of water or hot tea with honey.
Supplements: take one serving of a fiber/green superfood powder (mixed in) or five caplets of a super green formula (swallowed with) twelve-to-sixteen ounces of water or raw vegetable juice.
Advanced hygiene: for hands and nails, jab fingers into semisoft soap four or five times, and lather hands with soap for fifteen seconds, rubbing soap over cuticles and rinsing under water as warm as you can stand. Take another swab of semisoft soap into your hands, and wash your face.
Next, fill basin or sink with water as warm as you can stand, and add one-to-three tablespoons of table salt and one-to-three eyedroppers of iodine-based mineral solution. Swirl water. Dunk face into water and open eyes, blinking repeatedly under water.

Day 18

Upon Waking

Advanced hygiene: for hands and nails, jab fingers into semisoft soap four or five times, and lather hands with soap for fifteen seconds, rubbing soap over cuticles and rinsing under water as warm as you can stand. Take another swab of semisoft soap into your hands, and wash your face.

Next, fill basin or sink with water as warm as you can stand, and add one-to-three tablespoons of table salt and one-to-three eyedroppers of iodine-based mineral solution. Swirl water. Dunk face into water and open eyes, blinking repeatedly underwater. Keep eyes open under water for three seconds. After cleaning your eyes, put your face back in the water, and close your mouth while blowing bubbles out of your nose.

Supplements: take one serving of a fiber/green superfood powder (mixed in) or five caplets of a super green formula (swallowed with) twelve-to-sixteen ounces of water or raw vegetable juice. (See the GPRx Resource Guide, pages 346–347, for recommended products.)

Breakfast

Eggs Benedict (see appendix A, page 312, for recipe)

grilled onions and mushrooms

hot tea with honey

Supplements: take one or two whole food multivitamin caplets and one or two capsules of a probiotic/enzyme blend.

Lunch

Before eating, drink eight ounces of water.

During lunch, drink eight ounces of water or hot or iced fresh-brewed tea with honey.

almond butter and honey or jam sandwich on whole grain sprouted or sourdough bread

one apple

Supplements: take one or two whole food multivitamin caplets and one or two capsules of a probiotic/enzyme blend.

Dinner

Before eating, drink eight ounces of water.

During dinner, drink hot or iced fresh-brewed tea with honey.

Tomato Basil Soup (see appendix A, page 314, for recipe)

Chicken with Sun-Dried Tomatoes and Spinach (see appendix A, page 314, for recipe)

Garlic Mashed Potatoes (see appendix A, page 302, for recipe)

roasted peas and carrots

Supplements: take one or two whole food multivitamin caplets, one-to-three teaspoons or three-to-nine capsules of high omega-3 cod-liver oil, and one or two capsules of a probiotic/enzyme blend.

Snacks

yogurt and pineapple

Pepitas (see appendix A, page 269, for recipe)

chocolate protein whole food bar (see the GPRx Resource Guide, pages 329–330, for recommended products)

Drink eight-to-twelve ounces of water or hot or iced fresh-brewed tea with honey.

Before Bed

Drink eight-to-twelve ounces of water or hot tea with honey.

Supplements: take one serving of a fiber/green superfood powder (mixed in) or five caplets of a super green formula (swallowed with) twelve-to-sixteen ounces of water or raw vegetable juice.

Advanced hygiene: for hands and nails, jab fingers into semisoft soap four or five times, and lather hands with soap for fifteen seconds, rubbing soap over cuticles and rinsing under water as warm as you can stand. Take another swab of semisoft soap into your hands, and wash your face.

Next, fill basin or sink with water as warm as you can stand, and add one-to-three tablespoons of table salt and one-to-three eyedroppers of iodine-based mineral solution. Swirl water. Dunk face into water and open eyes, blinking repeatedly underwater. Keep eyes open under water for three seconds. After cleaning your eyes, put your face back in the water, and close your mouth while blowing bubbles out of your nose.

Day 19 (Partial Fast Day)

Upon Waking

Advanced hygiene: for hands and nails, jab fingers into semisoft soap four or five times, and lather hands with soap for fifteen seconds, rubbing soap over cuticles and rinsing under water as warm as you can stand. Take another swab of semisoft soap into your hands, and wash your face.

Next, fill basin or sink with water as warm as you can stand, and add one-to-three tablespoons of table salt and one-to-three eyedroppers of iodine-based mineral solution. Swirl water. Dunk face into water and open eyes, blinking repeatedly underwater. Keep eyes open under water for three seconds. After cleaning your eyes, put your face back in the water, and close your mouth while blowing bubbles out of your nose.

Supplements: take one serving of a fiber/green superfood powder (mixed in) or five caplets of a super green formula (swallowed with) twelve-to-sixteen ounces of water or raw vegetable juice. (See the GPRx Resource Guide, pages 346–347, for recommended products.)

Breakfast

none (partial fast day)

eight ounces of water

Lunch
   none (partial fast day)
   eight ounces of water

Dinner
   Before eating, drink eight ounces of water.
   During dinner, drink hot or iced fresh-brewed tea with honey.
   Wood-Grilled King Salmon (see appendix A, page 299, for recipe)
   asparagus
   cultured vegetables
   green salad
   Supplements: take whole food multivitamin caplets, one-to-three teaspoons or three-to-nine capsules of high omega-3 cod-liver oil, and one or two capsules of a probiotic/enzyme blend.

Snacks
   none (partial fast day)
   eight ounces of water

Before Bed
   Drink eight-to-twelve ounces of water or hot tea with honey.
   Supplements: take one serving of a fiber/green superfood powder (mixed in) or five caplets of a super green formula (swallowed with) twelve-to-sixteen ounces of water or raw vegetable juice.
   Advanced hygiene: for hands and nails, jab fingers into semisoft soap four or five times, and lather hands with soap for fifteen seconds, rubbing soap over cuticles and rinsing under water as warm as you can stand. Take another swab of semisoft soap into your hands, and wash your face.
   Next, fill basin or sink with water as warm as you can stand, and add one-to-three tablespoons of table salt and one-to-three eyedroppers of iodine-based mineral solution. Swirl water. Dunk face into water and open eyes, blinking repeatedly under water. Keep eyes open under water for three seconds. After cleaning your eyes, put your face back in the water, and close your mouth while blowing bubbles out of your nose. Come up from the water, and immerse your face in the water once again, gently taking water into your nostrils and expelling bubbles. Come up from the water, and blow your nose into facial tissue.

Day 20

Upon Waking
   Advanced hygiene: for hands and nails, jab fingers into semisoft soap four or five times, and lather hands with soap for fifteen seconds, rubbing soap over cuticles and rinsing under water as warm as you can stand. Take another swab of semisoft soap into your hands, and wash your face.

Next, fill basin or sink with water as warm as you can stand, and add one-to-three tablespoons of table salt and one-to-three eyedroppers of iodine-based mineral solution. Swirl water. Dunk face into water and open eyes, blinking repeatedly underwater. Keep eyes open under water for three seconds. After cleaning your eyes, put your face back in the water, and close your mouth while blowing bubbles out of your nose. Come up from the water, and immerse your face in the water once again, gently taking water into your nostrils and expelling bubbles. Come up from the water, and blow your nose into facial tissue. To cleanse the ears, use hydrogen peroxide and mineral-based ear drops, putting two or three drops into each ear and letting stand for sixty seconds. Tilt your head to expel the drops. (See the GPRx Resource Guide, page 349, for recommended advanced hygiene products.)

Supplements: take one serving of a fiber/green superfood powder (mixed in) or five caplets of a super green formula (swallowed with) twelve-to-sixteen ounces of water or raw vegetable juice. (See the GPRx Resource Guide, pages 346–347, for recommended products.)

Breakfast
Chicken King Omelet (see appendix A, page 282, for recipe)
grapefruit
hot tea with honey
Supplements: one or two whole food multivitamin caplets and one or two capsules of a probiotic/enzyme blend.

Lunch
Before eating, drink eight ounces of water.
During lunch, drink eight ounces of water or hot or iced fresh-brewed tea with honey.
Latin Style Orzo Salad (see appendix A, page 290, for recipe)
apple
Supplements: take one or two whole food multivitamin caplets and one or two capsules of a probiotic/enzyme blend.

Dinner
Before eating, drink eight ounces of water.
During dinner, drink hot or iced fresh-brewed tea with honey.
Italian Turkey Sausage and Peppers (see appendix A, page 313, for recipe)
Mushroom and Garden Vegetable Loaf (see appendix A, page 293, for recipe)
Supplements: take one or two whole food multivitamin caplets, one-to-three teaspoons or three-to-nine capsules of high omega-3 cod-liver oil, and one or two capsules of a probiotic/enzyme blend.

Snacks
baked corn chips and salsa and guacamole

apple-cinnamon fiber whole food bar (see the GPRx Resource Guide, pages 329–330, for recommended products)

Drink eight-to-twelve ounces of water or hot or iced fresh-brewed tea with honey.

Before Bed

Drink eight-to-twelve ounces of water or hot tea with honey.

Supplements: take one serving of a fiber/green superfood powder (mixed in) or five caplets of a super green formula (swallowed with) twelve-to-sixteen ounces of water or raw vegetable juice.

Advanced hygiene: for hands and nails, jab fingers into semisoft soap four or five times, and lather hands with soap for fifteen seconds, rubbing soap over cuticles and rinsing under water as warm as you can stand. Take another swab of semisoft soap into your hands, and wash your face.

Next, fill basin or sink with water as warm as you can stand, and add one-to-three tablespoons of table salt and one-to-three eyedroppers of iodine-based mineral solution. Swirl water. Dunk face into water and open eyes, blinking repeatedly underwater. Keep eyes open under water for three seconds. After cleaning your eyes, put your face back in the water, and close your mouth while blowing bubbles out of your nose. Come up from the water, and immerse your face in the water once again, gently taking water into your nostrils and expelling bubbles. Come up from the water, and blow your nose into facial tissue. To cleanse the ears, use hydrogen peroxide and mineral-based ear drops, putting two or three drops into each ear and letting stand for sixty seconds. Tilt your head to expel the drops.

Day 21

Upon Waking

Advanced hygiene: for hands and nails, jab fingers into semisoft soap four or five times, and lather hands with soap for fifteen seconds, rubbing soap over cuticles and rinsing under water as warm as you can stand. Take another swab of semisoft soap into your hands, and wash your face.

Next, fill basin or sink with water as warm as you can stand, and add one-to-three tablespoons of table salt and one-to-three eyedroppers of iodine-based mineral solution. Dunk face into water and open eyes, blinking repeatedly underwater. Keep eyes open under water for three seconds. After cleaning your eyes, put your face back in the water, and close your mouth while blowing bubbles out of your nose. Come up from the water, and immerse your nose in the water once again, gently taking water into your nostrils and expelling bubbles. Come up from the water, and blow your nose into facial tissue. To cleanse the ears, use hydrogen peroxide and mineral-based ear drops, putting two or three drops into each ear and letting stand for sixty seconds. Tilt your head to expel the drops. For the teeth, apply two or three drops of essential oil–based tooth drops to the toothbrush. This can be used to brush your teeth or added to existing toothpaste. After brushing your teeth, brush your tongue for fifteen seconds. (See the GPRx Resource Guide, page 349, for recommended advanced hygiene products.)

Supplements: take one serving of a fiber/green superfood powder (mixed in) or five caplets of a super green formula (swallowed with) twelve-to-sixteen ounces of water or raw vegetable juice. (See the GPRx Resource Guide, pages 346–347, for recommended products.)

Breakfast

hot tea with honey

Piña Colada Smoothie (see appendix A, page 313, for recipe) with two tablespoons of protein powder (optional)

Supplements: take one or two whole food multivitamin caplets and one or two capsules of a probiotic/enzyme blend.

Lunch

Before eating, drink eight ounces of water.

During lunch, drink eight ounces of water or hot or iced fresh-brewed tea with honey.

Beef Avocado Salad with Rosemary Dressing (see appendix A, page 316, for recipe)

Supplements: one or two whole food multivitamin caplets and one or two capsules of a probiotic/enzyme blend.

Dinner

Before eating, drink eight ounces of water.

During dinner, drink hot or iced fresh-brewed tea with honey.

Shepherd's Pie (see appendix A, page 315, for recipe)

green salad

Supplements: take one or two whole food multivitamin caplets, one-to-three teaspoons or three-to-nine capsules of high omega-3 cod-liver oil, and one or two capsules of a probiotic/enzyme blend.

Snacks

Blueberry Muffins and butter (see appendix A, page 272, for recipe)

cottage cheese with honey

Mango Berry smoothie mix blended in eight-to-twelve ounces of water

Drink eight-to-twelve ounces of water or hot or iced fresh-brewed tea with honey.

Before Bed

Drink eight-to-twelve ounces of water or hot tea with honey.

Supplements: take one serving of a fiber/green superfood powder (mixed in) or five caplets of a super green formula (swallowed with) twelve-to-sixteen ounces of water or raw vegetable juice.

Advanced hygiene: for hands and nails, jab fingers into semisoft soap four or five times, and lather hands with soap for fifteen seconds, rubbing soap over cuticles and rinsing under water as warm as you can stand. Take another swab of semisoft soap into your hands, and wash your face.

Next, fill basin or sink with water as warm as you can stand, and add one-to-three tablespoons of table salt and one-to-three eyedroppers of iodine-based mineral solution. Swirl water. Dunk face into water and open eyes, blinking repeatedly under water. Keep eyes open underwater for three seconds. After cleaning your eyes, put your face back in the water, and close your mouth while blowing bubbles out of your nose. Come up from the water, and immerse your nose in the water once again, gently taking water into your nostrils and expelling bubbles. Come up from the water, and blow your nose into facial tissue. To cleanse the ears, use hydrogen peroxide and mineral-based ear drops, putting two or three drops into each ear and letting stand for sixty seconds. Tilt your head to expel the drops. For the teeth, apply two or three drops of essential oil–based tooth drops to the toothbrush. This can be used to brush your teeth or added to existing toothpaste. After brushing your teeth, brush your tongue for fifteen seconds.

Key #4

Condition Your Body with Exercise and Body Therapies

Bodily exercise profits a little, but godliness is profitable for all things, having promise of the life that now is and of that which is to come.

—1 Timothy 4:8 (NKJV)

Ever since Joshua was born, sleep has been a precious commodity around our household. When Nicki was in the midst of her breast-feeding duties, I roused myself out of bed to help where I could and show my support.

On a few occasions, I flipped on the TV in the early morning hours just to see what was on. I think I saw more infomercials for abs than you can shake a credit card at. I viewed presentations for the Ab Rocker, the Ab Roller, the Ab Lounge, the Ab Sculptor, the Abslide, the Ab Trainer, the Ab Twister, and the Ab Works, just to name eight of the gazillion "ab" products out there. The infomercials slavishly followed the same script: as the camera focused on the bodybuilder's midsection, I was told that I could acquire the same killer, chiseled, washboard, twisted-steel, and rock-hard abs by making three easy payments of $39.95, plus shipping and handling.

It didn't take much for me to resist the pitch. Someone must be buying this stuff, however, though I'm not sure why anyone would fall for the idea that he or she could own a set of killer abs by exercising only five minutes a day for thirty days. From my observation, most people's idea of crunching has more to do with biting on snack chips than performing ab exercises.

I'll admit that it's a lot easier to reach for a bag of Fritos than to reach for gym clothes and engage in vigorous physical activity that raises the heart rate and induces the sweat glands to perspire. Exercising is like writing a book: everyone *wants* to have exercised, but no one wants to do the work.

What happens is that desire is often supplanted by reality. Our bodies get used to taking the path of least resistance, and that mind-set becomes entrenched in our lifestyles, which, for a majority of Americans, is Sedentary with a capital *S*. You see it every time you steer into a mall parking lot: people will drive in circles just so they can park one hundred yards closer to the mall entrance. They could have *walked* that short distance in less time than it took to find a more convenient parking place.

That behavior is an apt illustration of the curious country we live in. Americans own more gym memberships and exercise equipment than all other nations combined—and never have people gotten less use out of both. Every holiday season we pig out between Thanksgiving and Christmas, followed by guilt-filled New Year's resolutions to "get into shape this year," but we break those promises by Martin Luther King's birthday—or we "lose" our gym membership card.

Then we happen to see one of those infomercials for a high-tech workout contraption, and the guilt comes flooding back. *I've got to do something!* So you place the order, but you don't exercise while waiting six to eight weeks for delivery because, after all, you can't work out if you don't have the machine. After the UPS man lugs the heavy cardboard box inside your front door, several more weeks pass by before you have the time to put the machine together. You finally gather the energy to drag it to your laundry room, where you spend three hours assembling it.

You eventually get up and running, so to speak, but you don't pump your legs for too long because you don't want to wear yourself out—or overdo it. As time passes, however, you use your fancy treadmill to hang up semidry clothes from the dryer more often than you actually exercise on it.

Okay, so a lot of treadmills and home gym equipment are magnets for drying laundry instead of helping us raise our fitness levels. Even if that's been the case in the past, I urge you to jump on the exercise bandwagon. Keep in mind, however, that the road to fitness is paved with good intentions, and many of us encounter land mines along the way. We lose our resolve because consistent exercise is probably the number one most difficult thing for people to do.

Sometimes I wonder if the only exercise people get is jumping to the conclusion that they don't need to exercise. The body was meant to move: God designed us to lift, haul, stride, step, boost, drag, march, tread, run, kick, and heave with our limbs. There's a reason why the word *move* is close to *mobile* in the dictionary. God made us to be mobile people, and throughout history, people have walked miles and miles and performed manual labor in the fields and in the cities.

Today, at least in our Westernized culture, physical labor is an endangered species, and many of us put in our eight-plus hours inside office parks with cubicles that resemble chicken coops. There isn't much manual labor involved in answering e-mails, making phone calls, writing up TPS reports, studying sales figures, or sitting in your fifth meeting of the day.

Plopping your posterior down for hours on end—no matter how ergonomically correct the chair is—prompts a whole range of physical problems. As the shoulders slump, undue pressure is placed on the heart, and lung capacity diminishes. The back muscles tense to compensate for the imbalanced posture. Sitting on your posterior for hours on end creates chronic back pain, initiates headaches, and predisposes one to even *more* fatigue. Lower back pain is the number one cause of employee absenteeism in the workplace and can lead to injuries when trying to perform daily activities or enjoying your favorite hobby or sport.

The sitting position causes the stomach muscles to become slack and weak from underuse, and the internal organs are displaced downward, impairing their function. Knee and ankle joints become stiff, and muscles lose their tone. Physical inactivity is a surefire formula for adding weight to your "problem" areas.

Conditioning your body with exercise and body therapies, the fourth key to unlock your health potential, can help. I'm talking about more than just walking on a stationary treadmill several times a week and hitting a few Nautilus machines. In this chapter, I'll be introducing concepts like functional fitness, hydrotherapy, aromatherapy, and music therapy, as well as discussing the importance of getting adequate rest and sunlight, all core to the Great Physician's Rx for exercise and body therapies.

Taking a Step with Functional Fitness

Okay, we can all agree that we're busy. Careers are in full bloom, the kids are growing like weeds, and school and extracurricular activities are backing up like freeway lanes during rush hour. It would also be nice to resurrect the "date night" with that special person in our lives.

With our busy schedules, something has to give, and usually the first item to get crossed off the calendar is time reserved for exercise. We always figure we'll get around to getting in shape next week, next month, or next year. That way of thinking has to change. Choosing to go through life without exercise—and it's a choice, I might add—will result in a shortened life span and a lower quality of living. I've long said that eating healthy is only part of the equation when shooting for total physical health.

Nothing turns back the clock faster than a consistent regimen of exercise. Sure, aging is inevitable, and yes, Scripture tells us that it's "appointed for men to die once" (Heb. 9:27 NKJV). But those facts don't give us license to shuffle into old age, looking for a park bench to sit on. I believe we should exercise because God designed our bodies like finely tuned cars; if we never leave the garage, our batteries die. If we put our bodies through the paces, we add years to our lives—productive years that can be used in ministry or add value to the lives of others.

Where do you begin? By making a commitment to start exercising regularly, and if five or ten minutes a day is all you can spare in the beginning, that's a healthy start. You can look at increasing your exercise time once you establish that baseline.

From my viewpoint, people stop working out because they don't see immediate results. Exercise isn't like changing your diet to a healthy, more natural approach, which often offers quick changes in energy level and mental attitude. But exercise? That's the road less traveled, and many who step on the fitness path after years of inactivity feel like it's an exercise, all right—an exercise in futility. They see themselves like Sisyphus, doomed to ceaselessly roll a rock to the top of a mountain, only to witness the stone fall back from its own weight.

If you haven't darkened a gym door in years or have been lax about getting up off your duff and moving around, I have just the exercise program for you. It's called *functional fitness,* and it has helped me strengthen and improve the actions I perform every day, which helps my body stay agile, flexible, and resistant.

Functional fitness—also known as *purposeful training*—is catching on around the country, and I find it to be a welcome antidote to the more-is-better philosophy of one more plate on the Nautilus machine, one more level on the aerobics step, or one mile per hour faster on the treadmill. The idea behind functional fitness is to train movements, not muscles, in order to improve your balance and build up the body's core muscles. You may not have killer abs after a stint of functional fitness, but you'll be in better condition to tackle life's daily activities. This is a much more functional approach to exercise and perfect for people, including nearly all women, who aren't that interested in bulging biceps, ripped quads, or a six-pack of abs. They're more interested in having balance and functional health to perform in life.

In functional fitness, the no-pain, no-gain theory is out; exercises that give you strength and balance to carry three bags of groceries on an icy blacktop or bend over to pick up boxes out of the trunk are in. Functional exercise focuses on building a body capable of doing real-life activities in real-life positions, and it can be done by virtually everyone, regardless of present fitness level. These forms of moderate activity can significantly reduce the risk of heart disease, cancer, osteoporosis, and many other chronic diseases.

You're much less likely to injure yourself or throw your back out because you'll focus on doing real-life exercises in real-life positions, as opposed to lifting a certain amount of weight in an unnatural posture on a weight machine. The purpose of functional fitness is to train whole movements, not isolated muscles.

Functional fitness classes can now be found in exercise emporiums like LA Fitness, Bally Total Fitness, or the YMCA. Instructors hound you to focus more on technique than on how many "reps" you can do as they put you through a series of exercises that mimic everyday life. You can also perform functional fitness exercises in the privacy and comfort of your home anytime you want when you play a functional fitness video on your TV screen. (For more information on functional fitness products, please turn to The GPRx Resource Guide, page 327.)

The exercises are different in functional fitness. Squats—with feet apart, feet together, and one foot back with the other forward—are utilized. So are one-legged poses. But high-impact exercises like those found in aerobics or step classes aren't part of functional fitness. The functional fitness movements should be performed in a pain-free fashion with excellent control.

You can use simple household items like water bottles or cans of tomato sauce to do functional fitness, but those looking to take their physical fitness to a higher level can also employ dumbbells, mini trampolines, or stability balls—those large plastic balls you see in gyms—with their programs. Paul Chek, a rehabilitation and exercise specialist with more than twenty years of experience, uses a stability ball to help individuals improve their balance. For instance, he'll ask the individual to kneel on the ball and hold his balance while he tosses the person a small but heavy medicine ball. The individual not only strains to stay upright on the stability ball, but he also uses arm and stomach muscles to catch and toss the heavy medicine ball back to the trainer.

A Sample Functional Fitness Program

We begin with upper-body movements, which boost strength and flexibility. You can perform these exercises without weights, but feel free to add cans or small dumbbells for additional resistance. Attention: these movements should be done in a pain-free fashion, so if the movement hurts, stop immediately.

1. *Matrix upper body with pushing.* Begin with the *alternate overhead press.* Stand with your feet slightly more than shoulder-width apart. Keep your midsection straight and tight to protect your lower back. Fully extend each arm with palms facing upward (one at a time) toward the ceiling or sky as if you're pushing air upward. At the same time, bring the other hand down to shoulder level. If you can't lift your shoulder all the way up

because of injury or lack of motion in the joint, then do what you can. Perform five repetitions for each arm for a total of ten.

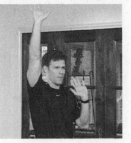 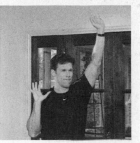

Alternate Overhead Presses

Next, do the *alternate diagonal press* using a Y pattern ten times, followed by the *alternate rotational push* in which you spin on your feet to one side into a slight lunge position. Push upward and forward like you're putting something on a high shelf. If you spin to the left, then push with the right hand while the left hand remains on your hip.

It should take about thirty seconds to do each of these exercises ten times.

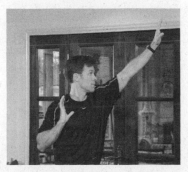 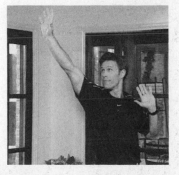

Alternate Diagonal Presses

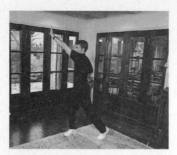
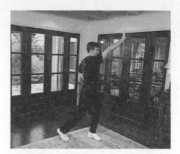

Alternate Rotational Pushes

2. *Matrix upper body with pulling.* The first exercise is a *bicep curl.* With both hands facing down and stretched out, curl each arm, one at a time, bending only at the elbow for a total of ten. Next, perform an *alternate upright row.* Using the same position, pull one elbow up toward the side at a time and toward the ceiling or sky. This motion is similar to pulling a lawnmower starting cord.

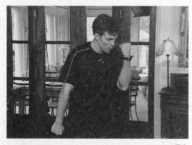
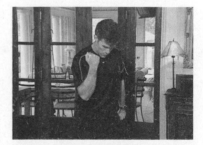

Bicep Curls

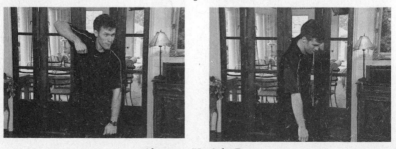

Alternate Upright Row

The final exercise in this series is called the *alternate rotation,* which is like putting an object on a high shelf. Spin on both feet into a slight lunge position toward each side. The difference is that when you spin to the left, you are taking an imaginary "handle" on the right side with your right hand and pulling it from the right all the way through to the left with an uppercut motion. Then spin to the right and do the same. Do these exercises for thirty seconds, then rest for fifteen seconds.

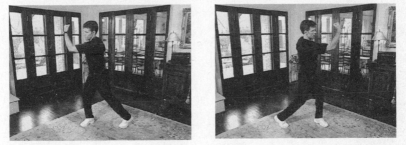

Alternate Rotation

3. *Squats.* Stand with your feet shoulder-width apart. Squat down as far as you comfortably can with palms facing down and open arms. Keep your back straight and feet flat throughout the entire movement. Go as low as you can control it, but don't overdo these squats if you feel pain. If you find these squats easy, however, use dumbbells or a medicine ball. Do this twenty times.

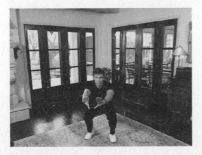
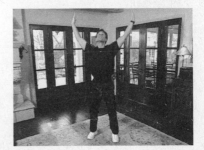

Squats

4. *Reaching lunges and overhead presses.* Begin by making a *reaching lunge forward* with the knee directly over the ankle. Try keeping your back leg straight at the same time. Do only four times. Next is a *reaching side lunge,* which is similar but to the side, keeping both feet facing forward. Reach down toward the side and touch the floor or ankle with both hands. Do each side twice. Finally, the *reaching wide lunge with the open hip* is a step backward and to the side in a 90-degree angle. While the front foot remains pointing forward, the other foot is at an angle, reaching down to that foot. Keep the front leg as straight as possible. Do four times total.

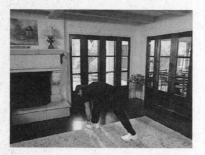 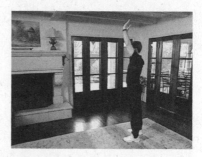

Reaching Lunge Forward

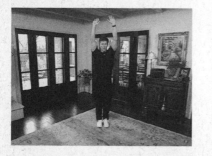 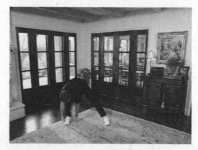

Reaching Side Lunge

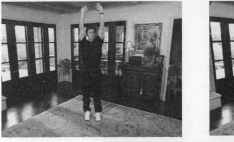

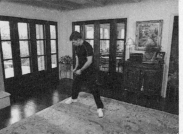

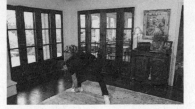

Reaching Side Lunge with Open Hip

5. *Alternate quad superman.* This exercise is done lying on your stomach or up on your hands and knees. Either way, lift up your right arm and extend while lifting your left leg into a fully extended position. Then do the opposite. Do each movement twenty times.

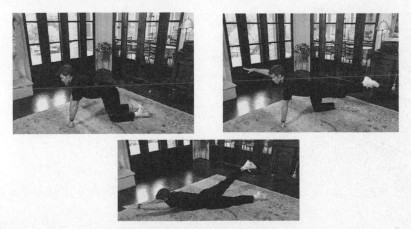

Alternate Quad Superman

6. *Push-ups.* Find a wall, sturdy counter, or stable chair. Or you can perform these push-ups the traditional way from the floor. Keep your back straight and curl your hips slightly forward to make your lower back lie flat. There should be no pressure or pain in the lower back during this movement. If you have trouble with wrist pain, try using push-up bars or handgrips that keep your wrists in a neutral position. Do twenty push-ups.

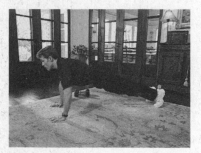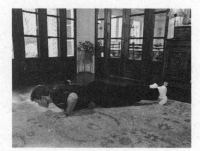

Push-Ups

7. *Rotation pumps.* This exercise involves stability, balance, and speed. Stand with your feet slightly wider than shoulder-width apart with knees slightly bent. Place your arms down with elbows bent at 90 degrees in front of you. Your hands are open and facing each other like you're holding on to an imaginary ten-pound medicine ball. Bend slightly forward and "crunch" your abdominal muscles. Then, keeping your elbows close and tight to your body, tense up your muscles and do quick rotations to each side, like you're moving the medicine ball back and forth to each side. Keep your lower back tight as you execute several full rotations. Do these exercises for thirty seconds.

Try to perform these functional exercises at least once a day or once in the morning and once in the evening, if possible. The advanced level is doing the entire program three times consecutively, morning and evening. Don't forget that functional fitness is designed to be part of a comprehensive lifestyle, which includes a healthy diet, nutritional supplementation, proper hygiene, deep-breathing exercises, and walking.

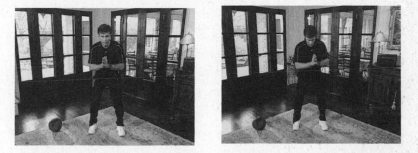

Rotation Pumps

"Conventional weight training isolates muscle groups, but it doesn't teach the muscle groups you're isolating to work with others," says Greg Roskopf, M.S., a biomechanics consultant with a company called Muscle Activation Techniques, who has worked with athletes from professional sports teams. "The key to functional exercise is integration. It's about teaching all the muscles to work together rather than isolating them to work independently."

What I like about functional fitness is that you don't have to lift weights or run on pavement. You don't have to be a bodybuilder or even a young person. By training movements instead of muscles, you can prevent lower back pain. Squats enhance functional fitness since they parallel movements such as bending over to pick something up, leaning forward to lift a heavy object, or sitting down and getting up from a chair.

Dips match the movement patterns of climbing stairs, walking up a steep hill, or trying to climb onto something from the ground. Functional fitness exercises can also be performed in a pool, where water resistance is three-dimensional.

A functional fitness program increases strength in the daily tasks of life and lowers the risk of injuries. If the last time you exercised was when the Berlin Wall came down, then functional fitness is a great place to start.

WALK, DON'T RUN

After hearing about functional fitness, now you know that you don't have to pump away on a futuristic-looking elliptical trainer to get your exercise jones. You don't have to sign up for a "spin class" on those newfangled bikes at the fitness club. And you don't have to bench-press humongous amounts of weight among the behemoth bodybuilders at Gold's Gym.

There's another route to fitness, and it's a low-impact one that just about anyone, any age, in any physical shape, can do. I'm talking about good old-fashioned walking, a highly acceptable form of exercise that requires no expensive equipment. In addition, walking can be done for any length of time, and the intensity can be adjusted according to age, health status, and fitness goals.

Walking, probably the most perfect exercise you can do, is a surprisingly effective strategy for long-term health. Those approaching retirement age will appreciate how this load-bearing exercise places a gentle strain on the hips and the rest of the body. According to the American Heart Association, vigorous activities that include brisk walking, and moderate activities that include walking for pleasure, can help reduce the following risk factors for heart disease:

- high blood pressure
- diabetes
- obesity and overweight
- high levels of triglycerides
- low levels of HDL (good cholesterol)

Walking imposes mild stress on the heart, which makes the heart work harder, which, in turn, helps build up the heart muscle. You can walk whenever it fits into your schedule: the crack of dawn before work, during the morning break, over the lunch hour, before dinner, or in the twilight hours. You can go at your own pace, your muscles don't need to recoup for twenty-four or forty-eight hours as they do after weightlifting, and it's an exercise that you can do every day. You can walk after eating a meal, and it's a superb social activity since walking is tailor-made for talking at the same time. It's a form of exercise you can do with someone of the opposite sex since strength and size don't count for much when it comes to walking. I enjoy taking walks with Nicki and Joshua and find it to be a great time of family fellowship.

For those with treadmills at home, walking is a way to burn calories and expend energy in the privacy of their homes. Some young mothers jump on the treadmill as soon as their kids go down for a nap. A home treadmill makes sense in a frigid climate or an area where you feel unsafe walking after dark, but walking outdoors in the fresh air and sunlight is always preferred.

You'd have to go the extra mile to find anything bad to say about walking. I will concede that walking on a treadmill can be boring, but that's why they hang TV monitors from the ceiling, right?

ALL ABOARD THE SLEEP TRAIN

When they said you don't realize what you've got until it's gone, I didn't know they were talking about sleep. Since Nicki and I are parents of a one-year old son, excuse me while I clear my throat and try to be serious about a serious topic—the role of sleep in our lives.

Nicki and I could be the poster couple—weary and haggard-looking—for America's sleep deficit because we count ourselves among the one hundred million Americans who get up in the morning without getting proper rest. Our excuse is that our baby boy hasn't quite gotten the hang of sleeping through the night. I also change time zones like people change their socks, so jet lag throws me for a loop.

Whether you possess a good excuse or not, the consequences of a sleep deficit are profound upon our culture: sleepy children daydream in the class-room, tired employees cost their companies billions in lost productivity each year, drivers falling asleep behind the wheel cause accidents that kill thousands annually, and interpersonal relationships become strained and often fracture when couples are too tired to deal with each other.

The root causes of our national sleep debt are overcrowded schedules, the desire to accomplish one more thing before retiring, and too much stimulation from watching TV in bed, which is a shame. Sleep and relaxation are basic necessities of life—right up there with diet and exercise in my book—but you'd never know it by the way we treat this foundation of good health. "Sleep plays a major role in preparing the body and brain for an alert, productive, psychologically, and physiologically healthy tomorrow," says Dr. James B. Maas, author of *Power Sleep*.[1]

This is as good a place as any to issue a wake-up call about the importance of sleep, a body therapy that is the most important nonnutrient you can incorporate into your healthy lifestyle. A good night's rest revitalizes tired bodies, gives us more energy, and helps us think more clearly throughout the day. Sleep experts say we have to shoot for the magic number of eight hours. Why eight hours? Because when people can control the amount of time they sleep, such as in a sleep laboratory, they naturally sleep eight hours in a twenty-four-hour period.

Twenty-four hours . . . the time it takes for the earth to spin on its axis and make one revolution. Our biological cycles normally follow the twenty-four-hour cycle of the sun, or what is known as a circadian rhythm. During this time, the body does things that we don't even know about, such as an automatic system that carries on functions of cleansing and rebuilding. The liver goes through a cleansing process between 11:00 p.m. and 1:00 a.m. If you're awake during that time, your liver will not cleanse properly. Take it from me: the liver is the one organ that receives the brunt of our poor lifestyle abuse. In addition, your body will not produce the right hormones if you don't sleep at the right times.

The problem is that most Americans haven't been getting eight hours of shut-eye for a long time. A century ago, long before David Letterman and Jay Leno began their stand-up monologues at 11:35 each evening, adults slept an average of nine hours a night, according to the National Sleep Foundation. Care to guess how long the average American adult sleeps each night in the present era?

The answer is a little less than seven hours, which is 20 percent less than our great-grandparents slept. If Joshua is cooperative, I get my eight hours, and when that joyful event happens, I feel refreshed and ready to go in the morning. When I get less than eight, I have to push through the day like millions of others, but I know I'm not firing on all cylinders.

I compensate by trying to follow the advice of my colleague, Dr. Joseph Mercola, who told me that one hour of sleep *before* midnight is equal to four hours of sleep after midnight. The formula makes sense to me. If I go to bed really late, say around 2:00 a.m., I just don't feel well for a couple of days. When I get to bed before midnight, I perform better the next day. I urge you to go to bed earlier, even if it's thirty minutes before you typically go to bed. If that means missing the local news on TV, you can catch up by reading the newspaper in the morning.

I know that as Joshua gets older, we'll be sticklers about getting him enough rest. I've come across research showing that a chronic lack of sleep among children hurts their performance inside and outside the classroom. Sleep-deprived teens also experience more emotional problems and are more prone to becoming obese adults. I'm well aware that teens, with their long days of class, after-school sports, and the usual tons of homework, are especially at risk for not getting enough rest. The National Sleep Foundation reports that high school students are averaging seven hours and twenty-four minutes each night when they should be receiving nine hours and fifteen minutes of sleep each night (meaning they should be in bed by 9:45 for a 7:00 a.m. wake-up call).[2] No wonder study halls are more known for students laying their heads on their desks than doing their math homework.

Researchers from the University of Chicago's Department of Medicine found that insufficient rest could make one old before his time. In one study, University of Chicago researchers restricted the sleeping habits of eleven young men (ages eighteen to twenty-seven) to four hours a night for six nights. The sleep-deprived men began experiencing metabolic and hormonal changes that doctors would usually see in patients older than sixty years of age. Researchers hypothesize that a lack of sleep hurts one's ability to metabolize carbohydrates (sugars and starches) and produce gland secretions. In fact, after just four nights of four hours of sleep, the men in the study consumed 35 percent more calories than they had on day one, with most of those excess calories coming from junk food loaded with sugar and fat. You could certainly say it appears that lack of sleep triggers cravings for the wrong foods. Fortunately the young men in the test group reversed those trends within one week by sleeping twelve hours a night.[3]

Science has demonstrated that sleep releases growth hormones that stimulate the growth and repair of damaged tissue. The more one sleeps deeply, the more growth hormones are released into the body's bloodstream. This is important, especially in middle age when the body releases lower amounts of growth hormone. University of Chicago researchers learned that a drop in growth hormone often leads to flabby stomachs and double chins.[4]

"Americans sleep the least of anyone in modern countries," Dr. Eve Van Cauter, a sleep researcher at the University of Chicago, said on ABC's *20/20* newsmagazine show. "And Americans are the most overweight and obese. Perhaps it's worth thinking about the possibility that we don't sleep enough, and therefore our appetites are unregulated."[5]

Sleep is good for the body and good for you. William Shakespeare wasn't too far off when he wrote four hundred years ago, "Sleep that knits up the ravell'd sleave of care . . . Chief nourisher in life's feast."

R AND R: REST AND RELAXATION

Most people, including me, never give the heart a second thought. The heart just keeps beating until the day we draw our final breath, right? Actually our hearts graphically design our need for rest because this important muscle *does* rest after each beat. After each contraction of the heart, known as the *systole,* there is a time of relaxation from the work that has been done. In medical terms, we call this the absolute refractory period—a time in the cardiac cycle when the heart *cannot* beat. During this period of relaxation, known as the *diastole,* the heart not only recovers, but it also refills with blood. The relaxation phase is long enough so that the heart's chambers can refill with the appropriate amount of blood. When the heart muscle finally contracts, it pumps nutrient-rich blood, which sustains each organ and vital function of the body, into the body's arteries.

Thus, the heart's cycle of rest is a shining example of the importance of balancing work and relaxation in our lives. We can all agree that our waking hours—the systole—require much energy, but in order to think clearly, do our jobs well, be attentive to others, and enjoy the day set before us, we must find times when we can rest. Without adequate relaxation, we cannot give our best or do our best. That's why our minds need an absolute refractory period— a time when we set aside what drives us and seek out peace and quiet instead.

That time of rest is supposed to come on the weekends, but Saturdays and Sundays have become wall-to-wall shopping-and-errands extravaganzas. The only chance to catch your breath comes on Sunday morning in the church pew, but most folks slip right back into the rat race minutes after shaking the pastor's hand and waving good-bye to the choir director.

When God created the earth and the heavens in six days, we're told that He rested on the seventh day. God wasn't worn out by His labors, of course, but I believe He rested to give us an example and to remind us that we were designed to work six days and rest on the seventh. Examples are evident throughout nature. When horses, mules, and oxen are worked ten, twelve, fourteen days straight, they break down. During World War II, the story goes, aircraft makers tried working Rosie the Riveter and Mac the Machinist seven days a week— and watched productivity plummet. Workers need a day off once a week.

Athletes understand that bodies need to recuperate. Triathletes are religious about not doing any swimming, biking, or running one day a week. NFL players always recuperate the day after a game, but football coaches never take *any* days off during the season. Guess who complains about burnout? Another example is seen in the tennis world. The Wimbledon tennis championship takes off the middle Sunday during the fortnight, which announcers now call a "quaint" tradition. Meanwhile, the other three Grand Slam tournaments— the French Open at Roland Garros, the U.S. Open, and the Australian Open—go for fourteen days straight, and even tennis fans have the blahs by the time the men's final is played on the second Sunday.

Spain is one country that provides a vivid example of the deleterious effects of lack of rest. The culprit is the afternoon siesta. I found out that the workday begins at 9:00 a.m., but everything shuts down for three hours in the middle of the afternoon, including all the stores and banks. Years ago, workers used to go home and eat lunch and snooze during the heat of the day, but today's long commutes make a trip home impractical. So the three-hour break is distinguished by extravagant multicourse lunches and a lot of sitting around and chatting before returning to work between four and five o'clock. The Spanish then conduct business and labor away until 8:00 p.m. before beginning the exodus home.

No self-respecting Spaniard would think of eating dinner before 10:00 p.m., and by the time things wind down, it's way after midnight when the Spaniards crawl into bed. The Spanish people sleep forty minutes fewer than the typical European. This deficit poses serious health effects, including greater physical and mental illness and higher numbers of accidents on the roadways and in the workplace.

In some ways, people in the United States aren't doing any better. One of the biggest mistakes this country has made in the last fifty years is relaxing the blue laws that prohibited most businesses from being open on Sundays. We shop until we literally drop. You can see it in the crowded mall parking lots on Sunday afternoons. That's why I tip my hat to Chick-fil-A, a fast-food eatery with more than 1,125 restaurants in thirty-seven states that closes down *all* its stores on Sundays.

A rest-filled Sunday (or Saturday, if that is when you take your day of rest, as I do) gives us a break from life's constant stresses. Scripture offers many examples. In Mark 6, Jesus recognized that to do God's work required periodic rest and renewal. After He sent out the twelve disciples two by two to tell others to turn from their sins, they returned to Jesus and told Him about all they had done and all they had said to the people they visited.

After hearing about their journeys, Jesus said, "Let's get away from the crowds for a while and rest" (Mark 6:31 NLT). In the next verse, we learn that there were so many people coming and going that they scarcely had time to eat, so they left "by boat" for a quiet spot.

"Every time we visit a lake and feel the boat gliding out into the water, we see the wisdom of Jesus," wrote medical doctors S. I. McMillen and David Stern in *None of These Diseases*. "Nothing shuts out the stresses of daily life like a boat gliding out on the water. Simple inactivity, however, is not rest. A couch-potato weekend is not refreshing. Twenty hours of TV, three bags of Doritos, and four liters of Coke will not get you ready to attack the next week. A rest that refreshes must calm the spirit *and* feed the soul."[6]

I've long felt that if you give God that one day of rest each week, He'll do greater things with the other six days than you can do in seven days. I constantly remind myself of this because I tend not to rest the way I should on Saturdays. In my quest to fulfill God's purpose for my life, which is to spread this wonderful message of health and hope, I always feel that every minute I'm not sharing this message means that people are suffering needlessly. Just as you do, I need to trust God that He'll do more with His six days, with me giving Him one, than I could do with my seven.

This concept must be very important to God because we read in Exodus 31:14–15 that anyone who worked on the Sabbath was to be killed. God, in His wisdom, rested on the seventh day and was refreshed, Scripture tells us.

I now understand much better than I used to the role of rest and relaxation, and I hope you do too.

A Breath of Fresh Sunlight

I'm going to talk about two things close to my heart that precipitate rest—deep breathing and sunbathing.

As for the former, I'm not talking about sitting cross-legged on a mat with your fingertips touching while you chant *ohmmm*. Instead, I'm talking about a technique that relaxes and refreshes the body in just five minutes. You'll feel calm, yet alert, after practicing deep breathing.

You begin by sitting in a comfortable chair and placing your feet flat on the floor. Although you don't have to shut your eyes, I find it's better to close them, which helps you pay close attention to the cadence of your breathing. Inhale slowly through your nose and allow a breath of air to completely fill your lungs. Most of the time, we don't completely fill the diaphragm with air because we're not aware that our lungs hang all the way toward the bottom of the rib cage. Instead of inflating the upper part of the lungs, concentrate on filling the lungs completely. Count to five as you breathe in, then hold your breath for several seconds before exhaling through your mouth for several more seconds. Visualize the diaphragm moving up and down to provide more room for your lungs to expand.

Repeat the process, but don't allow the mind to drift. Return your attention to your breathing, and you should feel better immediately because the oxygen you give your body is now moving rapidly through your bloodstream. Resist the urge to go on to something else. Deep-breathing techniques are a peaceful, powerful tool to calm your nervous system, slow down your heartbeat, and restore your energy.

You can take deep breathing one step further by sitting outside and drawing deep breaths in bright sunshine. My feelings on sunlight run counter to the conventional wisdom, which says the sun is bad for you. While it's true that a small segment of the population experience higher rates of melanoma and other forms of skin cancer, I believe that's more because they lack adequate nutrients in their diets, especially antioxidant-rich fruits, vegetables, and healthy fats. Think about it: before the modern era, people used to spend much more time outside—and they didn't get skin cancer in the rates we see today. How did the Israelites, who were enslaved for four hundred years, manage to be so healthy when they were breaking rocks and making bricks out of straw in the hot sun all day?

The reason we're having more skin cancer is not because we're getting too much sun. That can't be true because we're getting *far less* sun since so few people work outside these days. Getting sunlight is extremely important for our bodies because of the way the skin synthesizes vitamin D from the ultraviolet rays of sunlight. Exposure to the sun is a significant source of vitamin D (along with my favorite supplement, cod-liver oil) because sunlight provides many of us with our vitamin D requirement.

For instance, vitamin D plays a role in immunity and blood cell formation, and is also needed for adequate blood levels of insulin. I once heard a vitamin D expert say that more than 90 percent of Americans face a deficiency in vitamin D, so it's likely that you're among that group. You can meet your recommended daily allowance of vitamin D by sunbathing:

- one hour
- twice a week
- at noon
- near the equator
- in the nude

Very few can meet those parameters, which is why I recommend taking cod-liver oil as part of your daily diet *and* getting sunlight whenever possible. If you think about it, humans lived in harmony with the sun's heat and light for thousands of years, but in the last half century, we've become afraid of the sun. Worried moms lather their children in sunblock, while others prefer that they stay indoors and play on hot summer days.

While we should take steps to protect the skin from burning under the sun's rays, sunscreens with a sun protection factor (SPF) of 8 or greater will block ultraviolet rays that produce vitamin D. The National Institutes of Health (NIH) says that ten to fifteen minutes of sunlight allow adequate time for vitamin D synthesis to occur, after which (and not before) you can apply a natural sunscreen with an SPF of at least 15 to protect the skin or, better yet, apply extra-virgin coconut oil to your skin. At least twice weekly you should expose your face, arms, hands, and back to the sun to provide adequate vitamin D.

If you live in the Northeast, however, be aware that sunlight exposure from November through February is insufficient to produce significant vitamin D synthesis in the skin. Industrial pollution also decreases sun exposure, so if the sun comes out in the winter months, take yourself and the kids for a walk and soak up some rays.

The reason I'm making a big deal about sunlight and vitamin D is that vitamin D is actually not a vitamin but a critical hormone that helps regulate the health of more than thirty different tissues and organs, from the brain to the prostate. Vitamin D plays a role in regulating cell growth, the immune system, and blood pressure.

So now you can see why there aren't many healthier activities than sitting in a chair, closing your eyes, and taking deep breaths with a bright sun beating down on you.

THE WONDERS OF HYDROTHERAPY

Hydrotherapy is a fifty-cent word for using water to heal in various ways. Dozens of different treatments come in the forms of baths, showers, washings, wraps, and effusions, which is the pouring on of liquids.

My favorite hydrotherapy involves the therapeutic qualities of hot and cold showers and therapeutic baths. Cold water stimulates the body and boosts oxygen use in the cells. Hot water dilates blood vessels, which improves blood circulation, speeds the elimination of toxins, and transports more oxygen to the brain. I will often take a hot shower, but when I'm through washing, I'll switch off the hot water and allow my skin to be blasted by freezing cold water for sixty seconds. That'll wake you up in the morning!

I always wondered what it would be like to sit in an inferno-like sauna in some Norwegian woods, heating my body temperature up to a point where I thought I was being parboiled, and then run out of the sauna and dive into a blanket of fresh snow. Well, I found out one day after skiing in Vail, high in the Rocky Mountains. After soaking twenty minutes in a hot tub, I leaped into the snow like a crazy kid and made a snow angel. Then I sprinted back into the hot tub, and the scalding water felt like thousands of pins poking my skin. Now that's what I call invigorating!

Okay, call me wacko, but hydrotherapy is a proven but often overlooked treatment. While 99 percent of us take showers daily, when was the last time you took a lingering, hot bath? A fifteen- or twenty-minute soak up to your shoulders in 95- to 100-degree water will do wonders for frayed nerves and tense muscles after a harried day. A full bath is helpful for the bladder and urinary problems, mild colds, and low fevers. Adding essential oils or herbs softens and moisturizes the pores of the skin. Another form of bathing is a sitz bath, which involves sitting in a few inches of hot water that's touching the bottom, hips, and lower abdomen. Foot baths with healing herbs can be stimulating as well.

Our third president, Thomas Jefferson, soaked his feet in cold water every morning as a way of preventing colds. Until his death at the age of eighty-three, he said that he had a cold only every seven years or so. President Jefferson also battled intestinal problems, which he combated by sticking to a diet of green foods and periodic servings of red meat.

Recognition of the healing properties of water dates back much earlier than Jefferson's era, all the way to ancient times when the Greek physician Hippocrates prescribed bathing for its therapeutic effects. Later, the Romans constructed elaborate communal baths near natural hot springs and used aqueducts to carry water into their cities for their bathing palaces and stone bathing tubs. In their conquered lands, Roman baths were built in Bath, England; Baden-Baden, Germany; and Baden, Switzerland. (The German word *baden* means "bath.")

The Romans developed a sophisticated bathing culture for their time. After disrobing from their togas, the Romans rubbed oil onto their skin and moved to a warm room, where they would lie around and chat until it was time to enter the hot and steamy *caldarium*, which would be similar to a sauna or Turkish bath. While they sat and perspired, they scraped their skin with a curved metal tool, which removed much of their dead skin. Then it was time for the rinse cycle: a soak in a hot bath, followed by a quick dip in a cold bath.

Many of these bath emporiums were destroyed in the fall of Rome, and bathing fell out of favor during the Middle Ages. Queen Elizabeth I of England (1533–1603), it is said, insisted on bathing at least once a month, whether she needed it or not. As hygiene and sanitation improved in the Industrial Age, the well-heeled traveled for days to "take in the waters" at the first spas, a name that originated from the town of Spa, located in Belgium's Ardennes forest.

Today, hydrotherapy is an excellent way to increase energy and resistance to disease while improving body awareness. *The Encyclopedia of Natural Healing* outlines some basic principles of hydrotherapy:

1. Never use cold water on a body without warming the body first.
2. After cold application, do not dry parts of the body, but wipe off with the hand, except for areas with large concentrations of hair.
3. Dry parts of the body after warm and hot applications.
4. Reheat the body ten or fifteen minutes after cold applications.
5. Follow short treatments with active exercise.

In addition, cold baths should not be given to children or elderly people, and people with heart conditions should avoid saunas or hot baths.[7]

AROMATHERAPY AND MUSIC THERAPY

There are two other therapies that I want to introduce to you—aromatherapy and music therapy. The former involves the sense of smell, and the latter involves the sense of hearing.

Aromatherapy is a term coined by French chemist René Maurice Gattefossé more than seventy-five years ago when he used lavender oil to heal his burned hands without leaving any scars. In aromatherapy, essential oils are taken from plants, flowers, shrubs, trees, bushes, and seeds to be used in a variety of healing ways, and this healthy practice has been around since the days of Moses and the pharaohs.

For instance, the ancient Egyptians used aromatherapy oils for bathing, for massage, and for embalming their dead. In Exodus 30, the Lord told Moses to collect the choicest of spices—pure myrrh, cinnamon, sweet cane, and cassia—and mix them with olive oil to produce a "holy anointing oil." The brother of Jesus, James, wrote, "Is any one of you sick? He should call the elders of the church to pray over him and anoint him with oil in the name of the Lord" (James 5:14). A total of 188 references to precious oils, such as frankincense, galbanum, rosemary, hyssop, and spikenard, can be found in Scripture.

I believe significant health benefits can be derived from introducing essential oils to your skin and pores. Try rubbing a few drops of myrtle, coriander, hyssop, galbanum, or frankincense onto the palms, then cup your hands over your mouth and nose and inhale. Taking a deep breath will soothe the mind and invigorate the spirit.

An eyedropper or two of these essential oils into a hot bath will give you an opportunity to practice hydrotherapy and aromatherapy at the same time. You can also use essential oils in a compress or burn them in a diffuser. These essential oils stimulate the powerful sense of smell, and their pleasant odors can have a significant impact on how we feel. Smelling lavender, for instance, has been associated with relaxation.

I've rubbed some of these essential oils on the soles of my feet, and I've been amazed that I can taste cinnamon or peppermint oil on the tip of my tongue within twenty minutes. I recommend incorporating these essential oils found in the Bible on a daily basis. Whether you rub these oils into your skin or add them to your bath, you'll experience a renewed sense of health.

While aromatherapy is based on the sense of smell and touch, music therapy is all in the ears. I know I haven't spent much time describing how much I love music, but when I was heavily involved with the college group at First Baptist Church of Tallahassee during my Florida State days, I loved singing on the praise team. Before I got sick, I traveled with the college group and sang in church services, and I really wondered if the Lord was preparing me for a life in the worship ministry. Whenever I speak in churches these days, I show a music video of and play a song I cowrote with my good friend, worship pastor and recording artist Michael Neale, called "Faith Is a Place." (See the GPRx Resource Guide, page 350, to get your copy.)

Music therapy is the use of specific music to promote relaxation and healing. Research in music therapy supports its effectiveness in a wide variety of health-care and educational settings. Although most healing music is soft and soothing, it's up to your individual preferences as far as what is relaxing and therefore healing to you.

I'm not talking about "elevator music" but soothing arrangements that are calming and promote emotional healing from the stresses of the day. Listening to this type of music improves concentration and memory and thus can help hyperactive children stay focused.

When it comes to music therapy, I know what I like: contemporary Christian and praise and worship music. First of all, I am praising God through song, which is biblical. The psalmist declared, "Sing! Beat the tambourine. Play the sweet lyre and the harp. Sound the trumpet . . . for this is required by the laws of Israel; it is a law of the God of Jacob" (Ps. 81:2–4 NLT). The apostle Paul reminded us in Colossians 3:16 that we should "sing psalms, hymns and spiritual songs with gratitude in [our] hearts to God."

I like to listen to contemporary Christian music by artists such as Stephen Curtis Chapman, Casting Crowns, and Jeremy Camp. When I play one of their CDs, I feel my spirit come alive because there is something powerful about hearing God's Word put to song. Nicki shares my thirst for worship music as well. She loves Mercy Me and enjoys Casting Crowns and Jeremy Camp as much as I do.

You are never too young to enjoy music. In fact, when our son, Joshua, was a few months old, we couldn't get him to stop crying. I would hold him and sing to him, and he would become calm. Even now, if I can't get him to sleep, I play worship music in his room.

Any day now, I expect to catch him dancing in his crib.

For Further Study

For additional study on God's plan for exercise and body therapies, visit www.BiblicalHealthInstitute.com for a free introductory course called "Exercise and Body Therapies 101."

FUNCTIONAL FITNESS WORKS FOR ME
by Jason Kombrinck

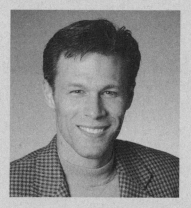

Athletics were a big part of my life growing up, and my father constantly encouraged me to do my best. His inspiration led me to excel in three sports throughout high school. During college I took Tae Kwon Do, was on the Florida State University Cheerleading Squad, and competed in natural body-building. Needless to say, I was very active.

A three-year battle with a sports injury led to me becoming a physical therapist. I learned to think in "functional" ways when working with patients. A patient doesn't need a goal of being able to perform three sets of ten-pound dumbbell curls. A functional (and reimbursable!) goal would be to pick up an object off the floor and put it on a shelf. These are real-life, practical movements that are of primary importance. These same principles are important to people who don't need rehab.

The typical person today often goes into a gym and sits down on many comfortable machines that totally eliminate the use of the "core" muscles. Getting away from the machine-dependent mindset and looking for ways to work on balance while using integrated muscle patterns is one of the main goals of Functional Fitness. I'm thirty-five years old and always looking for a way to "tweak" my workouts to make them more functional. It's fun and keeps things creative. A great example of a functional exercise would be to stand on one foot while bent over at the waist performing a dumbbell row with the opposite arm. Try it!

Other body therapies are important as well. I try to spend some time each day practicing deep-breathing techniques. People overlook its importance, because it's easy and available. This has been an energizing pursuit and can only bring health to our body's cells. I also try to get a little sunlight each day. Short walks in the sunshine during lunches or breaks have made a difference in my health. It's also a great time to think and pray.

Getting to bed earlier is obviously the hardest advice to follow, but when heeded it can make the next day seem like paradise. Having a hard time falling asleep? Try an Epsom salt bath. The magnesium in the salts is absorbed through the skin and will put you in total relaxation mode. It has worked well for me. Another one is the dry-heat sauna. I used to wonder why anyone would put themselves through the perceived torture, but it has become one of my favorite body therapies. It can work wonders in helping to get rid of toxins and impurities through the skin. The functional fitness philosophy and these body therapies have taken me to the next level in recovery and immune system strength. As you can see, they work for me.

THE GREAT PHYSICIAN'S Rx FOR CONDITIONING YOUR BODY WITH EXERCISE AND BODY THERAPIES

- *Make a commitment and an appointment to exercise at least three times a week.*

- *Incorporate five-to-ten minutes of functional fitness into your daily schedule.*

- Take a brisk walk and see how much better you feel at the end of the day.

- Make a conscious effort to practice deep breathing exercises once a day. Inflate your lungs to full and hold for several seconds before slowly exhaling.

- Go to sleep earlier, paying close attention to how much sleep you get before midnight. Do your best to get eight hours of sleep nightly. Remember that sleep is the most important nonnutrient thing you can do for your health.

- End your next shower by changing the water temperature to cool (or cold) and standing underneath the spray for one minute.

- Next Saturday or Sunday take a day of rest. Dedicate the day to the Lord, and do something fun and relaxing that you haven't done in a while. Make your rest day work-free, errand-free, and shop-free. Trust God that He'll do more with His six days than you can do with seven.

- Take a magazine (or this book!) and, during your next break from work, sit outside in a chair and face the sun. Soak up the rays for ten or fifteen minutes.

- Incorporate essential oils into your daily life.

- Play worship music in your home, in your car, or on your iPod. Focus on God's plan for your life.

THE GREAT PHYSICIAN'S Rx FOR WEEK #4

Day 22

Upon Waking

Advanced hygiene: by now you have read Key #3 on practicing advanced hygiene, and you have used the above method for several days in your morning routine. You will continue to use what you've learned, but I won't spell it out in detail every day. There will simply be a note saying "practice advanced hygiene." If you need a refresher on the directions, please see page 325.

Supplements: take one serving of a fiber/green superfood powder (mixed in) or five caplets of a super green formula (swallowed with) twelve-to-sixteen ounces of water or raw vegetable juice. (See the GPRx Resource Guide, pages 346–347, for recommended products.)

Exercise: perform functional fitness exercises for five minutes (one round of exercises found in Key #4, pages 138–145).

Breakfast

hot tea with honey (see the GPRx Resource Guide, page 339, for recommended tea blends)

Mocha Swiss Almond Smoothie (see appendix A, page 315, for recipe) with two tablespoons of protein powder (optional)

Supplements: take one or two whole food multivitamin caplets and one or two capsules of a probiotic/enzyme blend (see the GPRx Resource Guide, pages 345–348, for recommended products).

Lunch

Before eating, drink eight ounces of water.

During lunch, drink eight ounces of water or hot or iced fresh-brewed tea with honey.

Coconut Milk Soup (see appendix A, page 272, for recipe)

orange

Supplements: take one or two whole food multivitamin caplets and one or two capsules of a probiotic/enzyme blend.

Dinner

Before eating, drink eight ounces of water.

During dinner, drink hot or iced fresh-brewed tea with honey.

Southern Range Chicken Dinner (see appendix A, page 283, for recipe)

green salad

Supplements: take one or two whole food multivitamin caplets, one-to-three teaspoons or three-to-nine capsules of high omega-3 cod-liver oil (see the GPRx Resource Guide, pages 345–348, for recommended products), and one or two capsules of a probiotic/enzyme blend.

Snacks

Banana Bread and butter (see appendix A, page 312, for recipe)

raspberry super green whole food bar (with beta glucans from soluble oat fiber; see the GPRx Resource Guide, pages 329–330, for recommended products).

Drink eight-to-twelve ounces of water, or hot or iced fresh-brewed tea with honey.

Before Bed

Drink eight-to-twelve ounces of water or hot tea with honey.

Exercise: go for a walk outdoors.

Supplements: take one serving of a fiber/green superfood powder (mixed in) or five caplets of a super green formula (swallowed with) twelve-to-sixteen ounces of water or raw vegetable juice.

Advanced hygiene: practice advanced hygiene. See page 325 for guidance.

Day 23

Upon Waking

Advanced hygiene: practice advanced hygiene. See page 325 for guidance.

Supplements: take one serving of a fiber/green superfood powder (mixed in) or five caplets of a super green formula (swallowed with) twelve-to-sixteen ounces of water or raw vegetable juice. (See the GPRx Resource Guide, pages 346–347, for recommended products.)

Exercise: perform functional fitness exercises for five minutes (one round of exercises found in Key #4, pages 138–145) and do deep-breathing exercises for five minutes.

Body therapy: take a hot and cold shower. After a normal shower, alternate sixty seconds of water as hot as you can stand it, followed by sixty seconds of water as cold as you can stand it. Repeat cycle twice for a total of four minutes, finishing with cold.

Breakfast

hot tea with honey

Onion, Pepper, and Goat Cheese Omelet (see appendix A, page 267, for recipe)

whole grain sprouted or sourdough toast with butter

Supplements: take one or two whole food multivitamin caplets and one or two capsules of a probiotic/enzyme blend.

Lunch

Before eating, drink eight ounces of water.

During lunch, drink eight ounces of water or hot or iced fresh-brewed tea with honey.

Turkey and Goat Cheese Wrap

carrot sticks

Supplements: take one or two whole food multivitamin caplets and one or two capsules of a probiotic/enzyme blend.

Dinner

Before eating, drink eight ounces of water.

During dinner, drink hot or iced fresh-brewed tea with honey.

Goat Cheese Stuffed Free-Range Chicken Breast (see appendix A, page 298, for recipe)

R's House Salad (see appendix A, page 283, for recipe)

Supplements: take one or two whole food multivitamin caplets and one-to-three teaspoons or three-to-nine capsules of high omega-3 cod-liver oil and one or two capsules of a probiotic/enzyme blend.

Snacks

apple and almond butter

Crispy Pecans (see appendix A, page 270, for recipe)

vanilla protein whole food bar (see the GPRx Resource Guide, pages 329–330, for recommended products)

Drink eight-to-twelve ounces of water, or hot or iced fresh-brewed tea with honey.

Before Bed

Drink eight-to-twelve ounces of water or hot tea with honey.

Exercise: go for a short walk outdoors.

Supplements: take one serving of a fiber/green superfood powder (mixed in) or five caplets of a super green formula (swallowed with) twelve-to-sixteen ounces of water or raw vegetable juice.

Advanced hygiene: practice advanced hygiene. See page 325 for guidance.

Body therapy: spend ten minutes listening to soothing music before you retire.

Day 24

Upon Waking

Advanced hygiene: practice advanced hygiene. See page 325 for guidance.

Supplements: take one serving of a fiber/green superfood powder (mixed in) or five caplets of a super green formula (swallowed with) twelve-to-sixteen ounces of water or raw vegetable juice. (See the GPRx Resource Guide, pages 346–347, for recommended products.)

Exercise: perform functional fitness exercises for five minutes (two rounds of exercises found in Key #4, pages 138–145), or spend ten minutes on a mini trampoline, which is also known as a rebounder (see the GPRx Resource Guide, page 350, for recommended products). Finish with five minutes of deep-breathing exercises.

Supplements: take one serving of a fiber/green superfood combination mixed into twelve-to-sixteen ounces of water or raw vegetable juice.

Body therapy: get twenty minutes of direct sunlight.

Breakfast

Five Grain Porridge (see appendix A, page 273, for recipe) with two tablespoons of protein powder added after cooking

strawberries

hot tea with honey

Supplements: take one or two whole food multivitamin caplets and one or two capsules of a probiotic/enzyme blend.

Lunch

Before eating, drink eight ounces of water.

During lunch, drink eight ounces of water or hot or iced fresh-brewed tea with honey.

Green Chili (see appendix A, page 316, for recipe)

crackers (whole grain or flaxseed)

Supplements: take one or two whole food multivitamin caplets and one or two capsules of a probiotic/enzyme blend.

Dinner

Before eating, drink eight ounces of water.

During dinner, drink hot or iced fresh-brewed tea with honey.

Juicy Rosemary Baked Lamb (see appendix A, page 291, for recipe)

Warm Smile (see appendix A, page 288, for recipe)

green salad

Supplements: take one or two whole food multivitamin caplets, one-to-three teaspoons or three-to-nine capsules of high omega-3 cod-liver oil, and one or two capsules of a probiotic/enzyme blend.

Snacks

crackers (whole grain or flaxseed with sliced cheese)

apple

Mango Berry Smoothie mix (see the GPRx Resource Guide, page 329, for recommended products) blended in eight-to-twelve ounces of water

Drink eight to twelve ounces of water or hot or iced fresh-brewed tea with honey.

Before Bed

Drink eight-to twelve ounces of water or hot tea with honey.

Exercise: go for a walk outdoors or participate in a favorite sport or recreational activity.

Supplements: take one serving of a fiber/green superfood powder (mixed in) or five caplets of a super green formula (swallowed with) twelve-to-sixteen ounces of water or raw vegetable juice.

Body therapy: take a warm bath for fifteen minutes with one cup of Epsom salt added.

Advanced hygiene: practice advanced hygiene. See page 325 for guidance.

Sleep: go to bed by 11:30 p.m.

Day 25

Upon Waking

Advanced hygiene: practice advanced hygiene. See page 325 for guidance.

Supplements: take one serving of a fiber/green superfood powder (mixed in) or five caplets of a super green formula (swallowed with) twelve-to-sixteen ounces of water or raw vegetable juice. (See the GPRx Resource Guide, pages 346–347, for recommended products.)

Exercise: perform functional fitness exercises for fifteen minutes (three rounds of exercises found in Key #4, pages 138–145) or spend fifteen minutes on the rebounder. Finish with five minutes of deep-breathing exercises.

Body therapy: take a hot and cold shower. After a normal shower, alternate sixty seconds of water as hot as you can stand it, followed by sixty seconds of water as cold as you can stand it. Repeat cycle three times for a total of six minutes, finishing with cold.

Breakfast

hot tea with honey

Piña Colada Smoothie (see appendix A, page 313, for recipe) with two tablespoons of protein powder (optional)

Supplements: one or two whole food multivitamin caplets and one or two capsules of a probiotic/enzyme blend.

Lunch

Before eating, drink eight ounces of water.

During lunch, drink eight ounces of water or hot or iced fresh-brewed tea with honey.

Mushroom Soup (see appendix A, page 273, for recipe)

Jamaican Style Curried Chicken (see appendix A, page 292, for recipe)

Supplements: take one or two whole food multivitamin caplets and one or two capsules of a probiotic/enzyme blend.

Dinner

Before eating, drink eight ounces of water.

During dinner, drink hot or iced fresh-brewed tea with honey.

Salmon Lemon Sauté (see appendix A, page 284, for recipe)

Cinnamon Sweet Potatoes (see appendix A, page 285, for recipe)

green salad

Supplements: take one or two whole food multivitamin caplets, one-to-three teaspoons or three-to-nine capsules of high omega-3 cod-liver oil, and one or two capsules of a probiotic/enzyme blend.

Snacks

yogurt, honey, and berries

antioxidant fruit whole food bar (see the GPRx Resource Guide, pages 329–330, for recommended products)

Drink eight-to-twelve ounces of water or hot or iced fresh-brewed tea with honey.

Before Bed

Drink eight-to-twelve ounces of water or hot tea with honey.

Exercise: go for a walk outdoors or participate in a favorite sport or recreational activity.

Supplements: take one serving of a fiber/green superfood powder (mixed in) or five caplets of a super green formula (swallowed with) twelve-to-sixteen ounces of water or raw vegetable juice.

Advanced hygiene: practice advanced hygiene. See page 325 for guidance.

Body therapy: spend ten minutes listening to soothing music before you retire.

Sleep: go to bed by 11:15 p.m.

Day 26 (Partial Fast Day)

Upon Waking

Advanced hygiene: practice advanced hygiene. See page 325 for guidance.

Supplements: take one serving of a fiber/green superfood powder (mixed in) or five caplets of a super green formula (swallowed with) twelve-to-sixteen ounces of water or raw vegetable juice. (See the GPRx Resource Guide, pages 346–347, for recommended products.)

Exercise: perform functional fitness exercises for fifteen minutes (three rounds of exercises found in Key #4, pages 138–145) or spend fifteen minutes on the rebounder. Finish with five minutes of deep-breathing exercises.

Body therapy: get twenty minutes of direct sunlight.

Breakfast

none (partial fast day)

eight ounces of water

Lunch

none (partial fast day)

eight ounces of water

Dinner

Before eating, drink eight ounces of water.

During dinner, drink hot or iced fresh-brewed tea with honey.

Chicken Soup

cultured vegetables

green salad

Supplements: take one or two whole food multivitamin caplets, one-to-three teaspoons or three-to-nine capsules of high omega-3 cod-liver oil, and one or two capsules of a probiotic/enzyme blend.

Snacks
   none (partial fast day)
   eight ounces of water

Before Bed
   Drink eight-to-twelve ounces of water or hot tea with honey.
   Exercise: go for a walk outdoors or participate in a favorite sport or recreational activity.
   Supplements: take one serving of a fiber/green superfood powder (mixed in) or five caplets of a super green formula (swallowed with) twelve-to-sixteen ounces of water or raw vegetable juice.
   Body therapy: take a warm bath for fifteen minutes with eight drops of biblical essential oils added. (See the GPRx Resource Guide, page 350, for recommended products.)
   Advanced hygiene: practice advanced hygiene. See page 325 for guidance.
   Sleep: go to bed by 11:00 p.m.

Day 27 (Day of Rest)

Upon Waking
   Advanced hygiene: practice advanced hygiene. See page 325 for guidance.
   Supplements: take one serving of a fiber/green superfood powder (mixed in) or five caplets of a super green formula (swallowed with) twelve-to-sixteen ounces of water or raw vegetable juice. (See the GPRx Resource Guide, pages 346–347, for recommended products.)
   Exercise: do no formal exercise since it's a day of rest.
   Body therapies: do none since it's a rest day.

Breakfast
   Turkey Sausage Queen Omelet (see appendix A, page 285, for recipe)
   grapefruit or orange
   one piece of whole grain sprouted or sourdough toast and butter
   hot tea with honey
   Supplements: take one or two whole food multivitamin caplets and one or two capsules of a probiotic/enzyme blend.

Lunch
   Before eating, drink eight ounces of water.
   During lunch, drink eight ounces of water or hot or iced fresh-brewed tea with honey.
   roast beef sandwich on whole grain sourdough or sprouted bread
   apple
   Supplements: take one or two whole food multivitamin caplets and one or two casules of a probiotic/enzyme blend.

Dinner
   Before eating, drink eight ounces of water.

During dinner, drink hot or iced fresh-brewed tea with honey.

Soy Ginger Salmon (see appendix A, page 281, for recipe)

Blue Corn Posole (see appendix A, page 286, for recipe)

Italian Zucchini (see appendix A, page 286, for recipe)

Supplements: take one or two whole food multivitamin caplets, one-to-three teaspoons or three-to-nine capsules of high omega-3 cod-liver oil, and one or two capsules of a probiotic/enzyme blend.

Snacks

Healthy Trail Mix (see appendix A, page 271, for recipe)

yogurt and honey

chocolate protein whole food bar (see the GPRx Resource Guide, pages 329–330, for recommended products)

Drink eight-to-twelve ounces of water or hot or iced fresh-brewed tea with honey.

Before Bed

Drink eight-to-twelve ounces of water or hot tea with honey.

Exercise: do no formal exercise since it's a day of rest.

Body therapies: do none since it's a rest day.

Supplements: take one serving of a fiber/green superfood powder (mixed in) or five caplets of a super green formula (swallowed with) twelve-to-sixteen ounces of water or raw vegetable juice.

Advanced hygiene: practice advanced hygiene. See page 325 for guidance.

Sleep: go to bed by 11:00 p.m.

Day 28

Upon Waking

Advanced hygiene: practice advanced hygiene. See page 325 for guidance.

Supplements: take one serving of a fiber/green superfood powder (mixed in) or five caplets of a super green formula (swallowed with) twelve-to-sixteen ounces of water or raw vegetable juice. (See the GPRx Resource Guide, pages 346–347, for recommended products.)

Exercise: perform functional fitness exercises for fifteen minutes (three rounds of exercises found in Key #4, pages 138–145) or spend fifteen minutes on the rebounder. Finish with five minutes of deep-breathing exercises.

Body therapy: take a hot and cold shower. After normal shower, alternate sixty seconds of water as hot as you can stand it, followed by sixty seconds of water as cold as you can stand it. Repeat cycle four times for a total of eight minutes, finishing with cold.

Breakfast

poached eggs

Blueberry Muffins (see appendix A, page 272, for recipe)

hot tea with honey

Supplements: take one or two whole food multivitamin caplets and one or two capsules of a probiotic/enzyme blend.

Lunch

Before eating, drink eight ounces of water.

During lunch, drink eight ounces of water or hot or iced fresh-brewed tea with honey.

tuna salad on a bed of greens or on sprouted whole grain or sourdough bread

apple or pear

Supplements: take one or two whole food multivitamin caplets and one or two capsules of a probiotic/enzyme blend.

Dinner

Before eating, drink eight ounces of water.

During dinner, drink hot or iced fresh-brewed tea with honey.

Blackened Sea Bass (see appendix A, page 293, for recipe)

grilled asparagus

Supplements: take one or two whole food multivitamin caplets, one-to-three teaspoons or three-to-nine capsules of high omega-3 cod-liver oil, and one or two capsules of a probiotic/enzyme blend.

Snacks

apple-cinnamon fiber whole food bar (see the GPRx Resource Guide, pages 329–330, for recommended products)

Drink eight-to-twelve ounces of water or hot tea with honey.

Before Bed

Drink eight-to-twelve ounces of water or hot tea with honey.

Exercise: go for a walk outdoors or participate in a favorite sport or recreational activity.

Supplements: take one serving of a fiber/green superfood powder (mixed in) or five caplets of a super green formula (swallowed with) twelve-to-sixteen ounces of water or raw vegetable juice.

Advanced hygiene: practice advanced hygiene. See page 325 for guidance.

Body therapy: spend ten minutes listening to soothing music before you retire.

Sleep: go to bed by 10:30 p.m.

Key #5

Reduce Toxins in Your Environment

Let us purify ourselves from everything that contaminates body and spirit, perfecting holiness out of reverence for God.

—2 Corinthians 7:1

When it comes to dealing with toxins in your environment, I'm talking about more than separating your weekly trash for curbside recycling. This isn't about saving the whales or protecting the rain forest, or even reducing the destruction of the ozone layer, although these are good things. I'm referring to reducing the toxins in the personal environment *inside* your home: the air you breathe, the water you drink, the lotions and cosmetics you put on your skin, the products you use to clean your home, and the toothpaste you dab on your toothbrush. The reason we must pay attention to these mundane daily activities is that we live in a toxic world.

Just how toxic?

You may not want to know. In a study led by the Mount Sinai School of Medicine in New York, in collaboration with the Environmental Working Group and Commonweal, researchers at two major laboratories found an average of ninety-one industrial compounds, pollutants, and other chemicals in the blood and urine of nine volunteers.[1]

A partial listing of the contaminants found in the volunteer test group revealed that many of these toxins have been named as cancer-causing agents by the National Toxicology Program or the Environmental Protection Agency:

- **PCBs.** Polychlorinated biphenyls are a group of chemical compounds developed in the 1930s for making paint, ink, dye, hydraulic fluids, and electrical transformers, to name a few uses. Despite a worldwide ban in the late 1970s, concentrations of PCBs continue to be found in the fatty tissues of land animals and fish. Most farm-raised salmon are raised on pellets of ground-up fish that have absorbed PCBs from the environment.

- **Dioxins.** These organic compounds contain carbon, oxygen, and hydrogen and can be created naturally (from volcanoes and forest fires) or through the manufacturing of PVC products (plastic piping) or industrial chlorinated cleaners. This is another toxin that tends to accumulate in animals with high-fat contents such as fish and shellfish.

- **Furans.** These chemicals are country cousins to dioxins and PCBs, and although not as toxic, they are linked to problems with the endocrine (hormonal) system.

- **Metals.** Metallic particles of mercury, lead, arsenic, aluminum, and cadmium accumulate in the soft tissues of the body, which causes lowered IQs, developmental delays, and behavioral disorders. Mercury is especially prevalent in canned tuna, and arsenic can be found in tap water.

- **Asbestos.** Schools and office buildings constructed in the 1950s and 1960s were insulated with this cancer-causing material. Many asbestos-infested buildings have been carefully torn down, but problems persist with the buildings still standing since the insulation in ceilings and heat ducts can crumble and release asbestos particles into the air.

- **Organochlorine insecticides.** This is a long name for pesticides such as DDT and chlordane. DDT, widely used to kill mosquitoes after World War II, was found to cause thinning of the eggshells belonging to bald eagles, peregrine falcons, and brown pelicans, resulting in deformed or broken eggs. DDT is largely banned in this country, but environmental problems have persisted for decades.

- **Phthalates.** Pronounced THA-lates, these chemicals soften plastics and lengthen the shelf life of cosmetics, hair spray, mousses, and fragrances.

Phthalates harm the developing testes of males and damage the lungs, liver, and kidneys.

- **VOCs.** Volatile organic compounds, as well as semivolatile organic chemicals, are common petroleum-based chemicals present in many household products such as perfumes, aftershave lotions, toiletries, shampoos, household cleaners, furniture polishes, air fresheners, adhesives, foams, and plastics.

- **Chlorine.** Everyone who has ever swum in a municipal pool knows about chlorine, a chemical compound used as a disinfectant to kill, destroy, or control bacteria and algae. Chlorine is commonly used in municipal water supplies as well, and is found in household cleaners.

The nine volunteers in the Mount Sinai study did not work with chemicals on the job or live downwind from polluting smokestacks when they were scanned for 210 toxic substances. Of the 167 chemicals found in their blood and urine, 76 cause cancer in humans or animals, 94 are toxic to the brain and nervous system, and 79 cause birth defects or abnormal development in children. Scientists refer to this chemical residue as a person's *body burden*.

Although our bodies are designed to eliminate toxins, our immune systems have become overloaded to the point that they're on perpetual *Tilt!* What happens is that our bodies can absorb and excrete water-soluble chemical toxins just fine, but fat-soluble chemicals such as dioxins, phthalates, and chlorine are stored in our fatty tissues, where it takes months or years for these toxins to be eliminated from our systems.

I would love to know what my body burden is, but finding out would be an extremely expensive proposition unless I could participate in a scientific study. So what can we do to stay healthy and protect ourselves from an overloaded body burden? The editors at *Organic Style* magazine offer these excellent tips:

1. *Eat lean meats.* Consuming leaner meats is a good idea since fats in meat act as chemical magnets for toxins in the environment. I recommend consuming grass-fed or pastured beef or bison (as well as other healthy meat)

since these meats are naturally leaner and contain larger concentrations of nutrients and healthy fats.

2. *Stick with organic produce when possible. Organic Style* magazine quoted a study of children who ate only organic produce, and they had one-sixth the level of pesticides in their bodies, compared to those who consumed conventionally grown fruits and vegetables.

3. *Avoid certain types of fish and shellfish to lower your exposure to mercury.* As I've mentioned, canned tuna is a known culprit, and its consumption should be limited to two cans per week (unless you're pregnant, in which case you should restrict consumption to one can or less). Swordfish and king mackerel should be limited in consumption as well. You already know my feelings regarding shellfish, which is an unclean meat to begin with and contains a whole host of toxins.

4. *Use a water filter.* With all the chlorine swirling in today's tap water, a filter is a must. I'll have a lot more to say about water filtration later in this chapter.

5. *Air out your dry-cleaned clothes before bringing them into your house.* Around 80 percent of the dry cleaners in the United States use perchloroethylene, or perc, which does a wonderful job cleaning clothes but is a nasty chemical that has been linked to liver and kidney damage, as well as the Big C. Airing out your dry-cleaned clothes before bringing them indoors will dramatically reduce your exposure to this toxin.

6. *Vacuum often, using a machine with a high-efficiency particulate air (HEPA) filter because contaminants often cling to household dust.* These filters remove 99.97 percent of particles with a diameter greater than 0.3 microns.

7. *Steer clear of carpets and furniture treated with stain repellents, and get rid of chemical-laced household cleaners.* Use only natural cleaning products in your home. Most natural food stores carry them, or you can search online for them.[2]

I'll expand on some of these ideas as we talk about what you can do to reduce toxins in your environment, the fifth key in unlocking your health potential.

A GOOD SOAKING

I bet you take a shower once or twice a day—most people do. As I mentioned earlier, chlorine—when ingested—can be a potent toxin, which is one reason why drinking bottled water has become something of a fad. So we avoid drinking chlorinated water. Did you know that when you stand under a nozzle blast of steaming hot water for ten or fifteen minutes, you've absorbed chlorine through your skin—the equivalent of six to eight glasses of chlorinated water? That's how much chlorine the skin, whose pores are opened up by the beating of hot water, soaks up.

Scientists believe that the skin absorbs around 60 percent of everything applied to it, which is why the nicotine patch has been around for years and TV ads show relieved women—who weren't good at remembering to take their pills—explaining how easy and effective birth control can be with a hormone patch.

"Warm water causes the skin to act like a sponge," according to an article in the *Journal of Orthomolecular Medicine.* "One will absorb more chlorine in a ten-minute shower than by drinking eight glasses of the same water."

These days, municipal water treatment plants routinely treat their water supplies with chlorine, which is a potent bacteria-killing chemical. If you don't believe me, then watch what would happen if a friend forgot to add dechlorinator to his home aquarium. All his pet fish would die—rather quickly, I might add—if they swam in chlorinated water.

For the last two years, we've had a whole-house water filtration system that removes the chlorine and other impurities from the water *before* it enters our household pipes. That means Nicki and I can take showers and baths in chlorine-free water and confidently use it for drinking, for cooking, and for washing dishes and clothes. We didn't install a water softening system that uses salt or *adds* chemicals to the water, however. Instead, we use a carbon-based filtration system that allows us to enjoy filtered water from every tap inside our home.

Home-based water filtering systems are not cheap; they start at a thousand dollars for low-capacity versions and rise rapidly to five thousand dollars and more for larger homes. If money is an issue, then consider installing inexpensive water filters at your kitchen sink or purchasing a countertop water pitcher with a built in carbon-based filter for less than twenty dollars.

You can purify your shower water with an inexpensive carbon-block filter that you install on your showerhead. Another type of shower filter, called a kinetic degradation fluxion (KDF) unit, contains a special high-purity alloy that removes chlorine, heavy metals, and bacteria from the water. Once installed, these shower filters remove the toxic burden for a year until the filter needs to be changed. If you prefer to soak in a hot bath, bath filter balls float in the tub and reportedly remove 90 percent of the chlorine in the water. (For more information on water filtration products, please see the GPRx Resource Guide, page 353.)

Just as you don't want to bathe in chlorinated water, you definitely don't want to drink the stuff. While the addition of chlorine to our drinking water has greatly reduced the risk of waterborne diseases, people can taste the chemical aftertaste in their water, which is why drinking bottled water has become hip and popular.

The bottled water industry, which didn't exist when I was born in the mid-1970s, has matured into a huge $9 billion-a-year business. Today, sales of bottled water make it the number two beverage in the United States, right behind soft drinks. Gary Hemphill, a spokesman for the Beverage Marketing Corp., predicts that bottled water sales will overtake soft drinks in the next ten or fifteen years.[3]

Perrier, the fizzy French water, is credited with kicking off the water boom with its distinctive green bottles. Up until the mid-1970s, I'm told, it was inconceivable that anyone would *pay* for drinking water, but Perrier proved conventional wisdom wrong. Another French firm, Evian, made greater inroads into the U.S. market. By the early 1990s, the major soft drink manufacturers noticed that a new player on the block was cutting into their sales and profits.

So Coke and Pepsi decided, *If you can't beat them, join them.* In the mid-1990s, Coke launched its Dasani brand of bottled water while Pepsi responded with the introduction of Aquafina. With sizable marketing muscle behind them, Dasani and Aquafina have become the best-selling brands in the country, and these days, they rank well ahead of smaller companies like Poland Spring, Arrowhead, Deer Park, Crystal Geyser, and Ozarka. Heavy advertising has promoted an image of pristine alpine streams, fed from melting snowpack high in the mountains, producing water that is purer and healthier than the regular old tap variety.

But there's something you should know about Dasani and Aquafina that may influence your decision the next time you shop for a twenty-four-pack at a warehouse club. Not all brands of bottled water bring the same quality or chemical-free cleanliness to the table. Some critics claim that bottled water may be no safer or healthier than tap water, even though some of these trendy bottled brands sell for up to one thousand times the price of water from the tap. One of these critics, the World Wildlife Fund, commissioned a study on bottled water and found that all too often, bottled water differs from tap water only in the fact that it is distributed in plastic containers rather than delivered through copper pipes.

Dasani and Aquafina are purified water, which is essentially tap water that has gone through filtering processes. Brands such as Poland Spring, Arrowhead, and Deer Park are spring waters, which is water that comes from an underground source flowing naturally to the earth's surface. Voss, a chic water from Norway, hails from an aquifer. Other spring waters are mineral or artesian.

My feelings are that given a choice, you're better off purchasing bottled water from a natural spring source, although filtered tap water (Dasani and Aquafina, for example) is okay. Either source would be *far* better than drinking a soft drink or a heavily sugared tea drink. My favorite bottled water brands are Mountain Valley Spring Water, Trinity Springs Water, and Nariwa Water. All of these bottled waters come from natural springs and contain a high mineral content, making them highly alkaline. (For more information on my favorite bottled waters, see the GPRx Resource Guide, page 340.)

Let me reiterate how important it is to drink plenty of water throughout the day. Dr. Joseph Mercola recommends drinking one quart for every fifty pounds of body weight, so an average-sized adult weighing 150 pounds should drink three quarts (or ninety-six ounces) of water daily. Those weighing more than 200 pounds should drink one full gallon of water daily.[4]

I realize that is a *lot* of water, so let me make it simple: try to sip on water all day long. Keep a bottle of fresh water on your desk, as I do, and reach for a sip every now and then. This is one of the most important health habits you can have. Keep in mind that one reason we have so much toxic buildup—body burden—is that the body's filtration system isn't properly cleansed, and won't be until we drink water . . . and lots of it.

PLASTIC IS EVERYWHERE

There's a famous line from the late sixties film *The Graduate*, which stars Dustin Hoffman and features music from Simon and Garfunkel. Benjamin Braddock (Dustin Hoffman) has just graduated from a prestigious East Coast university and is wondering what to do with his life. A family friend sidles up to him and tells him that his future lies in . . . plastics.

Plastics? This prophetic dialogue occured in a 1967 movie, almost ten years before I was born, but if you look around people's homes and apartments these days, you'll see that plastic reigns in utilitarian ways. Low-cost, lightweight plastic, with its luminescent malleability, is found in everything from Ikea lamps to vinyl upholstery to PVC pipes under the kitchen sink. When it comes to items that store, hold, or cook our food, plastic is just as popular. Food containers, water jugs, baby bottles, and cling wrap are handy, inexpensive, and durable products to have around the home. Bottled water and many other beverages are sold in plastic containers.

But are plastic containers safe? After all, they're made out of petrochemicals, so does drinking water out of plastic bottles or scooping leftovers out of Tupperware expose one to, say, carcinogenic dioxins?

The Internet world has been flooded with e-mail missives warning readers about the dangers of dioxin carcinogens. One begins, "On Channel 2 this morning, they had a Dr. Edward Fujimoto from Castle Hospital on the program. He was talking about dioxins and how bad they are for us. He said that we should not be heating our food in the microwave using plastic containers." Another e-mail "health warning" states that researchers at Johns Hopkins University and Walter Reed Army Medical Center have issued an alert warning people not to freeze plastic water bottles with water in them because this releases dioxins from the plastic.

The Office of Communications and Public Affairs at Johns Hopkins Bloomberg School of Public Health felt compelled to release an interview with Rolf Halden, Ph.D., whose doctoral degree is in researching dioxin contamination in the environment.

When asked whether people should heed the e-mail warning that dioxins can be released by freezing water in plastic bottles, Dr. Halden said, "This is urban legend. Freezing actually works against the release of chemicals."[5]

So it's all right for people to drink out of plastic water bottles?

"First, people should be more concerned about the quality of the water they are drinking rather than the container it's coming from. Having said this, there is another group of chemicals, called phthalates, that are sometimes added to plastics to make them flexible and less brittle. Phthalates are environmental contaminants that can exhibit hormone-like behavior by acting as endocrine disruptors in humans and animals. If you heat up plastics, you could increase the leaching of phthalates from the containers into water and food."

The Johns Hopkins researcher said the safest thing to do would be to use only plastics that are specifically meant for cooking. Heat-resistant glass, like Corning Ware, ceramics, and good old stainless steel are even better. Dioxins are everywhere in the environment, he says. "Each of us already carries a certain body burden of dioxins regardless of how and what we eat. Paracelsus, the famous medieval alchemist, used to put it straight and simple: 'It's the dose that makes the poison.'"

Now, I've chosen not to have a microwave in the house because of my concern that microwaves radiate the food and absolutely alter it. There's an ongoing argument in the scientific community over whether microwave radiation is released in high enough levels to harm humans, but while the government and environmental activists debate on how much radiation you can be exposed to, I've decided that discretion is the better part of valor. Nicki and I have made the personal choice not to have a microwave in the house, nor would I stand in front of one while it was turned on. When we're in a hurry to heat something up, we use our toaster oven or our stove. I'd rather patiently wait for my food to be warmed up than have it irradiated by a microwave.

Discretion is why all of us should—when it's convenient—drink water from glasses instead of plastic bottles, buy condiments in glass containers instead of plastic, and store and cook food in glass, ceramic, or stainless steel. And while we're on the subject of cooking, you should avoid or minimize cooking with pots or pans that have nonstick coating. Nonstick coating gives off toxic chemicals, and when metal utensils are used to remove food from the nonstick surface, flakes of the coating break off and are consumed right along with the food. It's always best to cook with stainless steel cookware.

THE AIR WE BREATHE

Most people think air pollution is an outdoor problem. I can understand why you would think that way, especially if you live in a major city and look out upon a hazy skyline each day, knowing that millions of cars and industrial factories are belching tons of pollutants into the air. While seemingly not much can be done individually to combat smog and dirty air, you can take steps to clean the quality of your *indoor* air, which is swirling with toxic particles hazardous to your health.

Breathing recirculated air-conditioned air is a major culprit, especially in hot areas of the country like Florida, where I live. When it's hot outside, we breathe recirculated air around the clock: we sleep in air-conditioned homes, wake up and drive to work in a car with the air-conditioning cranked up, exit the employee parking lot, and step into a climate-controlled office building or commercial space. Eight or nine hours later, we retrace our steps by driving home in our air-conditioned cars to reach our air-conditioned homes. The American Lung Association estimates that we spend 90 percent of our time indoors, and that sounds right to me.

According to the U.S. Environmental Protection Agency, which reported the results of a five-year study that surveyed six hundred homes in six cities, peak concentrations of twenty toxic compounds were two hundred to five hundred times higher inside homes than outdoors.

Today's well-insulated homes and energy-efficient doors and windows are doing *too* good a job, trapping "used" air filled with harmful particles such as carbon dioxide, nitrogen dioxide, and pet dander. No doubt that airtight homes are one of the contributing factors to skyrocketing numbers of mold-related illnesses and insurance claims in recent years. Those living in mold-infested homes or apartments have been diagnosed with immunologic problems, impaired thyroid and adrenal function, chronic fatigue, and memory impairment. Declining indoor air quality has been linked to the rise of asthma and allergies, especially in children.

I'm not here to push the panic button, because healthy bodies fight off germs and toxins in amazing ways. But the prudent approach to health and wellness would be taking steps to drastically improve the air quality in our homes. Many of these ideas, which don't cost much money, simply involve a little planning and forethought:

1. *Open your doors and windows.* It's easy to get into a rut and forget to crack open a window during the day, but it's important to air out the house periodically, no matter what the temperature is outside. If it's summertime, open your doors and windows in the cool of the day—early in the morning and late in the evening. Let the fresh air flow through until it's too hot inside your home.

If it's freezing outside, wait until later in the morning to air things out. I'm certainly not one to brave the winter cold since temperatures in the sixties cause us to break out the sweaters in Florida. Even though I'm not very experienced with cold weather, I've been told by cold-weather veterans that opening windows for five minutes in frigid temperatures won't kill you. If you're fortunate to live in mild temperatures or a Mediterranean climate like San Diego, then let fresh air come in all day.

No matter how high or low the temperature is outside, I recommend that you sleep with a window cracked open. Even in Florida, where summer evening temperatures stay above 80 degrees, Nicki and I unbolt our windows at night to allow fresh air—albeit warm and humid—into our master bedroom. I've found that sleeping in climate-controlled, airtight cocoons—like hotel rooms that don't allow you to open windows—gives me headaches. I can tell the difference when I sleep with a window open.

During my recovery from illness, one of my health secrets was sleeping many a night in a motor home parked next to the ocean with the windows open. This allowed me to breathe not only fresh air, but fresh ocean air, which is that much better.

2. *Change your air-conditioning and heater filters more often.* You should check and change the filters on your air-conditioning and heating units every month or so. You would be surprised at the gunk that quickly builds up if you go for months between spot checks. All that gray stuff you see was circulating in your air! If you find that you need to wear a radioactive spacesuit with protective ski goggles before you pull off the filter screen so that the crud won't fall on your face, that might be a sign that you should change your air-conditioning filter more often.

Some popular filters can be rinsed to remove the particles, while others involve exchanging paperlike filters. I recommend spending a few dollars more and buying highly efficient filters that trap micron-size particles. Keep in mind that frequent upkeep and cleaning will result in much cleaner air flowing through your home.

3. *Check for mold.* Toxic mold has been discovered in old and new buildings and homes. If you detect a musty, earthy, or urine-scented odor, call a home inspector. Specks of black, brown, orange, pink, or green on walls, grout, or tile should be examined as well. Exposure to mold is a proven and serious health threat. Many high-end homes in Florida have been destroyed or required major remodeling due to black mold contamination.

4. *Purchase a good air purifier.* The Sharper Image glossy-stock catalogs popularized the Ionic Breeze air filters—the quiet, fanless purifiers that run room air through electrically charged plates to capture airborne particles. Sharper Image air filters continue to sell well, despite subpar ratings from *Consumer Reports* magazine. Meanwhile, dozens of air purifier companies are stepping into the market that Sharper Image created.

Air purifiers don't generally absorb gases, such as cigarette odors or perfumes, but they remove tiny airborne particles of dust, soot, pollen, mold, and dander. The most important thing to look for in an air purifier is the correct size for your room. Air purifiers are rated to clean only so much square footage, so if you have an open floor plan, you may need to purchase two or three units.

Nicki and I have set up four Pionair air treatment systems in our home: one in the family room, another in the living room, one in our master bedroom, and one in my home office. The Pionair filters organic odors, microbes, and molds without the use of fans, filters, or plates. I've found the Pionair system to be silent, and the only maintenance has been changing replacement modules once a year. (For more information about Pionair, see the GPRx Resource Guide, page 353.)

5. *Set out houseplants.* Did you know that houseplants can reduce toxins such as certain formaldehyde compounds within a hundred-square-foot radius? According to a study done by the National Aeronautics and Space Administration (NASA), many indoor plants absorb pollutants through their leaves and roots and convert them into breathable air. Within twenty-four hours, some plants can remove up to 87 percent of toxic indoor air.[6]

The general rule of thumb is that one houseplant will clean one hundred square feet of air. Among the indoor plants cultivated today, several show greater abilities to absorb chemicals than others. Houseplants such as the bamboo palm, the spider plant, dracaena, and weeping fig counteract airborne toxins. Other recommended plants include English ivy, ferns, Chinese evergreen, and ficus, but most healthy, mature indoor plants have the ability to absorb some amount of pollutants in the air. Houseplants are a win-win proposition: not only will they help clean up your indoor environment, but there's nothing more lovely and cheery than a room filled with beautiful green plants.

Please note that I'm talking about real plants, not imitation plants. Fake plants actually create more toxins in your environment instead of removing them. Houseplants can be great for your health and can provide you with the jungle motif that is so desirable these days.

6. *Consider buying a digital carbon monoxide detector.* If your home burns wood, kerosene, coal, charcoal, or propane or natural gas, consider purchasing a carbon monoxide detector, which can be easily found for less than fifty dollars. Carbon monoxide is a colorless and odorless gas. Because you can't see it, taste it,

or smell it, high concentrations of carbon monoxide can affect you before you even know it's there. Carbon monoxide is harmful because it depletes the ability of the blood to carry oxygen.

Another home-testing device to consider is one for radon, another colorless, odorless gas that can be carcinogenic. Home testing kits for carbon monoxide or radon can be purchased at home centers and hardware stores.

7. *Turn the furnace down when you have a fire going in the fireplace or stove.* The only time we use our fireplace in Florida is Christmas Day, when we crank up the air-conditioning full-blast so that it can get cool enough in the house to light a fire. Okay, so I'm pulling your leg, but I've been told that if you have a fire going in the home, you can probably lower the thermostat setting to 55 degrees or so and still be comfortable. Close all doors entering the room where the fireplace or stove is located, and allow the natural heat to permeate your living space. Be sure to crack open a window since fireplaces need oxygen. If the fireplace has an outside supply of air, opening a window is not needed.

8. *Store chemicals in a well-ventilated garage.* Cleaning products, wood and silver polishes, cans of paint, and liquid solvents don't belong inside the house. Store them in the garage or, preferably, in a backyard storage shed.

Go Natural with Housecleaning

Common household cleaners are amalgamations of potentially harmful chemicals and solvents, which we became particularly alert to when our son began crawling on our tile and hardwood floors and sliding his hands and knees along the surface. Given what we know about hitchhiking germs and toxins, there was some thought on our part that it would be safer for Joshua if we cleaned the floors—and the rest of the house—with natural cleaners. Our desire was to provide a clean, fresh-smelling home without exposing our son or ourselves to toxic materials. The Environmental Protection Agency (EPA) says that household cleansers and disinfectants, along with moth repellents and air fresheners, expose people to VOCs—volatile organic compounds—that can cause eye, nose, and throat irritation, as well as headaches and nausea.

We found that natural ingredients like vinegar, lemon juice, and baking soda, as well as commercially available natural cleansers, are excellent substances that make our home spick-and-span. Mr. Clean would turn green with envy if he saw how a solution of one cup vinegar and a pail of water would clean the bathtub, toilet, sink, countertops, appliances, stovetops, and floors in a jiffy. A vinegar-and-water solution is safe, way cheaper than the store-bought stuff, and doesn't leave a smelly residue. Adding a half-cup of vinegar to the rinse cycle in the washing machine will help clothes get rid of detergent traces. But don't clean marble countertops with vinegar and water because of vinegar's acidic properties.

Lemon juice will give a nice shine to brass and copper, and when mixed with olive oil, it works as a fine furniture polish. When you're finished with the lemon rinds, toss them into the garbage disposal. That'll freshen things up in the kitchen.

Baking soda works as a great cleanser in the bathroom. Just wet a sponge, sprinkle baking soda on it, and scrub toilets, sinks, and showers to your heart's content. A box of baking soda placed in refrigerators and freezers deodorizes unpleasant odors.

Too many over-the-counter cleaning products are harsh, abrasive, and potentially dangerous to the health of your family. By considering natural cleaning products, you'll dramatically lower the toxins inside your home. Some of the recommended alternatives available for purchase are AFM Safety Clean, Bon Ami Cleaning Powder, Brite, EarthRite All Surface Floor Cleaner, and Livos Avi-Soap Concentrate. (For more recommended cleaning products, see the GPRx Resource Guide, pages 352–353.)

NO GLOSSING OVER LIPSTICK

I have a simple rule that may surprise you: I will not put anything on my skin that I would not eat. Every time I make this statement before a live audience, I wonder if somebody will run home and spread moisturizing cream on his whole wheat sprouted bread and take a big bite. Actually, I'm not advising you to eat what you are currently using on your skin. I'm referring to using products that are much healthier for your skin, which, as I mentioned earlier, is very absorbent.

For those of you who are thinking I'm nuts right about now, here's an experiment you can try at home. Take a garlic clove and crush it. Then rub the crushed garlic on the soles of your feet. Within about twenty minutes, you may be running to the bathroom to brush your teeth because you'll smell garlic on your breath.

I've never met anyone who *intentionally* rubs crushed garlic on his skin, but I know plenty of women who run a tube of lipstick across their lips multiple times every single day. Many people are not aware of the toxic chemicals in their everyday cosmetics and toiletries. Products such as lipstick, lip gloss, lip conditioner, hair coloring, hair spray, shampoo, and soap routinely contain chemical solvents and phthalates, although you could never tell from reading the labels. Phthalates are chemicals with many industrial uses, including being used to preserve cosmetics and fragrances. Emerging scientific evidence is raising serious concerns, as certain phthalates have been shown to cause a wide range of adverse effects in laboratory animals, including reproductive and developmental harm, organ damage, endocrine disruption, and cancer. Representatives of the phthalate producers counter that human exposure levels are far below minimum safety levels set by U.S. regulatory agencies.

Our goal should be to minimize our exposure to potentially harmful toxins in our environment whenever and wherever we can. Natural cosmetics without phthalates can be found in progressive groceries and natural food stores, but they are becoming much more widely available in drugstores, supermarkets, and beauty stores in malls. I realize that sometimes you can't purchase cosmetics or other beauty aids that are totally healthy, but you can improve here and there. Nicki has integrated several healthy skin care products, such as toner and cleanser, but much to my chagrin, she still uses her favorite hair color, hair spray, and nail polish remover that are full of the usual toxic suspects. (I'm hoping that this chapter will convince her to try healthier alternatives.)

I think the group most affected by these chemicals is children. The other day I picked up a bottle of children's shampoo, and when I read the ingredient list, I didn't recognize a single one. This brings me to a label-reading hint: when buying food or skin or body care products, you should avoid those containing ingredients with really long names and lots of letters and numbers in them.

I've been sensitive in this area ever since I picked up a tube of a popular brand of toothpaste and noticed a warning in fine print: "If you accidentally swallow more than used for brushing, seek professional assistance or contact a Poison Control Center immediately."

What is that supposed to mean—*if you accidentally swallow more than used for brushing?* Does that mean eating toothpaste is dangerous enough to call the Poison Control Center? That's what the warning says.

And by the way, red, white, and blue stripes in your toothpaste are not made from fresh strawberries, coconut, and blueberries. Most commercially available toothpastes contain artificial sweeteners, potassium nitrate, sodium monofluorophosphate, and trace amounts of fluoride ion. Do these ingredients comprise a safe toothpaste for Joshua once his baby teeth fill in?

I don't think so, which is why we need to be very careful with our environment because the levels of the toxins that we're exposed to can make or break our health, especially where children are concerned. I have created a list of healthy environmental products, which are listed in the GPRx Resource Guide, pages 351–355.

In closing, let me be very clear that you most likely will not get sick immediately from drinking chlorinated water, breathing in recirculated air, using commercial household cleaners, rubbing chemical-laden shampoo in your hair, or even brushing your teeth with artificially flavored toothpaste, but the consistent use of these products can erode good health. By the time you notice symptoms, the damage may have already been done.

For Further Study

For additional study on God's plan for reducing toxins in your environment, visit www.BiblicalHealthInstitute.com for a free introductory course called "Reducing Toxins 101."

WATERING DOWN TOXINS IN OUR ENVIRONMENT
by Mike Donaldson

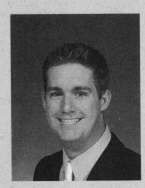

One of the best things I've done for my health in recent years was to rid my home of the dangerous toxins and chemicals that could keep me from maximizing my utmost health potential. Among the first changes I made was installing water filters in my shower and sink. I've seen an array of health benefits, including weight loss, increased energy, and drastically improved skin conditions. If this sounds too good to be true, let me explain.

City water contains chlorine, which affects the digestive system, immune system, and skin in adverse ways. Most people do not realize how much chlorine is actually in their water. Well, what if I told you that in most homes across the United States, the level of chlorine in the water would be considered unsafe to swim in? This would be a simple point to prove. Just purchase a common pool test kit from any hardware store for less than five dollars and test away.

You will find that the levels of chlorine in a large majority of homes are nearly double or more than the safe limit for a swimming pool. I know that if the chlorine tested high in my local pool, the lifeguard would blow his whistle, kick everyone out, make them shower, and adjust the chlorine level. Now don't get me wrong, we need chlorine in our water; otherwise our water would be about as safe as the water in a third-world country. What we need to do, however, is to remove the chlorine and other toxins before ingesting it or showering in it.

One negative effect of chlorine is that it kills digestive enzymes. This inhibits proper digestion, which can prevent one from maintaining optimal health or gaining or losing weight as needed. Since chlorine is a toxin, the body treats it as a hostile foreign invader. The defense mechanism responsible for reacting to these toxins is our immune system or, more specifically, our lymph nodes. When chlorine is introduced into our bodies, whether orally or topically, it filters into the bloodstream and into the lymph nodes.

A heavy burden is placed on our lymph nodes to filter these chemicals, which can cause chronic fatigue and a weakened immune system. If the immune system is busy filtering out chemicals that it was never meant to, then it can't be as efficient dispelling other disease-causing germs and viruses. This principle is the same for personal care products. There is no telling how great the wear and tear is on our bodies after a lifetime of using deodorants, shampoos, makeup, and other products containing these toxic chemicals.

Most people can't pronounce the ingredients in their favorite personal care products, much less know why they are in there, but most soap and shampoo products contain a chemical that helps them lather up more. These products need this chemical because chlorine in water prevents soap products from lathering up. We noticed that adding a shower filter made our soap and shampoo last a lot longer.

Our family noticed drastic differences in our health within two weeks of adding water filters in our home. For myself, I had more energy, less acne, and fewer allergies. My wife's psoriasis and my daughter's eczema cleared up almost overnight. Once we changed our lifestyle, we made sure that we let others know about it. We have seen many friends and family members experience the same benefits after removing the toxins in their environments.

Not everyone responds to our message, however. It saddens me that parents of children with skin problems like eczema can continue to fill prescriptions for drugs for their children's condition when all they may need to do is to filter their water and purchase natural soaps and skin care products.

Please know that it's impossible to remove all the toxins in our environment. Although we live in a fast-paced world that depends on many things harmful to our health, we can—and should—take steps to protect our loved ones and ourselves.

Our health and lives may depend on it.

 THE GREAT PHYSICIAN'S Rx FOR REDUCING TOXINS IN YOUR ENVIRONMENT

- *Consume organically produced food as much as possible.*

- *Improve indoor air quality by opening windows, changing air filters regularly, setting out houseplants, and buying an air filtration system.*

- *Drink only purified water.*

- *Shower in purified water.*

- *Use natural products for skin care, body care, hair care, cosmetics, and toothpaste.*

- *Don't heat food in plastic.*

- *Don't cook with nonstick cookware.*

- *Use natural cleaning products for your home, washing machine, and dishwasher.*

THE GREAT PHYSICIAN'S Rx FOR WEEK #5

Day 29

Upon Waking

Advanced hygiene: practice advanced hygiene. See page 325 for guidance.

Reduce toxins: open windows for one hour today. Make a plan to change air-conditioning or heating filters more regularly.

Supplements: take one serving of a fiber/green superfood powder (mixed in) or five caplets of a super green formula (swallowed with) twelve-to-sixteen ounces of water or raw vegetable juice. (See the GPRx Resource Guide, pages 346–347, for recommended products.)

Body therapy: take a hot and cold shower. After normal shower, alternate sixty seconds of water as hot as you can stand it, followed by sixty seconds of water as cold as you can stand it. Repeat cycle four times for a total of eight minutes, finishing with cold.

Exercise: perform functional fitness exercises for fifteen minutes (three rounds of exercises found in Key #4, pages 138–145) or spend fifteen minutes on the rebounder. Finish with ten minutes of deep-breathing exercises.

Breakfast

Berry Smoothie (see appendix A, page 304, for recipe) with two tablespoons of protein powder (optional)

hot tea with honey (see the GPRx Resource Guide, page 339, for recommended herbal tea blends)

Supplements: take one or two whole food multivitamin caplets and one or two capsules of a probiotic/enzyme blend (see the GPRx Resource Guide, pages 345–348, for recommended products).

Lunch

Before eating, drink eight ounces of water.

During lunch, drink eight ounces of water or hot or iced fresh-brewed tea with honey.

tuna salad on a bed of greens or on sprouted whole grain or sourdough bread

apple or pear

Supplements: take one or two whole food multivitamin caplets and one or two capsules of a probiotic/enzyme blend.

Dinner
Before eating, drink eight ounces of water.
During dinner, drink hot or iced fresh-brewed tea with honey.
Cajun Sauté Bowl (see appendix A, page 286, for recipe)
Curried Quinoa (see appendix A, page 287, for recipe)
green salad
Supplements: take one or two whole food multivitamin caplets, one-to-three teaspoons or three-to-nine capsules of high omega-3 cod-liver oil (see the GPRx Resource Guide, pages 345–346, for recommended products), and one or two capsules of probiotic/enzyme blend.

Snacks
raspberry super green whole food bar (see the GPRx Resource Guide, pages 329–330, for recommended products)
Drink eight-to-twelve-ounces of water or hot or iced fresh-brewed tea with honey.

Before Bed
Drink eight-to-twelve ounces of water or hot tea with honey.
Exercise: go for a walk outdoors or participate in a favorite sport or recreational activity.
Supplements: take one serving of a fiber/green superfood powder (mixed in) or five caplets of a super green formula (swallowed with) twelve-to-sixteen ounces of water or raw vegetable juice.
Advanced hygiene: practice advanced hygiene. See page 325 for guidance.
Body therapy: spend ten minutes listening to soothing music before you retire.
Sleep: go to bed by 10:30 p.m.

Day 30
Upon Waking
Advanced hygiene: practice advanced hygiene. See page 325 for guidance.
Reduce toxins: open windows for one hour today. Purchase three houseplants and place them in your living room and dining area.
Supplements: take one serving of a fiber/green superfood powder (mixed in) or five caplets of a super green formula (swallowed with) twelve-to-sixteen ounces of water or raw vegetable juice. (See the GPRx Resource Guide, pages 346–347, for recommended products.)
Body therapy: get twenty minutes of direct sunlight.
Exercise: perform functional fitness exercises for fifteen minutes (three rounds of exercises found in Key #4, pages 138–145), or spend fifteen minutes on the rebounder. Finish with ten minutes of deep-breathing exercises.

Breakfast
Easy Scrambled Eggs (see appendix A, page 317, for recipe)
bowl of strawberries

hot tea with honey

Supplements: take one or two whole food multivitamin caplets and one or two capsules of a probiotic/enzyme blend.

Lunch

Before eating, drink eight ounces of water.

During lunch, drink eight ounces of water or hot or iced fresh-brewed tea with honey.

Easy Lamb Stew (see appendix A, page 318, for recipe)

crackers (whole grain or flaxseed)

Supplements: take one or two whole food multivitamin caplets and one or two capsules of a probiotic/enzyme blend.

Dinner

Before eating, drink eight ounces of water.

During dinner, drink hot or iced fresh-brewed tea with honey.

Cilantro-Lime Halibut (see appendix A, page 302, for recipe)

sautéed asparagus and mushrooms

couscous

Supplements: take one or two whole food multivitamin caplets, one-to-three teaspoons or three-to-nine capsules of high omega-3 cod-live oil, and one or two capsules of a probiotic/enzyme blend.

Snacks

Cranberry Apple Crunch (see appendix A, page 317, for recipe)

Mango Berry Smoothie mix mixed in eight-to-twelve ounces of water

cottage cheese and pineapple

Drink eight to twelve ounces of water or hot or iced fresh-brewed tea with honey.

Before Bed

Drink eight-to-twelve ounces of water or hot tea with honey.

Exercise: go for a walk outdoors or participate in a favorite sport or recreational activity.

Supplements: take one serving of a fiber/green superfood powder (mixed in) or five caplets of a super green formula (swallowed with) twelve-to-sixteen ounces of water or raw vegetable juice.

Body therapy: take a warm bath for fifteen minutes with eight drops of biblical essential oils added.

Advanced hygiene: practice advanced hygiene. See page 325 for guidance.

Sleep: go to bed by 10:30 p.m.

Day 31

Upon Waking

Advanced hygiene: practice advanced hygiene. See page 325 for guidance.

Reduce toxins: open windows for one hour today. Purchase and install carbon-block shower filters for each shower in your home (if you're on city water). (See the GPRx Resource Guide, page 353, for recommended products.)

Supplements: take one serving of a fiber/green superfood powder (mixed in) or five caplets of a super green formula (swallowed with) twelve-to-sixteen ounces of water or raw vegetable juice. (See the GPRx Resource Guide, pages 346–347, for recommended products.)

Body therapy: take a hot and cold shower. After normal shower, alternate sixty seconds of water as hot as you can stand it, followed by sixty seconds of water as cold as you can stand it. Repeat cycle four times for a total of eight minutes, finishing with cold.

Exercise: perform functional fitness exercises for fifteen minutes (three rounds of exercises found in Key #4, pages 138–145) or spend fifteen minutes on the rebounder. Finish with ten minutes of deep-breathing exercises.

Breakfast

sprouted dry cereal with yogurt, goat's milk, or almond milk
banana
hot tea with honey
Supplements: take one or two whole food multivitamin caplets and one or two capsules of a probiotic/enzyme blend.

Lunch

Before eating, drink eight ounces of water.
During lunch, drink eight ounces of water or hot or iced fresh-brewed tea with honey.
Salmon and Mixed Greens (see appendix A, page 276, for recipe)
apple
Supplements: take one or two whole food multivitamin caplets and one or two capsules of a probiotic/enzyme blend.

Dinner

Before eating, drink eight ounces of water.
During dinner, drink hot or iced fresh-brewed tea with honey.
Nicki's Meatloaf (see appendix A, page 318, for recipe)
Smashed Potatoes with Shiitake Gravy (see appendix A, page 287, for recipe)
peas and carrots
Supplements: take one or two whole food multivitamin caplets, one-to-three teaspoons or three-to-nine capsules of high omega-3 cod-liver oil, and one or two capsules of a probiotic/enzyme blend.

Snacks

Blueberry Cobbler (see appendix A, page 319, for recipe)
vanilla protein whole food bar (with beta glucans from soluble oat fiber)
Drink eight-to-twelve ounces of water, or hot or iced fresh-brewed tea with honey.

Before Bed

Drink eight-to-twelve ounces of water or hot tea with honey.

Exercise: go for a walk outdoors or participate in a favorite sport or recreational activity.

Supplements: take one serving of a fiber/green superfood powder (mixed in) or five caplets of a super green formula (swallowed with) twelve-to-sixteen ounces of water or raw vegetable juice.

Advanced hygiene: practice advanced hygiene. See page 325 for guidance.

Body therapy: spend ten minutes listening to soothing music before you retire.

Sleep: go to bed by 10:30 p.m.

Day 32

Upon Waking

Advanced hygiene: practice advanced hygiene. See page 325 for guidance.

Reduce toxins: open windows for one hour today. Use natural soap and natural skin and body care products (shower gel, body creams, etc.). (See the GPRx Resource Guide, page 351, for recommended products.)

Supplements: take one serving of a fiber/green superfood powder (mixed in) or five caplets of a super green formula (swallowed with) twelve-to-sixteen ounces of water or raw vegetable juice. (See the GPRx Resource Guide, pages 346–347, for recommended products.)

Body therapy: get twenty minutes of direct sunlight.

Exercise: perform functional fitness exercises for fifteen minutes (three rounds of exercises found in Key #4, pages 138–145) or spend fifteen minutes on the rebounder. Finish with ten minutes of deep-breathing exercises.

Breakfast

Banana Peach Smoothie (see appendix A, page 320, for recipe) with two table-spoons protein powder (optional)

hot tea with honey

Supplements: take one or two whole food multivitamin caplets and one or two capsules of a probiotic/enzyme blend

Lunch

Before eating, drink eight ounces of water.

During lunch, drink eight ounces of water or hot or iced fresh-brewed tea with honey.

Marinated Raw Vegetables with Jack Cheese Wrap (see appendix A, page 289, for recipe)

Supplements: take one or two whole food multivitamin caplets and one or two capsules of a probiotic/enzyme blend.

Dinner

Before eating, drink eight ounces of water.

During dinner, drink hot or iced fresh-brewed tea with honey.

Herb Stir-Fried Chicken and Mixed Veggies (see appendix A, page 292, for recipe)

Sweet Potato Pie (see appendix A, page 319, for recipe)

Supplements: take one or two whole food multivitamin caplets, one-to-three teaspoons or three-to-nine capsules of high omega-3 cod-liver oil, and one or two capsules of a probiotic/enzyme blend.

Snacks

apple and carrots with almond butter

antioxidant fruit whole food bar (with beta glucans from soluble oat fiber)

Drink eight-to-twelve ounces of water or hot or iced fresh-brewed tea with honey.

Before Bed

Drink eight-to-twelve ounces of water or hot tea with honey.

Exercise: go for a walk outdoors or participate in a favorite sport or recreational activity.

Supplements: take one serving of a fiber/green superfood powder (mixed in) or five caplets of a super green formula (swallowed with) twelve-to-sixteen ounces of water or raw vegetable juice.

Body therapy: take a warm bath for fifteen minutes with eight drops of biblical essential oils added.

Advanced hygiene: practice advanced hygiene. See page 325 for guidance.

Sleep: go to bed by 10:30 p.m.

Day 33 (Partial Fast Day)

Upon Waking

Advanced hygiene: practice advanced hygiene. See page 325 for guidance.

Reduce toxins: open windows for one hour today. Use natural soap and natural skin and body care products (shower gel, body creams, etc.). (See the GPRx Resource Guide, page 351, for recommended products.)

Supplements: take one serving of a fiber/green superfood powder (mixed in) or five caplets of a super green formula (swallowed with) twelve-to-sixteen ounces of water or raw vegetable juice. (See the GPRx Resource Guide, pages 346–347, for recommended products.)

Body therapy: take a hot and cold shower. After normal shower, alternate sixty seconds of water as hot as you can stand it, followed by sixty seconds of water as cold as you can stand it. Repeat cycle four times for a total of eight minutes, finishing with cold.

Exercise: perform functional fitness exercises for fifteen minutes (three rounds of exercises are found in Key #4, pages 138–145) or spend fifteen minutes on the rebounder. Finish with ten minutes of deep-breathing exercises.

Breakfast

none (partial fast day)

eight ounces of water

Lunch

none (partial fast day)

eight ounces of water

Dinner

Before eating, drink eight ounces of water.

During dinner, drink hot or iced fresh-brewed tea with honey.

Soy Ginger Salmon (see appendix A, page 281, for recipe)

cultured vegetables

green salad

Supplements: one or two whole food multivitamin caplets, one-to-three teaspoons or three-to-nine capsules of high omega-3 cod-liver oil, and one or two capsules of a probiotic/enzyme blend.

Snacks

none (partial fast day)

eight ounces of water

Before Bed

Drink eight-to-twelve ounces of water or hot tea with honey.

Exercise: go for a walk outdoors or participate in a favorite sport or recreational activity.

Supplements: take one serving of a fiber/green superfood powder (mixed in) or five caplets of a super green formula (swallowed with) twelve-to-sixteen ounces of water or raw vegetable juice.

Advanced hygiene: practice advanced hygiene. See page 325 for guidance.

Body therapy: spend ten minutes listening to soothing music before you retire.

Sleep: go to bed by 10:30 p.m.

Day 34 (Day of Rest)

Upon Waking

Advanced hygiene: practice advanced hygiene. See page 325 for guidance.

Reduce toxins: open windows for one hour today. Use natural soap and natural skin and body care products (shower gel, body creams, etc.). Purchase and use natural toothpaste. (See the GPRx Resource Guide, pages 351–352, for recommended products.)

Supplements: take one serving of a fiber/green superfood powder (mixed in) or five caplets of a super green formula (swallowed with) twelve-to-sixteen ounces of water or raw vegetable juice. (See the GPRx Resource Guide, pages 346–347, for recommended products.)

Exercise: do no formal exercise since it's a day of rest.

Body therapies: do none since it's a rest day.

Breakfast
     Vegetable Frittata (see appendix A, page 274, for recipe)
     grapefruit or orange
     hot tea with honey
     Supplements: take one or two whole food multivitamin caplets and one or two
capsules of a probiotic/enzyme blend.

Lunch
     Before eating, drink eight ounces of water.
     During lunch, drink eight ounces of water or hot or iced fresh-brewed tea with honey.
     All-Day Beef Stew (see appendix A, page 274, for recipe)
     crackers (whole grain or flaxseed)
     carrots
     Supplements: take one or two whole food multivitamin caplets and one or two
capsules of a probiotic/enzyme blend.

Dinner
     Before eating, drink eight ounces of water.
     During dinner, drink hot or iced fresh-brewed tea with honey.
     Ginger Tamari Bowl with Chicken (see appendix A, page 288, for recipe)
     Italian Salad (see appendix A, page 277, for recipe)
     Supplements: Take one or two whole food multivitamin caplets, one-to-three
teaspoons or three-to-nine capsules of high omega-3 cod-liver oil, and one or two
capsules of a probiotic/enzyme blend.

Snacks
     chocolate protein whole food bar (see the GPRx Resource Guide, pages 329–330,
for recommended brands)
     apple
     Drink eight-to-twelve ounces of water or hot or iced fresh-brewed tea with honey.

Before Bed
     Drink eight-to-twelve ounces of water or hot tea with honey.
     Exercise: do no formal exercise since it's a day of rest.
     Body therapies: do none since it's a rest day.
     Supplements: take one serving of a fiber/green superfood powder (mixed in) or five
caplets of a super green formula (swallowed with) twelve-to-sixteen ounces of water or raw
vegetable juice.
     Advanced hygiene: practice advanced hygiene. See page 325 for guidance.
     Sleep: go to bed by 10:30 p.m.

Day 35

Upon Waking

Advanced hygiene: practice advanced hygiene. See page 325 for guidance.

Reduce Toxins: open windows for one hour today. Use natural soap and natural skin and body care products (shower gel, body creams, etc.). Use natural facial care products. Use natural toothpaste. Purchase and use natural hair care products, such as shampoo, conditioner, gel, mousse, and hairspray. (See the GPRx Resource Guide, pages 351–352, for recommended products.)

Supplements: take one serving of a fiber/green superfood powder (mixed in) or five caplets of a super green formula (swallowed with) twelve-to-sixteen ounces of water or raw vegetable juice. (See the GPRx Resource Guide, pages 346–347, for recommended products.)

Body therapy: get twenty minutes of direct sunlight.

Exercise: perform functional fitness exercises for fifteen minutes (three rounds of exercises found in Key #4, pages 138–145) or spend fifteen minutes on the rebounder. Finish with ten minutes of deep-breathing exercises.

Breakfast

hot tea with honey
Easy Soft/Hard-Boiled Eggs (see appendix A, page 320, for recipe)
Five Grain Porridge (see appendix A, page 273, for recipe)
Supplements: take one or two whole food multivitamin caplets and one or two capsules of a probiotic/enzyme blend.

Lunch

Before eating, drink eight ounces of water.
During lunch, drink eight ounces of water or hot or iced fresh-brewed tea with honey.
Salad Nicoise (see appendix A, page 275, for recipe)
Supplements: take one or two whole food multivitamin caplets and one or two capsules of a probiotic/enzyme blend.

Dinner

Before eating, drink eight ounces of water.
During dinner, drink hot or iced fresh-brewed tea with honey.
ground bison patties with grilled onions and mushrooms
Millet Corn Casserole (see appendix A, page 280, for recipe)
green beans
Supplements: one or two whole food multivitamin caplets, one-to-three teaspoons or three-to-nine capsules of high omega-3 cod-liver oil, and one to three capsules of a probiotic/enzyme blend.

Snacks

baked corn chips with cheese, salsa, guacamole, or hummus

apple-cinnamon fiber whole food bar (see the GPRx Resource Guide, pages 329–330, for recommended products)

Drink eight-to-twelve ounces of water or hot or iced fresh-brewed tea with honey.

Before Bed

Drink eight-to-twelve ounces of water or hot tea with honey.

Exercise: go for a walk outdoors or participate in a favorite sport or recreational activity.

Supplements: take one serving of a fiber/green superfood powder (mixed in) or five caplets of a super green formula (swallowed with) twelve-to-sixteen ounces of water or raw vegetable juice.

Body therapy: take a warm bath for fifteen minutes with eight drops of biblical essential oils added.

Advanced hygiene: practice advanced hygiene. See page 325 for guidance.

Sleep: go to bed by 10:30 p.m.

Key #6

Avoid Deadly Emotions

A cheerful heart is good medicine, but a crushed spirit dries up the bones.

—Proverbs 17:22

Interstate 95 is the main north-to-south superhighway along the eastern seaboard, extending 1,907 miles from Houlton, Maine, to its terminus in Miami.

Florida has more miles of I-95 pavement than any other state, and at certain times of the year, we have more drivers over the age of sixty than any stretch of four-lane highway in the United States. Between Thanksgiving and New Year's Day, traffic on I-95 becomes a virtual parking lot as the retiree crowd— "snowbirds," we call them—arrive from points north in their Caddies and RVs.

When gridlock slows traffic to a crawl, I admit to becoming impatient and wishing I were somewhere else. Some of my Floridian brethren pound their dashboards in frustration and send the snowbirds one-finger salutes, causing heads to bob while verbal brickbats are tossed back and forth between the drivers. Tempers flare but usually fail to crest the boiling point, although I've seen the confrontations escalate to classic cases of road rage on occasion.

The shaking of clenched fists and swerving in and out of traffic lanes rev up the body's production of a hormone called cortisol, which puts the drivers' bodies on high alert. Blood vessels constrict and divert the flow of blood from leisurely processes like digestion to quick-acting muscles in the arms and legs, where an energy burst could be needed. The heart races to keep up with the frenzied motion, and the hyper-alertness causes all sorts of anxiety.

These angry drivers fail to realize that even if they ate healthy, took all the right supplements, practiced advanced hygiene, exercised faithfully, and removed every toxin from their environment, none of those healthy practices would matter if they were too riled up or stressed out behind the wheel. Instead of motoring down the highway on all cylinders, they are careening down a blind alley named Sickness. When frustrated people harbor resentment and unforgiveness, nurse grudges, or seek revenge, their overstimulated bodies produce the same toxins as they would have if they binged on the worst junk food.

Anger, acrimony, apprehension, agitation, anxiety, and alarm are deadly emotions, and when you experience any of these feelings—whether justified or not—the efficiency of your immune system decreases noticeably for six hours. (This is the same amount of time your immune system shuts down when you eat large amounts of sugar.) So if you're one of those people on your way to work while motoring down I-95, minding your business while biting into a Krispy Kreme, only to become unglued by fifty-mile-per-hour senior citizens clogging up the road, your immune system could be shot for the whole day. Welcome to the Angry Doughnut Crowd!

Flying off the handle piles stress on the immune system like a bricklayer adding another row of bricks to a wall. Unless your attitude changes, you will become an unhealthy individual overnight. Stress is demonstrably a key source for a variety of ills: hypertension, elevated heartbeat, headaches, and hormonal imbalances in the body. Anger and hostility rev up blood pressure and cortisol levels, a precursor to heart disease. Guilt follows people around like an iron ball chained to their leg. Fear has a remarkable way of generating evidence to support itself. Tension caused by work-related or family-related stress compounds physical problems. What's becoming more and more apparent to researchers is that emotions are powerful forces within the human mind that clearly affect the body and the soul.

My friend, Don Colbert, M.D., author of the fine book *Deadly Emotions*, says that an emotional roller coaster saps a person of both physical and psychological health, which often leaves body and mind depleted of energy and strength. Dr. Colbert points out that medical studies dealing with unhealthy emotions show that:

- the mind and the body are linked, which means how you feel emotionally can determine how you feel physically;
- certain emotions release hormones into the body that can trigger the development of a host of diseases;
- researchers have directly and scientifically linked deadly emotions to hypertension, cardiovascular disease, and diseases related to the immune system;
- those fighting depression have an increased risk of developing cancer and heart disease; and
- emotions such as anxiety and fear have been linked to heart palpitations, irritable bowel syndrome, tension headaches, and other diseases.

Deadly emotions alter the chemistry of your body, and unchecked emotions can be a pervasive force in determining your daily behavior. Eating while under stress causes the liver's bile tubes to narrow, which blocks bile from reaching the small intestine, where food is waiting to be digested. This is not healthy for the body. An old proverb states it well: "What you are eating is not nearly as important as what's eating you."

That's wise advice, but it's been my experience that when stress overwhelms people's lives, they tend to fall off the healthy food wagon. When life overwhelms them like a tidal wave, they revert to old habits: nibbling on sweets or oily chips, raiding the refrigerator, or ordering in. They hunt down extremely pleasurable foods filled with fat and sugar—Belgian chocolates or Ben & Jerry's Cherry Garcia Ice Cream—to dampen stress and ameliorate symptoms of depression. They eat all the wrong foods to take their minds off their troubles.

Dr. Nick Yphantides, the San Diego family physician who weighed 467 pounds (introduced in Key #1), said that when he was at his heaviest, a thunderbolt of terrible news turned over his applecart. It happened at the age of thirty when his declining health prompted him to submit to a battery of tests. A statement from the urologist stunned him: "Nick, I'm afraid you have testicular cancer."

Dr. Nick maintained his composure inside the doctor's office, but on the drive home, he sobbed like a child who had lost his mother. His extended kin—Nick grew up in a big, fat Greek family—greeted him at his parents' home. Few could look him in the eye, and the mood inside the living room was as somber as a funeral.

After an hour of hugs, tears, and taking phone calls, Nick couldn't stand the stress any longer. Saying he needed some fresh air, he left the house and went for a drive—to visit the Colonel.

Colonel Sanders, the courtly southern gentleman with a white suit and black string tie who founded Kentucky Fried Chicken, was waiting for him with open arms. He welcomed Nick inside and offered him a five-piece, extra-crispy chicken dinner with all the trimmings—mashed potatoes, gravy, corn on the cob, and two biscuits. Eating the double-breaded fried chicken with eleven secret herbs and spices, Nick said, provided a heaping helping of emotional comfort when he needed it most. Dr. Nick found solace in a box of fried chicken and assorted sides at a time when he was forced to face his mortality head-on.

Many of us turn to comfort food—deep-fried catfish, chicken potpie, country-fried steak, and macaroni and cheese—when life is at its most stressful. We have no trouble justifying our actions: we feel intense pressure at work or at home, our interpersonal relationships are marked by bitter acrimony, the car has broken down for the second time in a month, or the family has experienced one financial reversal after another.

Turning to a diet of comfort food, junk food, or gooey desserts is going backward, not forward, on the road to becoming healthy. Instead of these rich foods taking your mind off your troubles, they only compound them, which creates more emotional distress.

STRESS TEST

A superb explanation of stress is found in the book *Margin: Restoring Emotional, Physical, Financial and Time Reserves to Overloaded Lives,* written in the early 1990s by Richard Swenson, M.D. Traveling through a stressful life without margin, says Dr. Swenson, is like being thirty minutes late for your son's basketball game because you were twenty minutes late getting out of a meeting because you were ten minutes late getting back from lunch.[1]

I can certainly relate. I'm a very busy, very driven person, and when things go wrong at work, I get stressed to the point that I feel like I've been hit with a solid punch below the belt. On rare occasions, when worry and anxiety really set in, I get the chills. A recent example occurred when I got word that a local TV station planned to run a negative story on my book, *The Maker's Diet*. The thought that people who didn't know me or my heart would criticize me left me feeling very upset.

When the story aired, I couldn't bear to watch because my stomach was tied up in knots. After the story ran, however, a friend who'd watched the piece told me that it wasn't nearly as bad as either of us expected.

Later, after I had time to reflect, I was reminded of three lessons that day:

1. When God calls you to your life's work and you boldly proclaim His name in areas of darkness, you will experience great opposition.
2. Anxiety, worry, and fear are not only detrimental to your health, but nine times out of ten, the very things you were anxious, nervous, or fearful about don't turn out to be as bad as you thought they'd be.
3. We are commanded to forgive those who hurt us, and with God's help, we can forgive.

While I've been better at reminding myself not to stress out since God gave me my health back, it's been tough letting things go. Dr. Swenson says that we can reduce stress in our lives by adding margin around the edges, much like there is a margin around the type found on the pages of this book. If my publisher, Thomas Nelson, completely covered this page with lines of type from top to bottom, you'd find reading *The Great Physician's Rx for Health and Wellness* aesthetically displeasing, hard to comprehend, and somewhat unruly.

Adding margin, therefore, is a cushion one builds in beyond what is necessary to face life's routines. Margin is the space that exists between us and our limits. When flying from West Palm Beach to Tulsa, Oklahoma, I wouldn't want Delta to schedule only five minutes to change planes in Atlanta, the world's busiest airport. A much greater margin of error is needed.

In the same way, a lack of margin leads to unhealthy stress, and distressed folks cannot be fully effective or fully healthy. Adding margin, however, means erecting a hedge of protection to our lives: scheduling more time to complete tasks (instead of trying to complete so many chores in a short time) and carving out more time with those we love the most (instead of giving them our leftovers).

Listen, I know this is easier said than done. Stuff happens, and "life is just one darn thing after another," as Mark Twain once said. My share of personal health setbacks, business crises, adjustments to married life, and starting a family have thrown me for a loop. In fact, as every first-time father knows, the challenges of taking care of a newborn can be overwhelming. I haven't forgotten the time when Joshua was two months old, and Nicki left me to care for him while she ran some errands. She was breast-feeding at the time, and for some reason, she did not leave me with a bottle. As soon as the garage door went down and she pulled out of the driveway, Joshua began to wail, and there wasn't a thing I could do to get him to stop crying. Every minute of Joshua's full-throated crying seemed like an hour.

When I tried Nicki's cell phone, it was turned off. Of course. When I attempted to reach my mother for some advice on what to do, she wasn't home. As my newborn son screamed and screamed, my heart pounded, and it was more than I could bear. All I could do was pray. Five or ten minutes later, Joshua stopped crying, and eventually Nicki came home, and everything returned to normal again. These days, Nicki recounts this story with a chuckle, telling our friends that I am the father who can't watch his son for five minutes without panicking.

Hey, even the smallest challenge can bring intense stress and pressure. When life seems to be crashing down on my shoulders, I try to remember that God is in control, and I look to Him as the source of peace and contentment. Jesus declared, ". . . don't worry about everyday life . . . Look at the birds. They don't need to plant or harvest or put food in barns because your heavenly Father feeds them. And you are far more valuable to him than they are. Can all your worries add a single moment to your life? Of course not." (Matt. 6:25a, 26–27 NLT).

All too often, things I worry about that *could* happen wind up not happening anyway, as was the case with that TV story about *The Maker's Diet.* Yet I always seem to be running from one crisis to another. The same week I was attempting to finish this book, I was scheduled to speak at a student chapel on the Oral Roberts University campus, followed by a speaking engagement at Lindsay Roberts's women's conference, followed by giving several talks during a weeklong Caribbean cruise with Charles Stanley's In Touch ministries.

The night before I took off for Tulsa, Oklahoma, my cell phone died, and my computer crashed, leaving me without a vital Internet connection for research and interacting with my editor. Knowing that my manuscript was due in ten days, I was understandably uptight and feared the worst. At nine o'clock that night, I knew that I couldn't get my Blackberry cell phone/palm-sized computer or my laptop computer fixed before my departure. I fumed as the stress mounted, and then I snapped at Nicki, which I immediately regretted.

To my surprise, I was able to get a computer tech to make a house call, and within an hour, my Blackberry and computer were running again. As everything was turning back to normal, I asked God and Nicki for forgiveness, knowing that what should have been a manageable situation had become a bad time for me and those around me. Everything could have been avoided if I had just trusted God and not acted anxiously about anything.

A great passage of Scripture that I repeat to myself during stressful situations has been Philippians 4:6–7 (NKJV): "Be anxious for nothing, but in everything by prayer and supplication, with thanksgiving, let your requests be made known to God; and the peace of God, which surpasses all understanding, will guard your hearts and minds through Christ Jesus."

Repeating those verses has been a stress reducer for me, and another short verse from God's Word calms roiling waters: "My yoke is easy and My burden is light" (Matt. 11:30 NKJV).

AN UNFORGIVING HEART

There's another emotion that God calls a sin and causes great bodily harm and shortens one's life span—an unforgiving heart. Going through life without forgiving people who have hurt you is like running the marathon with a fifty-pound weighted vest. I believe that an underlying factor in some chronic, incurable illnesses is unforgiveness. The irony is that I've met people who've told me how angry they were about someone or some situation, but when I asked them to describe what happened, they had a hard time articulating what they were so angry about. By allowing their antagonism to fester, however, their unforgiving hearts turned hard with bitterness, which is why they were bothered so much by the situation.

I learned a lot about the importance of forgiving others during a breakfast meeting with Bruce Wilkinson, author of *The Prayer of Jabez*. During the course of our conversation, he asserted that people who harbor unforgiveness in their hearts develop all sorts of problems that keep them from reaching their full potential. I nodded my head in agreement. Then Dr. Wilkinson asked me a bold question: "Jordan, is there anyone in your life you need to forgive?"

"No, I'm a pretty easygoing person," I blurted, probably a bit too glibly. "I don't hold any grudges."

Dr. Wilkinson leaned back in his chair with a knowing look on his face. "I don't believe you," he said, placing his arms behind his head.

"Really, I don't," I insisted. "I'm fine."

Dr. Wilkinson let that thought hang in the air, which gave me time to reflect on what he said. The more I thought about it . . . "Yes, there have been some people who have hurt me," I confided, "but I've moved on. I've forgiven them."

"I don't believe you," Dr. Wilkinson declared.

Maybe he was right . . . there was that person who . . . and that other guy . . . "Okay, there are a couple of people. But I forgive them."

"It's not that simple," Dr. Wilkinson asserted.

"Then how do I forgive somebody?"

"Here is a practical way I teach people how to forgive," said the founder of Walk Thru the Bible ministries. "A great way to forgive somebody is to take a white sheet of paper and write down the name of the person you need to forgive at the top. Ask the Lord to show you grievances that person has caused you, and then write down the things that person did to cause you pain. I can tell you from experience that once you start remembering those things, your emotions will rise to the surface, but that's okay. That's just a sign that you haven't forgiven them yet."

"What do I do after I've written these names down and what they did against me?" I wondered.

"Once your list is complete, you need to look at each person's name and say, 'I forgive you for . . . ,' and say out loud what they did to hurt you. Then ask God to cleanse you of your past unforgiveness. By the time you've reached this step, you'll be heading down the road to recovery. After you've completed your list, you should cut up the paper or burn it."

Later, when I had a private moment, I contemplated whom I should start with. Without revealing too much personal detail, I wrote down the names of a couple of doctors who told me that my illness was my fault. I moved on to the names of relatives and friends who said they would be there for me when I got sick, but I never heard from them again. Then there were names of mean people who had been especially critical of my first two books, *Patient, Heal Thyself* and *The Maker's Diet*. Some roasted me in flaming posts on the Internet.

Bruce Wilkinson was right: there were more people than I would have thought. After I dealt with each person, I bowed my head and asked God to help me forgive these people just as He forgives me for my sins. I prayed with a contrite heart, seeking His mercy and forgiveness. When I was finished, I ripped the paper into pieces and tossed them into the wastebasket of history.

I shared this forgiveness message at a conference recently, and a young woman contacted me afterward to say, "Jordan, I did the forgiveness thing that you talked about, and it was awesome. I took out a sheet of paper and wrote down all of the areas I had to forgive this person for. Doing this was tough and emotional, but I felt like a huge weight was lifted off my shoulders when I was done. Then I folded the piece of paper up, stuck it in an envelope, and mailed it to the person who hurt me."

"Mailed it to the person who hurt you? That's not forgiveness," I told her. "That's revenge."

Psychologist Robert Enright of the University of Wisconsin is a proponent of *therapeutic forgiveness,* which teaches injured parties to forgive their offenders. He points to studies showing that forgiving others reduces stress-producing anger and improves mental, emotional, and physical health.

Fred Luskin, Ph.D., works with the Stanford University Forgiveness Project—further proof that the benefit of forgiveness is attracting scientific inquiry—and he points to two primary reasons that forgiveness is important:

1. *Forgiveness reduces chronic stress.* Dr. Luskin says that chronic stress triggers negative physical changes that increase blood pressure and heart rate and decrease immune function, all harbingers of disease.

2. *Forgiveness increases one's sense of control.* By forgiving someone, you feel in control. You're less likely to panic, and you develop emotional confidence to get through any difficulty. Feeling helpless, on the other hand, leads to illness.

Experts such as Dr. Luskin note that the first step to forgiving someone else involves taking responsibility for how you feel. Rather than rehashing your grievances—which is like falling down a rabbit hole—focus on what you're grateful for and those you love as well as their love for you.[2]

I understand that it's difficult to appreciate the good in life, and that I have no idea regarding the depth of pain that you may have experienced. Some of you have been deeply hurt by parents, spouses, siblings, close friends, bosses, and neighbors in ways I can't even imagine. No matter how badly you've been hurt, though, unforgiveness will cause your health to suffer and, more important, will separate you from your heavenly Father. Always remember Matthew 6:14–15 (NKJV): "If you forgive men their trespasses, your heavenly Father will also forgive you. But if you do not forgive men their trespasses, neither will your Father forgive your trespasses."

Just because you forgive others doesn't mean you'll forget the pain they caused you. But if you truly forgive them, I'm confident that the next time you think of them, you'll remember the day that you received victory. I think by now you know what I'm getting at: God wants you to deal with your emotions so that you can lead a much healthier life on behalf of the kingdom.

Sometimes, though, the hardest person to forgive is yourself. Maybe there's something in your past that you deeply regret. An abortion. An affair. A divorce. An estranged son or daughter.

Somehow and some way you'll have to find it in your power to forgive yourself. Perhaps you need to see a counselor or your pastor. Anything that I could say here may come across as trite, but I urge you to take an active step so that you can put the past in the past and keep it there.

You know, the Lord promised to forget our sins "as far as the east is from the west" (Ps. 103:12 NKJV). He said that, I believe, because He understands human nature: we have a built-in tendency not to let go or forgive ourselves because we're sure that we don't deserve any better.

We don't deserve salvation either, but Jesus said when we come to Him like little children and accept Him, He wipes away our tears and our past sins— sins that He took with Him to the cross. "If we confess our sins to him, he is faithful and just to forgive us and to cleanse us from every wrong," wrote John (1 John 1:9 NLT). The next time you feel as if you can't forgive yourself, remember that the Lord of creation has already forgiven you for all the sins you have ever committed and will commit. Your relationship with God is secure. Confess your unforgiving heart, and then let it go.

A MERRY HEART

We've been talking a great deal about negative emotions and their effects on the body, but the flip side of the coin is that positive emotions such as love, acceptance, and laughter are a fragrant balm to the soul. I love the King James Version of the verse I used to open this chapter: "A merry heart doeth good like a medicine" (Prov. 17:22).

Laughter is good medicine. A good belly laugh is the equivalent of internal jogging. Humor allows people to forget what ails them. A Loma Linda

University study on the effect of laughter shows that hilarity and mirth release endorphins—the body's painkillers—and lower blood pressure. I don't think we've reached the point where doctors are going to turn their surgical bays into Comedy Central, but they might tell patients to go home and watch *Seinfeld, Saturday Night Live,* or *Dumb and Dumber* as word gets out regarding the therapeutic benefits of good, clean laughter.

Having positive emotions of laughter, love, and acceptance filling your sails is as healing as implementing the first five keys of *The Great Physician's Rx for Health and Wellness.* I believe if we can get a handle on these deadly emotions, we can truly walk in God's full potential for our lives.

For Further Study

For additional study on avoiding deadly emotions, visit www.BiblicalHealthInstitute.com for a free introductory course called "Emotional Health 101."

LET GO AND LET GOD
by Denise Kennedy

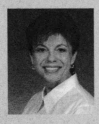

I grew up in a close-knit family with two brothers and a sister. Dad and mom were healthy individuals who ate right and enjoyed their morning walks together. I don't remember Dad ever missing a day of work, and while we were growing up, he seemed immune from our childhood colds and flus. I put my father on a pedestal.

That's why it was a surprise a couple of years ago when I received a phone call informing me that Dad had suffered a stroke. How could that happen to such a strong, self-sufficient person, even though he was in his late seventies? A knot formed in my stomach as I waited for the next call dealing with his progress. I just *knew* he would be fine. The following day, however, the doctor told me that I'd better head home—Dad wasn't going to make it.

This couldn't be true! The knot in my stomach turned to nausea as I packed for my trip. My stomach was so upset that when I ate a light lunch on the airplane, I got immediately sick. Good thing the fasten seatbelt sign was off because I barely made it to the bathroom in time.

When I finally walked into Dad's hospital room, I was not prepared for what I saw. I steadied myself as I drew near to his bed. My once-invincible father had been reduced to a frail, lifeless form. He looked hideous because a hole had been drilled in the top of his head with draining tubes exposed.

My siblings explained that Dad had gone through two brain surgeries to relieve pressure and fluid from around the skull. For the next several days, we took turns sitting by his bed waiting . . . waiting for him to come back to us. Day after day, we talked and prayed.

As the days turned into weeks, I adjusted to the trauma, but fear and anxiety remained my constant companions. I suffered severe diarrhea for days, as well as stomach cramps and weight loss. This happened despite the fact that I ate healthy, took nutritional supplements, and found time to exercise. I was always known as the "health nut" in the family, yet I had all the symptoms of a sick person. Why did I feel that way?

What I came to learn was that when I allowed fear and anger to dominate my mind, my body and spirit were affected as well—they could not be disconnected from one another. My sickness and symptoms were manifestations of the fear poisoning me on the inside. I had to find a way to deal with these negative emotions and not let them control me.

I eventually came through this experience by "letting go and letting God" take my emotional burdens. Jesus said to come unto Him, all who were weary and carried heavy burdens, and He would give them rest. I gave my emotional burdens to the Lord because I could not control these hurdles—but I could control my reaction to them.

The rest of my story is nothing less than miraculous. My dad *did* wake up, and even though it took months of physical therapy, he recovered from his stroke 100 percent, which amazed me and my family, as well as his doctors and nurses.

What I learned is that when Dad became seriously ill, I could not control the outcome, but I needn't react in fear because God is the author of life . . . and death. When I let go and let God be in control, my health dramatically improved, and my feelings of anxiousness evaporated.

THE GREAT PHYSICIAN'S Rx FOR AVOIDING DEADLY EMOTIONS

- *Do your best to avoid stress, anxiety, and anger.*

- *Don't sweat the small stuff.*

- *Don't eat when you're sad, scared, or ticked off.*

- *Trust God when you face circumstances that cause you to worry or become anxious.*

- *Practice forgiveness every day, and forgive those who hurt you.*

- *Look for ways to laugh every day.*

THE GREAT PHYSICIAN'S Rx FOR WEEK #6

Day 36

Upon Waking

Advanced hygiene: practice advanced hygiene. See page 325 for guidance.

Reduce toxins: open windows for one hour today. Use natural soap and natural skin and body care products (shower gel, body creams, etc.). Use natural facial care products. Use natural toothpaste. Use natural hair care products such as shampoo, conditioner, gel, mousse, and hairspray.

Supplements: take one serving of a fiber/green superfood powder (mixed in) or five caplets of a super green formula (swallowed with) twelve-to-sixteen ounces of water or raw vegetable juice. (See the GPRx Resource Guide, pages 346–347, for recommended products.)

Body therapy: get twenty minutes of direct sunlight.

Exercise: perform functional fitness exercises for fifteen minutes (three rounds of exercises found in Key #4, pages 138–145) or spend fifteen minutes on the rebounder. Finish with ten minutes of deep-breathing exercises.

Emotional health: when you face a circumstance that would usually cause you to worry, repeat the following: "Lord, I trust You. I cast my cares upon You, and I believe that You're going to take care of [insert your current situation]." Confess that throughout the day whenever you think about your circumstance.

Breakfast

Berry Smoothie (see appendix A, page 304, for recipe) with two tablespoons of protein powder (optional)

hot tea with honey (see the GPRx Resource Guide, page 339, for recommended herbal tea blends)

Supplements: take one or two whole food multivitamin caplets (see the GPRx Resource Guide, page 345, for recommended products) and one or two capsules of a probiotic/enzyme blend (see The GPRx Resource Guide, pages 347–348, for recommended products).

Lunch

Before eating, drink eight ounces of water.

During lunch, drink eight ounces of water or hot or iced fresh-brewed tea with honey.

tuna salad on a bed of greens or on sprouted whole grain or sourdough bread

apple or pear

Supplements: take one or two whole food multivitamin caplets and one or two capsules of a probiotic/enzyme blend.

Dinner
Before eating, drink eight ounces of water.
During dinner, drink hot or iced fresh-brewed tea with honey.
Stuffed Free-Range Turkey Breast (see appendix A, page 294, for recipe)
brown rice
grilled asparagus
green salad
Supplements: take one or two whole food multivitamin caplets, one-to-three teaspoons or three-to-nine capsules of high omega-3 cod-liver oil (see the GPRx Resource Guide, pages 345–348, for recommended products), and one or two capsules of a probiotic/enzyme blend.

Snacks
yogurt and pineapple
raspberry super green whole food bar (with beta glucans from soluble oat fiber; see the GPRx Resource Guide, pages 329–330, for recommended products)
Drink eight-to-twelve ounces of water or hot or iced fresh-brewed tea with honey.

Before Bed
Drink eight-to-twelve ounces of water or hot tea with honey.
Exercise: go for a walk outdoors or participate in a favorite sport or recreational activity.
Supplements: take one serving of a fiber/green superfood powder (mixed in) or five caplets of a super green formula (swallowed with) twelve-to-sixteen ounces of water or raw vegetable juice.)
Body therapy: take a warm bath for fifteen minutes with eight drops of biblical essential oils added.
Advanced hygiene: practice advanced hygiene. See page 325 for guidance.
Sleep: go to bed by 10:30 p.m.

Day 37
Upon Waking
Advanced hygiene: practice advanced hygiene. See page 325 for guidance.
Reduce toxins: open windows for one hour today. Use natural soap and natural skin and body care products (shower gel, body creams, etc.). Use natural facial care products. Use natural toothpaste. Use natural hair care products such as shampoo, conditioner, gel, mousse, and hairspray.
Supplements: take one serving of a fiber/green superfood powder (mixed in) or five caplets of a super green formula (swallowed with) twelve-to-sixteen ounces of water or raw vegetable juice. (See the GPRx Resource Guide, pages 346–347, for recommended products.)
Exercise: perform functional fitness exercises for fifteen minutes (three rounds of

exercises found in Key #4, pages 138–145) or spend fifteen minutes on the rebounder. Finish with ten minutes of deep-breathing exercises.

Body therapy: take a hot and cold shower. After your normal shower, alternate sixty seconds of water as hot as you can stand it, followed by sixty seconds of water as cold as you can stand it. Repeat cycle four times for a total of eight minutes, finishing with cold.

Emotional health: when you face a circumstance that would usually cause you to worry, repeat the following: "Lord, I trust You. I cast my cares upon You, and I believe that You're going to take care of [insert your current situation]." Confess that throughout the day whenever you think about your circumstance.

Breakfast

Garden Herb Omelet (see appendix A, page 267, for recipe)
grapefruit
hot tea with honey
Supplements: take one or two whole food multivitamin caplets and one or two capsules of a probiotic/enzyme blend.

Lunch

Before eating, drink eight ounces of water.
During lunch, drink eight ounces of water or hot or iced fresh-breewed tea with honey.
Red Meat Chili (see appendix A, page 305, for recipe)
brown rice
peas and carrots
Supplements: take one or two whole food multivitamin caplets and one or two capsules of a probiotic/enzyme blend.

Dinner

Before eating, drink eight ounces of water.
During dinner, drink hot or iced fresh-brewed tea with honey.
Halibut with Coconut Curry Roasted Nori Rolls (see appendix A, page 297, for recipe)
sautéed asparagus and mushrooms
Rosemary Quinoa Salad
Supplements: take one or two whole food multivitamin caplets, one-to-three teaspoons or three-to-nine capsules of high omega-3 cod-liver oil, and one or two capsules of a probiotic/enzyme blend.

Snacks

cottage cheese and pineapple
Tropical Smoothie mix (with beta glucans from soluble oat fiber; see the GPRx Resource Guide, page 329, for recommended products) blended in eight-to-twelve ounces of water
Crispy Almonds (see appendix A, page 270, for recipe)
Drink eight-to-twelve ounces of water or hot or iced fresh-brewed tea with honey.

Before Bed

Drink eight-to-twelve ounces of water or hot tea with honey.

Exercise: go for a walk outdoors or participate in a favorite sport or recreational activity.

Supplements: take one serving of a fiber/green superfood powder (mixed in) or five caplets of a super green formula (swallowed with) twelve-to-sixteen ounces of water or raw vegetable juice.

Advanced hygiene: practice advanced hygiene. See page 325 for guidance.

Emotional health: ask the Lord to bring to your mind someone you need to forgive. Take out a sheet of paper and write the person's name at the top. Try to remember each specific action that person did against you that brought you pain. Write down the following: "I forgive [insert person's name] for [insert the action he or she did against you]." After you fill up the paper, tear it up or burn it, and ask God to give you the strength to truly forgive that person.

Body therapy: spend ten minutes listening to soothing music before retiring.

Sleep: go to bed by 10:30 p.m.

Day 38

Upon Waking

Advanced hygiene: practice advanced hygiene. See page 325 for guidance.

Reduce toxins: open windows for one hour today. Use natural soap and natural skin and body care products (shower gel, body creams, etc.). Use natural facial care products. Use natural toothpaste. Use natural hair care products such as shampoo, conditioner, gel, mousse, and hairspray.

Supplements: take one serving of a fiber/green superfood powder (mixed in) or five caplets of a super green formula (swallowed with) twelve-to-sixteen ounces of water or raw vegetable juice. (See the GPRx Resource Guide, pages 346–347, for recommended products.)

Exercise: perform functional fitness exercises for fifteen minutes (three rounds of exercises found in Key #4, pages 138–145) or spend fifteen minutes on the rebounder. Finish with ten minutes of deep-breathing exercises.

Body therapy: get twenty minutes of direct sunlight.

Emotional health: when you face a circumstance that would usually cause you to worry, repeat the following: "Lord, I trust You. I cast my cares upon You, and I believe that You're going to take care of [insert your current situation]." Confess that throughout the day whenever you think about your circumstance.

Breakfast

sprouted dry cereal with yogurt, goat's milk, or almond milk

banana

hot tea with honey

Supplements: take one or two whole food multivitamin caplets and one or two capsules of a probiotic/enzyme blend.

Lunch

Before eating, drink eight ounces of water.

During lunch, drink eight ounces of water or hot or iced fresh-brewed tea with honey.

Thai Express Bowl with Chicken (see appendix A, page 288, for recipe)

Supplements: take one or two whole food multivitamin caplets and one or two capsules of a probiotic/enzyme blend.

Dinner

Before eating, drink eight ounces of water.

During dinner, drink hot or iced fresh-brewed tea with honey.

Oven-Roasted Koshered Veal

Garlic Mashed Potatoes (see appendix A, page 302, for recipe)

peas and carrots

Supplements: take one or two whole food multivitamin caplets, one-to-three teaspoons or three-to-nine capsules of high omega-3 cod-liver oil, and one or two capsules of a probiotic/enzyme blend.

Snacks

crackers, cheese, and fruit

vanilla protein whole food bar (see the GPRx Resource Guide, pages 329–330, for recommended products)

Drink eight-to-twelve ounces of water or hot or iced fresh-brewed tea with honey.

Before Bed

Drink eight-to-twelve ounces of water, or hot tea with honey.

Exercise: go for a walk outdoors or participate in a favorite sport or recreational activity.

Supplements: take one serving of a fiber/green superfood powder (mixed in) or five caplets of a super green formula (swallowed with) twelve-to-sixteen ounces of water or raw vegetable juice.

Advanced hygiene: practice advanced hygiene. See page 325 for guidance.

Emotional health: ask the Lord to bring to your mind someone you need to forgive. Take out a sheet of paper and write the person's name at the top. Try to remember each specific action that person did against you that brought you pain. Write down the following: "I forgive [insert person's name] for [insert the action he or she did against you]." After you fill up the paper, tear it up or burn it, and ask God to give you the strength to truly forgive that person.

Body therapy: take a warm bath for fifteen minutes with eight drops of biblical essential oils added.

Sleep: go to bed by 10:30 p.m.

Day 39

Upon Waking

Advanced hygiene: practice advanced hygiene. See page 325 for guidance.

Reduce toxins: open windows for one hour today. Use natural soap and natural skin and body care products (shower gel, body creams, etc.). Use natural facial care products. Use natural toothpaste. Use natural hair care products such as shampoo, conditioner, gel, mousse, and hairspray.

Supplements: take one serving of a fiber/green superfood powder (mixed in) or five caplets of a super green formula (swallowed with) twelve-to-sixteen ounces of water or raw vegetable juice. (See the GPRx Resource Guide, pages 346–347, for recommended products.)

Exercise: perform functional fitness exercises for fifteen minutes (three rounds of exercises found in Key #4, pages 138–145) or spend fifteen minutes on the rebounder. Finish with ten minutes of deep-breathing exercises.

Body therapy: take a hot and cold shower. After your normal shower, alternate sixty seconds of water as hot as you can stand it, followed by sixty seconds of water as cold as you can stand it. Repeat cycle four times for a total of eight minutes, finishing with cold.

Emotional health: when you face a circumstance that would usually cause you to worry, repeat the following: "Lord, I trust You. I cast my cares upon You, and I believe that You're going to take care of [insert your current situation]." Confess that throughout the day whenever you think about your circumstance.

Breakfast

Banana Peach Smoothie (see appendix A, page 320), with two tablespoons protein powder (optional)

hot tea with honey

Supplements: take one or two whole food multivitamin caplets and one or two capsules of a probiotic/enzyme blend.

Lunch

Before eating, drink eight ounces of water.

During lunch, drink eight ounces of water or hot or iced fresh-brewed tea with honey.

roast beef on sprouted whole grain or sourdough bread

Supplements: take one or two whole food multivitamin caplets and one or two capsules of a probiotic/enzyme blend.

Dinner

Before eating, drink eight ounces of water.

During dinner, drink hot or iced fresh-brewed tea with honey.

Roasted Pastured Chicken (see appendix A, page 320, for recipe)

steamed broccoli

sweet potato

Lentil Salad (see appendix A, page 275, for recipe)

Supplements: take one or two whole food multivitamin caplets, one-to-three teaspoons or three-to-nine capsules of high omega-3 cod-liver oil, and one or two capsules of a probiotic/enzyme blend.

Snacks

apple and carrots with almond butter

berry smoothie mix mixed in eight-to-twelve ounces of water (see the GPRx Resource Guide, page 329, for recommended products).

Zesty Popcorn (see appendix A, page 321, for recipe)

Drink eight-to-twelve ounces of water or hot or iced fresh-brewed tea with honey.

Before Bed

Drink eight-to-twelve ounces of water or hot tea with honey.

Exercise: go for a walk outdoors or participate in a favorite sport or recreational activity.

Supplements: take one serving of a fiber/green superfood powder (mixed in) or five caplets of a super green formula (swallowed with) twelve-to-sixteen ounces of water or raw vegetable juice.

Advanced hygiene: practice advanced hygiene. See page 325 for guidance.

Emotional health: ask the Lord to bring to your mind someone you need to forgive. Take out a sheet of paper and write the person's name at the top. Try to remember each specific action that person did against you that brought you pain. Write down the following: "I forgive [insert person's name] for [insert the action he or she did against you]." After you fill up the paper, tear it up or burn it, and ask God to give you the strength to truly forgive that person.

Body therapy: spend ten minutes listening to soothing music before you retire.

Sleep: go to bed by 10:30 p.m.

Day 40 (Partial Fast Day)

Upon Waking

Advanced hygiene: practice advanced hygiene. See page 325 for guidance.

Reduce toxins: open windows for one hour today. Use natural soap and natural skin and body care products (shower gel, body creams, etc.). Use natural facial care products. Use natural toothpaste. Use natural hair care products such as shampoo, conditioner, gel, mousse, and hairspray.

Supplements: take one serving of a fiber/green superfood powder (mixed in) or five caplets of a super green formula (swallowed with) twelve-to-sixteen ounces of water or raw vegetable juice. (See the GPRx Resource Guide, pages 346–347, for recommended products.)

Exercise: perform functional fitness exercises for fifteen minutes (three rounds of exercises found in Key #4, pages 138–145) or spend fifteen minutes on the rebounder. Finish with ten minutes of deep-breathing exercises.

Body therapy: get twenty minutes of direct sunlight.

Emotional health: when you face a circumstance that would usually cause you to worry, repeat the following: "Lord, I trust You. I cast my cares upon You, and I believe that You're going to take care of [insert your current situation]." Confess that throughout the day whenever you think about your circumstance.

Breakfast

none (partial fast day)

eight ounces of water

Supplements: take one or two whole food multivitamin caplets and one or two capsules of a probiotic/enzyme blend.

Lunch

none (partial fast day)

eight ounces of water

Supplements: take one or two whole food multivitamin caplets and one or two capsules of a probiotic/enzyme blend.

Dinner

Before eating, drink eight ounces of water.

During dinner, drink hot or iced fresh-brewed tea with honey.

Chicken Soup (see appendix A, page 269, for recipe)

cultured vegetables

green salad

Supplements: take one or two whole food multivitamin caplets, one-to-three teaspoons or three-to-nine capsules of high omega-3 cod-liver oil, and one or two capsules of a probiotic/enzyme blend.

Snacks

none (partial fast day)

eight ounces of water

Before Bed

Drink eight-to-twelve ounces of water or hot tea with honey.

Exercise: go for a walk outdoors or participate in a favorite sport or recreational activity.

Supplements: take one serving of a fiber/green superfood powder (mixed in) or five caplets of a super green formula (swallowed with) twelve-to-sixteen ounces of water or raw vegetable juice.

Advanced hygiene: practice advanced hygiene. See page 325 for guidance.

Emotional health: ask the Lord to bring to your mind someone you need to forgive. Take out a sheet of paper and write the person's name at the top. Try to remember each specific action that person did against you that brought you pain. Write down the following: "I forgive [insert person's name] for [insert the action he or she did against you]." After you fill up the paper, tear it up or burn it, and ask God to give you the strength to truly forgive that person.

Body therapy: take a warm bath for fifteen minutes with eight drops of biblical essential oils added.

Sleep: go to bed by 10:30 p.m.

Day 41 (Day of Rest)

Upon Waking

Advanced hygiene: practice advanced hygiene. See page 325 for guidance.

Reduce toxins: open windows for one hour today. Use natural soap and natural skin and body care products (shower gel, body creams, etc.). Use natural facial care products. Use natural toothpaste. Use natural hair care products such as shampoo, conditioner, gel, mousse, and hairspray.

Supplements: take one serving of a fiber/green superfood powder (mixed in) or five caplets of a super green formula (swallowed with) twelve-to-sixteen ounces of water or raw vegetable juice. (See the GPRx Resource Guide, pages 346–347, for recommended products.)

Exercise: do no formal exercise since it's a day of rest.

Body therapies: do none since it's a rest day.

Emotional health: when you face a circumstance that would usually cause you to worry, repeat the following: "Lord, I trust You. I cast my cares upon You, and I believe that You're going to take care of [insert your current situation]." Confess that throughout the day whenever you think about your circumstance.

Breakfast

Zucchini Frittata (see appendix A, page 274, for recipe)
Easy French Toast (see appendix A, page 321, for recipe)
hot tea with honey
Supplements: take one or two whole food multivitamin caplets and one or two capsules of a probiotic/enzyme blend.

Lunch

Before eating, drink eight ounces of water.
During lunch, drink eight ounces of water or hot or iced fresh-brewed tea with honey.
Chicken Soup
crackers (whole grain or flaxseed)
Supplements: take one or two whole food multivitamin caplets and one or two capsules of a probiotic/enzyme blend.

Dinner

Before eating, drink eight ounces of water.
During dinner, drink hot or iced fresh-brewed tea with honey.
Marinated Baked Salmon with Capers (see appendix A, page 290, for recipe)
Easy Sautéed Greens (see appendix A, page 321, for recipe)
Simple Beans (see appendix A, page 276, for recipe)
green salad
Supplements: take one or two whole food multivitamin caplets, one-to-three teaspoons or three-to-nine capsules of high omega-3 cod-liver oil, and one or two capsules of a probiotic/enzyme blend.

Snacks

Healthy Trail Mix (see appendix A, page 271, for recipe)
yogurt and berries
Drink eight-to-twelve ounces of water or hot or iced fresh-brewed tea with honey.

Before Bed

Drink eight-to-twelve ounces of water or hot tea with honey.

Exercise: go for a walk outdoors or participate in a favorite sport or recreational activity.

Supplements: take one serving of a fiber/green superfood powder (mixed in) or five caplets of a super green formula (swallowed with) twelve-to-sixteen ounces of water or raw vegetable juice.

Advanced hygiene: practice advanced hygiene. See page 325 for guidance.

Emotional health: ask the Lord to bring to your mind someone you need to forgive. Take out a sheet of paper and write the person's name at the top. Try to remember each specific action that person did against you that brought you pain. Write down the following: "I forgive [insert person's name] for [insert the action he or she did against you]." After you fill up the paper, tear it up or burn it, and ask God to give you the strength to truly forgive that person.

Body therapy: spend ten minutes listening to soothing music before you retire.

Sleep: go to bed by 10:30 p.m.

Day 42

Upon Waking

Advanced hygiene: practice advanced hygiene. See page 325 for guidance.

Reduce toxins: open windows for one hour today. Use natural soap and natural skin and body care products (shower gel, body creams, etc.). Use natural facial care products. Use natural toothpaste. Use natural hair care products such as shampoo, conditioner, gel, mousse, and hairspray.

Supplements: take one serving of a fiber/green superfood powder (mixed in) or five caplets of a super green formula (swallowed with) twelve-to-sixteen ounces of water or raw vegetable juice. (See the GPRx Resource Guide, pages 346–347, for recommended products.)

Exercise: perform functional fitness exercises for fifteen minutes (three rounds of exercises found in Key #4, pages 138–145) or spend fifteen minutes on the rebounder. Finish with ten minutes of deep-breathing exercises.

Body therapy: get twenty minutes of direct sunlight.

Emotional health: when you face a circumstance that would usually cause you to worry, repeat the following: "Lord, I trust You. I cast my cares upon You, and I believe that You're going to take care of [insert your current situation]." Confess that throughout the day whenever you think about your circumstance.

Breakfast

Easy Oatmeal with two tablespoons of protein powder after cooking (see appendix A, page 306, for recipe) one cup blueberries

hot tea with honey

Supplements: take one or two whole food multivitamin caplets and one or two capsules of a probiotic/enzyme blend.

Lunch

Before eating, drink eight ounces of water.

During dinner, drink hot or iced fresh-brewed tea with honey.

Warm Chicken Supreme Salad (see appendix A, page 281, for recipe)

Supplements: take one or two whole food multivitamin caplets and one or two capsules of a probiotic/enzyme blend.

Dinner

Before eating, drink eight ounces of water.

During dinner, drink hot or iced fresh-brewed tea with honey.

Lamb Chops (see appendix A, page 277, for recipe)

baked potato

green beans

Supplements: take one or two whole food multivitamin caplets, one-to-three teaspoons or three-to-nine capsules of high omega-3 cod-livewr oil, and one or two capsules of a probiotic/enzyme blend.

Snacks

baked corn chips with cheese, salsa, guacamole, or hummus

chocolate protein whole food bar (see the GPRx Resource Guide, pages 329–330, for recommended products)

Drink eight-to-twelve ounces of water or hot or iced fresh-brewed tea with honey.

Before Bed

Drink eight-to-twelve ounces of water or hot tea with honey.

Exercise: go for a walk outdoors or participate in a favorite sport or recreational activity.

Supplements: take one serving of a fiber/green superfood powder (mixed in) or five caplets of a super green formula (swallowed with) twelve-to-sixteen ounces of water or raw vegetable juice.

Advanced hygiene: practice advanced hygiene. See page 325 for guidance.

Emotional health: ask the Lord to bring to your mind someone you need to forgive. Take out a sheet of paper and write the person's name at the top. Try to remember each specific action that person did against you that brought you pain. Write down the following: "I forgive [insert person's name] for [insert the action he or she did against you]." After you fill up the paper, tear it up or burn it, and ask God to give you the strength to truly forgive that person.

Body therapy: take a warm bath for fifteen minutes with eight drops of biblical essential oils added.

Sleep: go to bed by 10:30 p.m.

Key #7

Live a Life of Prayer and Purpose

The effective, fervent prayer of a righteous man avails much.

—James 5:16 (NKJV)

Prayer is the foundation of a healthy life, linking your mind, body, and spirit to God. Prayer is two-way communication with our Creator, the God of the universe. There's power in prayer: "The prayer offered in faith will make the sick person well" (James 5:15). I sure found that out in the midst of my health challenges.

Prayer is how we talk to God. There is no greater source of power than talking to the One who made us. Prayer is not a formality. Prayer is not about religion. Prayer is about a relationship—the hotline to heaven. We can talk to God anytime, anywhere, for any reason. He is always there to listen, and He always has our best interests at heart because we are His children.

There was something about facing my mortality that made prayer seem very real to me. When my health spun out of control and tumbled into a free fall, I didn't have much else to hang on to but the Lord. In my darkest hour, I spoke with Him constantly. At times I felt as if I heard God's voice in reply, while on other occasions, He directed me to Scriptures that seemed particularly relevant to my dire situation.

What God was teaching me was to listen to Him. Jesus said, "My sheep listen to my voice" (John 10:27), and I count myself among His flock. Another Scripture seemed particularly apt for my situation: "Blessed is the man who listens to me, watching daily at my doors, waiting at my doorway.

For whoever finds me finds life and receives favor from the LORD" (Prov. 8:34–35).

Sometimes when I prayed, the Lord put things on my heart that I hadn't even thought about before I started. Sometimes He didn't answer my prayers in the way I expected Him to, but He transformed my heart to align with His. In living a healthy, purpose-filled life, prayer is the most powerful tool that we possess. Prayer connects the entire person—mind, body, and spirit—to God. Through prayer, God takes away our guilt, shame, bitterness, and anger and gives us a brand-new start. We can eat organic whole foods, supplement our diet with whole food supplements, practice good hygiene, reduce toxins, and exercise, but if the spirit is not where it needs to be with God, then we will never be completely healthy. Talking to our Maker through prayer is the foundation for optimal health and makes us whole. After all, God's love and grace are our greatest foods for mind, body, and spirit.

The seventh key to unlocking your health potential is living a life of prayer and purpose. Prayer will confirm your purpose, and it will give you the perseverance to complete it. Seal all that you do with the power of prayer, and watch your life become more than you ever thought possible.

PRAYING FOR A HEALTHY LIFESTYLE

"Prayer must be foundational to every Christian endeavor," wrote Germaine Copeland, author of *Prayers That Avail Much*.[1] Her book contains more than 150 prayers covering just about every situation under the sun: living free from worry, conquering the thought life, knowing God's will, experiencing protection for travel, finding a mate, having peace in a troubled marriage, conducting successful meetings, and being delivered from poor habits. I was particularly drawn to Mrs. Copeland's prayer for "victory in a healthy lifestyle," which went like this:

> Lord, thank You for declaring Your plans for me—plans to prosper me and not to harm me, plans to give me hope and a future. I choose to

renew my mind to Your plans for a healthy lifestyle . . . My body is for the Lord. So here is what I want to do with Your help, Father God. I choose to take my everyday, ordinary life—my sleeping, eating, going-to-work, and walking-around life—and place it before You as an offering. Embracing what You do for me is the best I can do for You.[2]

If you feel drawn to ask God to give you discipline to make changes in how you live and how you eat, or to exercise consistently, I urge you to get on your knees today. Prayer is imperative! R. A. Torrey, an American evangelist born in the nineteenth century, said that James 4:2—"You do not have, because you do not ask God"—contains the secret to the poverty and powerlessness of the average Christian. Your life can change today, but only if you pray. Do not underestimate the power of communicating with your heavenly Father. When you pray and open up to God, you allow Him to fill your heart with Scripture, where He can speak to you in the stillness of the moment and transform your life simultaneously.

I can assure you that prayer works; God listened and answered my prayers as well as those of righteous people like my parents and those in my church family. But don't take my word for it. Dr. Joseph Mercola, author of *Total Health Program*, regularly reviews scientific studies that demonstrate the efficacy of prayer. "There appears to be no question that prayer works," said Dr. Mercola. "We have many studies now that document that. The science is very solid in excellent peer-reviewed publications. It makes no logical sense to me why someone would not utilize this resource."[3]

If you're wondering how to react to the message of *The Great Physician's Rx for Health and Wellness*, I urge you to first pray for God's purpose for your life, which is often a catalyst to making major health-related changes. I believe that people who live a life of purpose live longer and live better because they are more likely to take good care of their bodies. They have a goal—to serve God—because they believe He wants to use them.

Our Maker created you for a purpose, and unveiling that purpose is crucial to your well-being. His Word declares that His purposes "will bring health to your body and nourishment to your bones" if you follow Him (Prov. 3:8). So when you live for a divine purpose, you reap divine health. That's good news!

If you're not living a life of purpose, however, you're like a lamp that's not plugged into a power source. No matter how hard you try, you cannot do anything to brighten a dark room. That's not the way to go through life. After all, what are we here for if we're not making a difference in the lives of other people—our spouses, our children, our family members, our friends, and our neighbors?

THE SEARCH FOR SIGNIFICANCE

"Living a life of purpose" is a buzz phrase these days because of a certain book you've probably read or heard about—*The Purpose-Driven Life* by Rick Warren, pastor of Saddleback Church in Lake Forest, California. You may not be aware of this, but *The Purpose-Driven Life* is the biggest-selling hardback book in U.S. history. Around twenty-five million copies have been purchased in the last three years, which says to me that Rick's book has touched a raw nerve in the popular culture. To give you an idea of just how big those sales numbers are, *The Purpose-Driven Life* has sold more copies than *The Da Vinci Code, South Beach Diet*, and Bill and Hillary Clinton's autobiographies combined.[4]

The Purpose-Driven Life is about the search for significance—something we can all identify with. The desire to count for something lies deep within all our hearts, if you strip away enough layers. In the movie *Saving Private Ryan*, when an elderly James Ryan totters toward a particular gravesite on the green lawns perched above the Normandy beachhead, he ponders the Big Question: "Have I led a good life?" He might as well have been asking, "Did I matter? Did I live a life of purpose?"

"Lack of something to feel important about is almost the greatest tragedy a man may have," engineer Arthur E. Morgan once said. That's the feeling Rick Warren tapped into when he wrote *The Purpose-Driven Life*, teaching us that God created every person for a purpose and gave us unique personalities and talents for a reason—to fit into His master plan. When you realize what that purpose is and live it out every day, you'll find fulfillment in life.

When God took me through two years of horrible sickness before restoring my health, I came out of that experience knowing what my purpose was in life: sharing God's message of health and hope so that people wouldn't have to go through what I did. Everything else that I do today is icing—made with raw honey, of course—on the cake. I can't wait to get up in the morning, hoping that I have the privilege of communicating life-changing principles of good health with one person, one thousand people, or even millions that day through television.

If you say to yourself, *I'm not sure I have a purpose*, you would be wrong. If there is air in your lungs, you have a purpose; it's ingrained in your being. If you haven't found your purpose yet, search your heart. What makes you feel alive? What are you passionate about? The joys of family? The arts? Teaching others?

Your purpose is waiting to be discovered. Pinpoint your passions, and you'll uncover your purpose. Keep in mind that God gives us different desires, different dreams, and different talents for a reason because we are all part of one body. Having a purpose will give you something to live for.

Ninety-four-year-old Italian operatic composer Gian Carlo Menotti, who once said that a man becomes wise only when he begins to calculate the approximate depth of his ignorance, spoke a greater truth when he declared, "Hell begins on that day when God grants us a clear vision of all that we might have achieved, of all the gifts we wasted, of all that we might have done that we did not do."[5]

Heaven begins, I believe, after we find our purpose. Whenever I speak before audiences, I like to say, "If you find your passion, then you'll know that your talent gives you the power to live your purpose." Dr. John Maxwell, a renowned leadership expert and best-selling author, said it even better. He made this remarkable assertion about purpose when I recently heard him speak at my home church in Palm Beach Gardens, Florida. John said, "I'm going to make a statement of prayer that you should repeat after me: I want to make a difference . . . with people who want to make a difference . . . doing something that makes a difference . . . at a time that makes a difference."

We all want to make a difference in life. No one wants to travel ten, twenty, or thirty years down the road and say, "Man, I just wasted the only life I'll ever have." I'm afraid that I run into people every day who aren't aware that they are letting life's opportunities pass them by, or they're passing through without knowing what their purpose is.

Don't think that you have to preach before millions or become a missionary to AIDS-ravaged Africa to be effective for the Lord. You can make a difference in your own circle of friends and acquaintances, and you can make a difference with other people who want to make a difference. You can make a difference in your own family.

For instance, if you're a young mother who's cooped up with young ones underfoot all day long but who prepares meals using fresh, organic ingredients and goes to great lengths to keep your family healthy, you are a heroine to me. If you're a father who takes the kids to the park and plays soccer with them instead of driving them to McDonald's for a Happy Meal, you're a hero to me.

My hope is that you will incorporate the seven keys of *The Great Physician's Rx for Health and Wellness* into your life as well as the lives of your family members. I can assure you that you have family, friends, and acquaintances waiting—or maybe dying—for somebody like you to share with them these seven keys to health and wellness.

Surely you know someone who could benefit from eating the right foods, taking the right supplements, practicing advanced hygiene, conditioning his body with exercise and body therapies, reducing toxins in his environment, and avoiding deadly emotions. You probably know someone who eats totally the wrong way—someone who frequents a fast-food restaurant as often as Morgan Spurlock did in *Super Size Me*.[6] You probably know someone whose health is going downhill fast. Are there people in your community, in your church, in your workplace, or in your *family* who are suffering needlessly from illness due to poor diet and lifestyle?

God has put on my heart a mission to transform the health of His people one life at a time. At the end of this chapter, I will give you several great opportunities to share this message of *The Great Physician's Rx for Health and Wellness* with others.

THE MIRACLE OF LIFE

I believe God is still in the business of working miracles. He demonstrated another health miracle after I married the love of my life, Nicki, in 1999. I think we were rushing through a hail of organic rice at the church steps when we heard a well-meaning friend shout, "So, when you are going to have children?"

Nicki and I were not exactly the youngest of brides and grooms when we married—I was twenty-four, and she was twenty-eight, but we had a little time on our side before starting a family. After a year or two of settling into our marriage, we thought we were ready for come what may, so we decided to try in earnest. That was the fun part.

The not-so-fun-part was the crushing disappointment we experienced when Nicki didn't become pregnant. We were among the one in ten married couples in whom infertility was rearing its ugly head. Month after month passed by without a positive home pregnancy test, so after two-and-a-half years of trying, we decided to visit our family physician. That was not easy because we knew he would refer us to a fertility specialist who would probably suggest medication and surgery.

There's some background that you should know before we go too much farther. If you had asked Nicki when we met whether she thought she ate well, she would have given you a wholehearted nod signifying a "yes." I soon learned that her idea of "eating well" meant snacking on a whole bag of strawberry-flavored Twizzlers while sipping from a tall glass of sweet tea, which had enough sugar to feed an army. Naturally she learned about my passion for health while we dated, and by the time I proposed, she had bought into the program. Her one weakness, however, was consuming too many carbohydrates, particularly sugars and starches, which probably raised her insulin levels and may have led to a hormonal imbalance, not a good thing if you're trying to get pregnant.

Back to our infertility troubles. After two-and-a-half years of trying, we were emotionally worn out from the stress and feelings of failure. During the summer of 2003, I was also dealing with the heavy responsibility of writing *The Maker's Diet*, which contains many of the foundational health principles found in *The Great Physician's Rx for Health and Wellness*.

Since I was living and breathing this "eat right" stuff morning, noon, and night, I pleaded with my wife, "Nicki, why don't you just *try* the Maker's Diet for forty days?"

I'll never forget her reply: "Jordan, I eat healthy, but I'm not going to be a radical like you."

A few days later, we had an appointment with the fertility specialist, who promised to give us the results of a battery of tests performed on both of us.

"Nicki, I have some bad news," he began. "From the best we can determine, you've never ovulated, and you certainly aren't ovulating now."

The news stunned us. If Nicki wasn't ovulating, then it was impossible for her to conceive a child. A woman's ability to produce an egg each month is central to the equation.

"Now, you're probably wondering why you're not ovulating," the doctor continued, as if he were reading our minds. "My suspicion is that you have endometriosis, which is the presence of tissue similar to the uterine lining in locations outside the uterus, such as the ovaries, fallopian tubes, and abdominal cavity. We can operate on you to fix this condition, but the procedure comes with no guarantees that you will become pregnant."

"What kind of surgery are we talking about?" I asked.

"This would require an outpatient surgery and a couple of days of recovery, and then we'll see what happens," replied the physician.

Nicki and I were scheduled to go on a cruise to Alaska with In Touch Ministries and Dr. Charles Stanley. We wondered whether we should proceed with the surgery prior to the cruise, but then Nicki ran into a friend who had just gone through the same procedure.

When Nicki explained that her doctor said the recovery time would be a couple of days, her friend replied, "Two days? Forget it. Try more like a week."

We didn't have enough time for Nicki to recuperate before the cruise, so we postponed the surgery until after the trip.

We flew cross-country to Seattle, where we boarded our ship, the MS *Amsterdam*, bound for Alaskan waters. Steaming past icy glaciers and the beautiful fjords of Alaska's Inside Passage was just what our harried lives needed. We ate extremely healthy meals on-board the luxury liner, and during one enchanted evening, I asked Nicki to give the forty-day Maker's Diet a try. "If you're not pregnant in three months, then we'll go ahead with the surgery. But let's try the Maker's Diet. I'll do it with you," I promised.

Nicki, much to my happiness, agreed to go on the Maker's Diet. After we flew back to Florida, I invited three couples to join us on the forty-day Maker's Diet health experience, figuring that it would be a bonding experience. Besides, I joked to Nicki, misery loves company.

The eight of us had a great time, fellowshipping together, keeping one another accountable, and eating one meal a week together. Midway through our experience, we agreed that we could write our own book: *101 Ways to Eat Berries and Never Get Sick of Them.*

Nicki, who is a trained CPA, was very good at following through with details, so when it came to tracking with the Maker's Diet, she stuck with the program. "I'm definitely feeling better," she said as we neared the end of the first month. On the infertility front, however, nothing was happening, even though forty days had passed. Suddenly a ray of hope appeared: Nicki was late with her period.

"Have you done one of those home pregnancy tests?" I asked her.

"Not yet," she replied.

Nicki retreated to the bathroom to perform the pregnancy test, and when she came out, she displayed the hugest grin. "I think we're pregnant," she said, holding up a stick with blue lines.

"That's incredible!" I exclaimed, hugging Nicki closely. Nicki then said, "Let's not tell anybody until the end of the first trimester, just to be sure." We had a friend who had lost her baby to miscarriage around the eighth week.

"You're probably right, sweetie."

I lasted a whole ten minutes. I quickly called my parents, unable to contain the news any longer. "Nicki's pregnant! We're going to have a baby!" I blurted. Oh, well, I had never been one to keep secrets, but in my defense, God had worked a miracle, and I trusted that He was going to see this thing through.

Around eight months later, on May 29, 2004, Joshua Michael Rubin joined this world, and we became proud parents. To us, that is an amazing story by itself, but when Nicki went back and paged through her food diary, she realized that we conceived Joshua on the fortieth day of the Maker's Diet forty-day health experience! Stories like this confirm that God has a plan for Nicki and me, and He has a plan for you—and a purpose for your life. I'm not guaranteeing that if you undertake the Great Physician's Rx of seven weeks of wellness that miraculous things will happen to you and your loved ones, although they often do. But I will tell you that if you treat your body as God meant for you to treat it—like a temple of the Holy Spirit—God will honor that. Like I joked before, eating healthy doesn't make you any more of a Christian, but it usually allows you to live a fuller, more abundant life in service to the Lord.

God gave you a free will. You are not a robot. You are free to make choices— to steal or not to steal, to cheat or not to cheat on your taxes, to accept Jesus or walk away. You also have a choice when it comes to what you put into your mouth to eat. You have a choice to augment your diet with nutritional supplements because you've heard that today's foods lack the nutrients that they contained a hundred or more years ago. You have a choice about whether you get off your duff and exercise and get some sun. You have a choice about what time you go to bed and whether you rest on the Sabbath.

God makes no guarantees what tomorrow will bring; I learned that truth of Scripture when I was a nineteen-year-old skeleton whose body had wasted away to 104 pounds. Now He's restored my health and graciously allowed me to take part in His mission to transform the health of the church and reach out to others with a health message from which all people can benefit.

I believe that God is calling us to be healthy at such a time as this. People everywhere are experiencing one major health crisis after another. Heart disease, cancer, and diabetes are robbing us of many productive years. The need is great, and the time is now. Can you commit to being a modern-day

Daniel by going against the grain? Are you bold enough to say, "I'm not going to do what everyone is doing"?

You can make a difference. Here's how:

- You can transform your health by committing to seven weeks of wellness using the principles contained in the very book you're holding.
- You can transform the health of your family. (To provide daily account-ability and encouragement, visit www.GreatPhysiciansRx.com and register for a free online daily newsletter.)
- You can transform the health of your friends and neighbors by facili-tating a seven-week small group. A free online training and facilitator's guide can be found at www.GreatPhysicansRx.com.
- You can transform the health of your church by bringing a Biblical Health Coach to share God's health plan. Visit www.GreatPhysiciansRx.com, and click on the *Bring the health message to your church* icon for more information on beginning a health revival in your church.
- You can transform the health of your place of business or a community organization by bringing a Health Coach to share practical steps on improving the wellness of every employee or member. Visit www.GreatPhysiciansRx.com, and click on the *Bring the health message to your organization* icon.

I have developed a program that trains health-minded individuals to become Health Coaches and transform the health of their city or region. To enroll in this forty-hour online training and certification program, visit www.BiblicalHealthInstitute.com and register today.

In addition, you and your entire city can embark on the "Seven Weeks of Wellness" program, which teams up churches, ministries, natural food stores, health fairs, Christian and secular bookstores, Christian radio stations, health talk radio programs, doctors, health practitioners, restaurants, gyms, and spas to take the health of your city to the next level. To see how thousands of lives in your city can change in just seven weeks, visit www.7weeksofwellness.com.

God is raising up folks like you to help Him on His mission, but while the harvest is plentiful, the workers are few, as it says in Scripture. That's why I want you to consider becoming a small-group facilitator and teaching others about *The Great Physician's Rx for Health and Wellness.*

If you feel called to the health ministry, we have started the Biblical Health Institute, which is a fully accredited online learning institute that will equip you, train you, and give you everything you need to help others live a healthy life. You can find more details by visiting www.BiblicalHealthInstitute.com.

You can make a difference today. Even the simple act of giving a friend or loved one a copy of *The Great Physician's Rx for Health and Wellness* could add years of healthy living to his or her life. What would that be worth?

But it all starts with you. I urge you to follow the Great Physician's prescription today. I've yet to meet anyone who regretted becoming healthier, and you won't either.

A FINAL PRAYER

I know I may have been a bit long-winded in this final Key, but that's a reflection of my deep passion for the topic of living a healthy life and getting that message out to God's people.

In the last few years, I've been afforded the humbling opportunity to speak around the country, including churches on Sunday mornings, and when I speak before church congregations, I often include Deuteronomy 30:19–20 (NKJV), which goes like this:

> I call heaven and earth as witnesses today against you, that I have set before you life and death, blessing and cursing; therefore choose life, that both you and your descendants may live; that you may love the LORD your God, that you may obey His voice, and that you may cling to Him, for He is your life and the length of your days; and that you may dwell in the land which the LORD swore to your fathers, to Abraham, Isaac, and Jacob, to give them.

Do you want those promises? I hope you do, because it's time for us to stand up as God's children and once again become that city on a hill—a peculiar people set apart for God and His great purpose.

Whenever I'm in a church setting, I usually finish my talks with a prayer because of my desire to give proper respect, honor, and glory to God—our rescuer, our strong tower, and our durable defense. I also ask those who are suffering from a health challenge—cancer, heart disease, diabetes, obesity, or whatever—to stand up so that I can pray for them.

I'm going to close the book in the same way, except I'm going to pray for you. So, with all humility before the Lord Jesus Christ, in whose name I pray, allow me to do that:

Heavenly Father, I praise You that we are fearfully and wonderfully made. But You know what, Lord? Many of us are not extremely healthy right now, but I want to thank You for the health that we do have. I want to thank You that You have sustained us. You are our rock and our fortress. The righteous run in, and we are safe.

Lord, I pray right now for Your healing touch. You say in Exodus 15:26 that You are the God who heals. You say that You spoke Your Word and healed our diseases. And I pray right now that You would send Your healing touch, Lord God, and that You would provide abundant and long life to Your children. And with that long life, we would satisfy You and show You our salvation. Lord God, I pray for all manner of sickness—physical, mental, spiritual, and emotional—and I pray right now that You would plant a seed . . . a seed of faith, a lifeline that will turn around any illnesses of those reading this book for Your glory.

And Lord, I pray that everyone reading this book will realize that You have given us the most wonderful precious gift of all—Your son Jesus. And You also gave us a physical body to live a life on earth as it is in heaven. May each and every one of us take personal responsibility and stewardship and give what You already own back to You. May we present our bodies as a holy sacrifice acceptable unto You as a spiritual act of worship.

I thank You Lord God that You have great plans for us, to prosper us and not to harm us, and that You will restore health unto us and heal our wounds. I ask all of this in the precious name of Jesus the Messiah. Amen.

For Further Study

For additional study on living a life of prayer and purpose, visit www.BiblicalHealthInstitute.com for a free introductory course called "Prayer and Purpose 101."

FINDING PURPOSE IN MY HEART

by Andrew Mincy

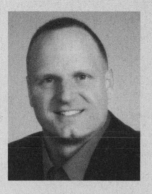

I have no idea where I came from. I know nothing about my biological father or mother. My whole life has been like that. A search. A quest to find where I came from.

I'm told that I lived in an orphanage for a year or so, where my name was Charlie, before my adoptive parents took me home with them in the early 1970s. I grew up in Nashville, Tennessee, not really fitting in, not knowing where I came from. My mother and father gave me love and did their best to raise me in a nice home, but I couldn't see my reflection in my adoptive parents. Every child reflects his or her parents in certain ways, but because I didn't know where I came from, the toughest thing about growing up as an adopted child was figuring out why I was born—what my purpose on Earth was.

My parents sent me to the good private Christian school from the first to ninth grades, but we weren't a churchgoing family, and I never heard my teachers talking about who Jesus was the entire time I was there. I drifted through adolescence and attended college at Florida State University. I heard my share of "turn-or-burn" messages from campus pastors, but that turned me off.

During my senior year, I was hired as the assistant strength and conditioning coach for the Seminole football team. One evening, the team was invited to hear an evangelist speak in the team's film room, and when he shared the Gospel, for some reason, the light came on that night. I realized that I had a void in my heart that I had been desperately trying to fill with the things of the world. Only Christ could fill that void.

That night, God's love got me. I realized that if I was the only person left on this Earth, Jesus would have gone to the Cross just for me—His love and mercy for me were that great. It wasn't the nails that held Him on the Cross that day, it was His love for me.

That night, on October 13, 1993, I gave my heart to Christ by speaking a simple prayer. I was twenty-two years old. Although I never knew my biological father, I now knew my heavenly father. He handpicked me. He chose me. Now I could see my reflection in my father. I knew who I was, and *whose* I was. I found my place in Christ. I had been adopted a second time (Romans 8:15).

Two weeks later, I was asked to speak to a youth group in Tallahassee about how I accepted Christ into my heart. Now, there's something you need to know about me. I had never spoken in public before. I was shy of speaking publicly. Whenever I had a group presentation in school, I called in sick that day or made sure someone else was speaking on my behalf.

So it was to my surprise that when I was introduced to speak before a room of two hundred rambunctious teens, something came over me—a certain boldness that I can't describe. I shared my story in greater and more dramatic detail than I have here, and half of the youth group gave their hearts to Christ that day. That day I found my gift, or talent. I found that intangible that could only be given from God. Just as a singer finds his or her voice, I found what God had placed on the inside of me.

Ever since then, I've known exactly what God created me to do. These days, I speak for a living, and I know I'm living a life of prayer and purpose. These days I tell audiences that God has a plan and a purpose for their lives.

So if you're wondering what your purpose is, I urge you to examine your heart. Find your gift, and you'll fulfill your purpose. When you find and use your natural gift or talent, God will bless everything it touches. And you will know it.

You know why? Because then you are living your life for God, not yourself. Your life is not about you—it's about Christ in you and through you. God is waiting for you to discover a powerful purpose that will shape your life.

Knowing where you come from is critical so that you can know where you are going. Many people spend their time chasing dreams in their hearts, but they neglect the very thing that God created them to do. God is waiting for you to discover his powerful purpose that will shape your life. Once you find that, you will find true success in all that you do.

THE GREAT PHYSICIAN'S Rx FOR LIVING A LIFE OF PRAYER AND PURPOSE

- *Pray continually.*

- *Confess God's promises the first thing upon waking and the last thing before you retire.*

- *Find God's purpose for your life and live it.*

- *Be an agent of change in your life, the life of your family, the life of your church, the life of your organization, the life of your community, and the life of your region.*

THE GREAT PHYSICIAN'S Rx FOR WEEK #7

Day 43

Upon Waking

Prayer: thank God because this is the day that the Lord has made. Rejoice and be glad in it. Thank Him for the breath in your lungs and the life in your body. Pray and confess the following Scripture out loud:

Our Father in heaven,
Hallowed be Your name.
Your kingdom come.
Your will be done
On earth as it is in heaven.
Give us this day our daily bread.
And forgive us our debts,
As we forgive our debtors.
And do not lead us into temptation,
But deliver us from the evil one.
For Yours is the kingdom and the power and the glory forever. Amen.
(Matt. 6:9–13 NKJV)

Purpose: ask the Lord to give you an opportunity to add significance to someone's life today. Watch for that opportunity. Ask God to use you this day for His intended purpose.

Advanced hygiene: practice advanced hygiene. See page 325 for guidance.

Reduce toxins: open windows for one hour today. Use natural soap and natural skin and body care products (shower gel, body creams, etc.). Use natural facial care products. Use natural toothpaste. Use natural hair care products such as shampoo, conditioner, gel, mousse, and hairspray.

Supplements: take one serving of a fiber/green superfood powder (mixed in) or five caplets of a super green formula (swallowed with) twelve-to-sixteen ounces of water or raw vegetable juice. (See the GPRx Resource Guide, pages 346–347, for recommended products.)

Body therapy: get twenty minutes of direct sunlight.

Exercise: perform functional fitness exercises for fifteen minutes (three rounds of exercises found in Key #4, pages 138–145) or spend fifteen minutes on the rebounder. Finish with ten minutes of deep-breathing exercises.

Emotional health: when you face a circumstance that would usually cause you to worry, repeat the following: "Lord, I trust You. I cast my cares upon You, and I believe that You're going to take care of [insert your current situation]." Confess that throughout the day whenever you think about your circumstance.

Breakfast

Creamsicle Smoothie (see appendix A, page 322, for recipe) with two tablespoons of protein powder (optional)

hot tea with honey (see the GPRx Resource Guide, page 339, for recommended herbal tea blends)

Supplements: take one or two whole food multivitamin caplets and one or two capsules of a probiotic/enzyme blend (see the GPRx Resource Guide, pages 345–348, for recommended products).

Lunch

Before eating, drink eight ounces of water.

During lunch, drink eight ounces of water or hot or iced fresh-brewed tea with honey.

salmon salad on a bed of greens or on sprouted whole grain or sourdough bread

apple or pear

Supplements: take one or two whole food multivitamin caplets and one or two capsules of a probiotic/enzyme blend.

Dinner

Before eating, drink eight ounces of water.

During dinner, drink hot or iced fresh-brewed tea with honey.

Rare-Seared Tuna with Brown Rice (see appendix A, page 300, for recipe)

grilled asparagus, mushrooms, and onions

Italian Salad (see appendix A, page 277, for recipe)

Supplements: take one or two whole food multivitamin caplets, one-to-three teaspoons or three-to-nine caplsules of high omega-3 cod-liver oil (see the GPRx Resource Guide, pages 345–346, for recommended products), and one or two capsules of a probiotic/enzyme blend.

Snacks

apple-cinnamon fiber whole food bar (with beta glucans from soluble oat fiber; see the GPRx Resource Guide, pages 329–330, for recommended products)

piece of fruit

Drink eight-to-twelve ounces of water or hot or iced fresh-brewed tea with honey.

Before Bed

Drink eight-to-twelve ounces of water or hot tea with honey.

Exercise: go for a walk outdoors or participate in a favorite sport or recreational activity.

Supplements: take one serving of a fiber/green superfood powder (mixed in) or five caplets of a super green formula (swallowed with) twelve-to-sixteen ounces of water or raw vegetable juice.

Body therapy: take a warm bath for fifteen minutes with eight drops of biblical essential oils added.

Advanced hygiene: practice advanced hygiene. See page 325 for guidance.

Emotional health (only applicable if there are still people you need to forgive): ask the Lord to bring to your mind someone you need to forgive. Take out a sheet of paper and write the person's name at the top. Try to remember each specific action that person did against you that brought you pain. Write down the following: "I forgive [insert person's name] for [insert the action he or she did against you]." After you fill up the paper, tear it up or burn it, and ask God to give you the strength to truly forgive that person.

Purpose: ask yourself this question: "Did I live a life of purpose today?" What did you do to add value to someone else's life today? Commit to living a day of purpose tomorrow.

Prayer: thank God for this day, asking Him to give you a restoring night's rest and a fresh start tomorrow. Thank Him for His steadfast love that never ceases and His mercies new every morning. Pray and confess the following Scripture out loud:

> *Who shall separate us from the love of Christ? Shall tribulation, or distress, or persecution, or famine, or nakedness, or peril, or sword? . . . Yet in all these things we are more than conquerors through Him who loved us. For I am persuaded that neither death nor life, nor angels nor principalities nor powers, nor things present nor things to come, nor height nor depth, nor any other created thing, shall be able to separate us from the love of God which is in Christ Jesus our Lord.* (Rom. 8:35, 37–39 NKJV)

Sleep: go to bed by 10:30 p.m.

Day 44

Upon Waking

Prayer: thank God because this is the day that the Lord has made. Rejoice and be glad in it. Thank Him for the breath in your lungs and the life in your body. Pray and confess the following Scripture out loud:

> *He who dwells in the secret place of the Most High shall abide under the shadow of the Almighty. I will say of the LORD, "He is my refuge and my fortress; my God, in Him I will trust." Surely He shall deliver me from the snare of the fowler and from the perilous pestilence. He shall cover me with His feathers, and under His wings I shall take refuge; His truth shall be my shield and buckler. I*

shall not be afraid of the terror by night, nor of the arrow that flies by day, nor of the pestilence that walks in darkness, nor of the destruction that lays waste at noonday. A thousand may fall at my side, and ten thousand at my right hand; but it shall not come near me. Only with my eyes shall I look and see the reward of the wicked. Because I have made the LORD, who is my refuge, even the Most High, my dwelling place, no evil shall befall me, nor shall any plague come near my dwelling; for He shall give His angels charge over me, to keep me in all my ways. In their hands shall they bear me up, lest I dash my foot against a stone. I shall tread upon the lion and the cobra, the young lion and the serpent I shall trample underfoot. Because I have set my love upon Him, therefore He will deliver me; He will set me on high, because I have known His name. I shall call upon Him, and He will answer me. He will be with me in trouble; He will deliver me and honor me. With long life He will satisfy me, and show me His salvation. (adapted from Psalm 91 NKJV, in the first person)

Purpose: ask the Lord to give you an opportunity to add significance to someone's life today. Watch for that opportunity. Ask God to use you this day for His intended purpose.

Advanced hygiene: practice advanced hygiene. See page 325 for guidance.

Reduce toxins: open windows for one hour today. Use natural soap and natural skin and body care products (shower gel, body creams, etc.). Use natural facial care products. Use natural toothpaste. Use natural hair care products such as shampoo, conditioner, gel, mousse, and hairspray.

Supplements: take one serving of a fiber/green superfood powder (mixed in) or five caplets of a super green formula (swallowed with) twelve-to-sixteen ounces of water or raw vegetable juice. (See the GPRx Resource Guide, pages 346–347, for recommended products.)

Exercise: perform functional fitness exercises for fifteen minutes (three rounds of exercises found in Key #4, pages 138–145) or spend fifteen minutes on the rebounder. Finish with ten minutes of deep-breathing exercises.

Body therapy: take a hot and cold shower. After normal shower, alternate sixty seconds of water as hot as you can stand it, followed by sixty seconds of water as cold as you can stand it. Repeat cycle four times for a total of eight minutes, finishing with cold.

Emotional health: when you face a circumstance that would usually cause you to worry, repeat the following: "Lord, I trust You. I cast my cares upon You, and I believe that You're going to take care of [insert your current situation]." Confess that throughout the day whenever you think about your circumstance.

Breakfast
two soft-boiled eggs
one piece of whole grain sprouted or sourdough toast and butter
grapefruit
hot tea with honey

Supplements: take one or two whole food multivitamin caplets and one or two capsules of a probiotic/enzyme blend.

Lunch

Before eating, drink eight ounces of water.

During lunch, drink eight ounces of water or hot or iced fresh-brewed tea with honey.

Tropical Chicken and Vegetable Kabobs (see appendix A, page 289, for recipe)

Supplements: take one or two whole food multivitamin caplets and one or two capsules of a probiotic/enzyme blend.

Dinner

Before eating, drink eight ounces of water.

During dinner, drink hot or iced fresh-brewed tea with honey.

Wood-Grilled Buffalo Tenderloin (see appendix A, page 300, for recipe)

sautéed asparagus and mushrooms

green salad

Simple Lentils (see appendix A, page 278, for recipe)

Supplements: take one or two whole food multivitamin caplets, one-to-three teaspoons or three-to-nine capsules of high omega-3 cod-liver oil, and one or two capsules of a probiotic/enzyme blend.

Snacks

cottage cheese and pineapple

berry smoothie mix blended with eight-to-twelve ounces of water (see the GPRx Resource Guide, page 329, for recommended products).

Crispy Walnuts (see appendix A, page 270, for recipe for Crispy Almonds)

Drink eight-to-twelve ounces of water or hot or iced fresh-brewed tea with honey.

Before Bed

Drink eight-to-twelve ounces of water or hot tea with honey.

Exercise: go for a walk outdoors or participate in a favorite sport or recreational activity.

Supplements: take one serving of a fiber/green superfood powder (mixed in) or five caplets of a super green formula (swallowed with) twelve-to-sixteen ounces of water or raw vegetable juice.

Advanced hygiene: practice advanced hygiene. See page 325 for guidance.

Emotional health (only applicable if there are still people you need to forgive): ask the Lord to bring to your mind someone you need to forgive. Take out a sheet of paper and write the person's name at the top. Try to remember each specific action that person did against you that brought you pain. Write down the following: "I forgive [insert person's name] for [insert the action he or she did against you]." After you fill up the paper, tear it up or burn it, and ask God to give you the strength to truly forgive that person.

Purpose: ask yourself this question: "Did I live a life of purpose today?" What did you do to add value to someone else's life today? Commit to living a day of purpose tomorrow.

Prayer: thank God for this day, asking Him to give you a restoring night's rest and a fresh start tomorrow. Thank Him for His steadfast love that never ceases and His mercies that are new every morning. Pray and confess the following Scripture out loud:

> *Love is patient, love is kind and is not jealous; loves does not brag and is not arrogant, does not act unbecomingly; it does not seek its own, is not provoked, does not take into account a wrong suffered, does not rejoice in unrighteousness, but rejoices with the truth; bears all things, believes all things, hopes all things, endures all things. Love never fails.* (1 Cor. 13:4–8 NASB)

Body therapy: spend ten minutes listening to soothing music before you retire.
Sleep: go to bed by 10:30 p.m.

Day 45

Upon Waking

Prayer: thank God because this is the day that the Lord has made. Rejoice and be glad in it. Thank Him for the breath in your lungs and the life in your body. Pray and confess the following Scripture out loud:

> *I put on the whole armor of God, that I may be able to withstand in the evil day, and having done all, to stand. I stand therefore, having girded my waist with truth, having put on the breastplate of righteousness, and having shod my feet with the preparation of the gospel of peace; above all, taking the shield of faith with which I will be able to quench all the fiery darts of the wicked one. And I take the helmet of salvation, and the sword of the Spirit, which is the word of God; praying always with all prayer and supplication in the Spirit, being watchful to this end with all perseverance and supplication for all the saints.* (adapted from Ephesians 6:13–18 NKJV, in first person)

Purpose: ask the Lord to give you an opportunity to add significance to someone's life today. Watch for that opportunity. Ask God to use you this day for His intended purpose.

Advanced hygiene: practice advanced hygiene. See page 325 for guidance.

Reduce toxins: open windows for one hour today. Use natural soap and natural skin and body care products (shower gel, body creams, etc.). Use natural facial care products. Use natural toothpaste. Use natural hair care products such as shampoo, conditioner, gel, mousse, and hairspray.

Supplements: take one serving of a fiber/green superfood powder (mixed in) or five caplets of a super green formula (swallowed with) twelve-to-sixteen ounces of water or raw vegetable juice. (See the GPRx Resource Guide, pages 346–347, for recommended products.)

Exercise: perform functional fitness exercises for fifteen minutes (three rounds of exercises found in Key #4, pages 138–145) or spend fifteen minutes on the rebounder. Finish with ten minutes of deep-breathing exercises.

Body therapy: get twenty minutes of direct sunlight.

Emotional health: when you face a circumstance that would usually cause you to worry, repeat the following: "Lord, I trust You. I cast my cares upon You, and I believe that You're going to take care of [insert your current situation]." Confess that throughout the day whenever you think about your circumstance.

Breakfast

sprouted dry cereal with yogurt, goat's milk, or almond milk

banana

hot tea with honey

Supplements: take one or two whole food multivitamin caplets and one or two capsules of a probiotic/enzyme blend.

Lunch

Before eating, drink eight ounces of water.

During lunch, drink eight ounces of water or hot or iced fresh-brewed tea with honey.

Oriental Salmon Salad (see appendix A, page 303, for recipe)

apple

Supplements: take one or two whole food multivitamin caplets and one or two capsules of a probiotic/enzyme blend.

Dinner

Before eating, drink eight ounces of water.

During dinner, drink hot or iced fresh-brewed tea with honey.

Thai-Spiced Steak and Vegetables (see appendix A, page 295, for recipe)

Easy Brown Rice (see appendix A, page 278, for recipe)

Miso Soup (see appendix A, page 278, for recipe)

Supplements: take one or two whole food multivitamin caplets, one-to-three teaspoons or three-to-nine capsules of high omega-3 cod-liver oil, and one or two capsules of a probiotic/enzyme blend.

Snacks

crackers, cheese, and fruit

raspberry super green whole food bar (see the GPRx Resource Guide, pages 329–330, for recommended products)

Drink eight-to-twelve ounces of water or hot or iced fresh-brewed tea with honey.

Before Bed

Drink eight-to-twelve ounces of water or hot tea with honey.

Exercise: go for a walk outdoors or participate in a favorite sport or recreational activity.

Supplements: take one serving of a fiber/green superfood powder (mixed in) or five caplets of a super green formula (swallowed with) twelve-to-sixteen ounces of water or raw vegetable juice.

Advanced hygiene: practice advanced hygiene. See page 325 for guidance.

Emotional health (only applicable if there are still people you need to forgive): ask the Lord to bring to your mind someone you need to forgive. Take out a sheet of paper and write the person's name at the top. Try to remember each specific action that person did against you that brought you pain. Write down the following: "I forgive [insert person's name] for [insert the action he or she did against you]." After you fill up the paper, tear it up or burn it, and ask God to give you the strength to truly forgive that person.

Body therapy: take a warm bath for fifteen minutes with eight drops of biblical essential oils added.

Purpose: ask yourself this question: "Did I live a life of purpose today?" What did you do to add value to someone else's life today? Commit to living a day of purpose tomorrow.

Prayer: thank God for this day, asking Him to give you a restoring night's rest and a fresh start tomorrow. Thank Him for His steadfast love that never ceases and His mercies that are new every morning. Pray and confess the following Scripture out loud:

> *Rejoice in the Lord always. Again I will say, rejoice! Let your gentleness be known to all men. The Lord is at hand. Be anxious for nothing, but in everything by prayer and supplication, with thanksgiving, let your requests be made known to God; and the peace of God, which surpasses all understanding, will guard your hearts and minds through Christ Jesus . . . Finally, brethren, whatever things are true, whatever things are noble, whatever things are just, whatever things are pure, whatever things are lovely, whatever things are of good report, if there is any virtue and if there is anything praiseworthy—meditate on these things . . . Not that I speak in regard to need, for I have learned in whatever state I am, to be content: I know how to be abased, and I know how to abound. Everywhere and in all things I have learned both to be full and to be hungry, both to abound and to suffer need. I can do all things through Christ who strengthens me . . . And my God shall supply all your need according to His riches in glory by Christ Jesus.* (Phil. 4:4–8, 11–13, 19 NKJV)

Sleep: go to bed by 10:30 p.m.

Day 46

Upon Waking

Prayer: thank God because this is the day that the Lord has made. Rejoice and be glad in it. Thank Him for the breath in your lungs and the life in your body. Pray and confess the following Scripture out loud:

Our Father in heaven,
Hallowed be Your name.
Your kingdom come.
Your will be done
On earth as it is in heaven.
Give us this day our daily bread.
And forgive us our debts,
As we forgive our debtors.
And do not lead us into temptation,
But deliver us from the evil one.
For Yours is the kingdom and the power and the glory forever. Amen.
(Matt. 6:9–13 NKJV)

Purpose: ask the Lord to give you an opportunity to add significance to someone's life today. Watch for that opportunity. Ask God to use you this day for His intended purpose.

Advanced hygiene: practice advanced hygiene. See page 325 for guidance.

Reduce toxins: open windows for one hour today. Use natural soap and natural skin and body care products (shower gel, body creams, etc.). Use natural facial care products. Use natural toothpaste. Use natural hair care products such as shampoo, conditioner, gel, mousse, and hairspray.

Supplements: take one serving of a fiber/green superfood powder (mixed in) or five caplets of a super green formula (swallowed with) twelve-to-sixteen ounces of water or raw vegetable juice. (See the GPRx Resource Guide, pages 346–347, for recommended products.)

Exercise: perform functional fitness exercises for fifteen minutes (three rounds of exercises found in Key #4, pages 138–145) or spend fifteen minutes on the rebounder. Finish with ten minutes of deep-breathing exercises.

Body therapy: take a hot and cold shower. After normal shower, alternate sixty seconds of water as hot as you can stand it, followed by sixty seconds of water as cold as you can stand it. Repeat cycle four times for a total of eight minutes, finishing with cold.

Emotional health: when you face a circumstance that would usually cause you to worry, repeat the following: "Lord, I trust You. I cast my cares upon You, and I believe that You're going to take care of [insert your current situation]." Confess that throughout the day whenever you think about your circumstance.

Breakfast

Banana Peach Smoothie (see appendix A, page 320, for recipe) with two tablespoons protein powder (optional)

hot tea with honey

Supplements: take one or two whole food multivitamin caplets and one or two capsules of a probiotic/enzyme blend.

Lunch

Before eating, drink eight ounces of water.

During lunch, drink eight ounces of water or hot or iced fresh-brewed tea with honey.

Turkey and Goat Cheese Wrap

grapes

Supplements: take one or two whole food multivitamin caplets and one or two capsules of a probiotic/enzyme blend.

Dinner

Before eating, drink eight ounces of water.

During dinner, drink hot or iced fresh-brewed tea with honey.

Herb-Baked Salmon with Creamed-Style Spinach

steamed broccoli

green salad

Supplements: take one or two whole food multivitamin caplets, one-to-three teaspoons or three-to-nine capsules of high omega-3 cod-liver oil, and one or two capsules of a probiotic/enzyme blend.

Snacks

apple and carrots with almond butter

tropical smoothie mix blended in eight-to-twelve ounces of water (see the GPRx Resource Guide, page 329, for recommended products)

Ginger Muffins with butter (see appendix A, page 272, for recipe)

Drink eight-to-twelve ounces of water or hot or iced fresh-brewed tea with honey.

Before Bed

Drink eight-to-twelve ounces of water or hot tea with honey.

Exercise: go for a walk outdoors or participate in a favorite sport or recreational activity.

Supplements: take one serving of a fiber/green superfood powder (mixed in) or five caplets of a super green formula (swallowed with) twelve-to-sixteen ounces of water or raw vegetable juice.

Advanced hygiene: practice advanced hygiene. See page 325 for guidance.

Emotional health (only applicable if there are still people you need to forgive): ask the Lord to bring to your mind someone you need to forgive. Take out a sheet of paper and write the person's name at the top. Try to remember each specific action that person did against you that brought you pain. Write down the following: "I forgive [insert person's name] for [insert the action he or she did against you]." After you fill up the paper, tear it up or burn it, and ask God to give you the strength to truly forgive that person.

Purpose: ask yourself this question: "Did I live a life of purpose today?" What did you do to add value to someone else's life today? Commit to living a day of purpose tomorrow.

Prayer: thank God for this day, asking Him to give you a restoring night's rest and a fresh start tomorrow. Thank Him for His steadfast love that never ceases and His mercies that are new every morning. Pray and confess the following Scripture out loud:

> *Who shall separate us from the love of Christ? Shall tribulation, or distress, or persecution, or famine, or nakedness, or peril, or sword? . . . Yet in all these things we are more than conquerors through Him who loved us. For I am persuaded that neither death nor life, nor angels nor principalities nor powers, nor things present nor things to come, nor height nor depth, nor any other created thing, shall be able to separate us from the love of God which is in Christ Jesus our Lord.* (Rom. 8:35, 37–39 NJKV)

Body therapy: spend ten minutes listening to soothing music before you retire.
Sleep: go to bed by 10:30 p.m.

Day 47 (Partial Fast Day)

Upon Waking
Prayer: thank God because this is the day that the Lord has made. Rejoice and be glad in it. Thank Him for the breath in your lungs and the life in your body. Pray and confess the following Scripture out loud:

> *Is this not the fast that I have chosen: to loose the bonds of wickedness, to undo the heavy burdens, to let the oppressed go free, and that you break every yoke? Is it not to share your bread with the hungry, and that you bring to your house the poor who are cast out; when you see the naked, that you cover him, and not hide yourself from your own flesh? Then your light shall break forth like the morning, your healing shall spring forth speedily, and your righteousness shall go before you; the glory of the LORD shall be your rear guard. Then you shall call, and the LORD will answer; you shall cry, and He will say, "Here I am."* (Isa. 58:6–9 NKJV)

Purpose: ask the Lord to give you an opportunity to add significance to someone's life today. Watch for that opportunity. Ask God to use you this day for His intended purpose.
Advanced hygiene: practice advanced hygiene. See page 325 for guidance.
Reduce toxins: open windows for one hour today. Use natural soap and natural skin and body care products (shower gel, body creams, etc.). Use natural facial care products. Use natural toothpaste. Use natural hair care products such as shampoo, conditioner, gel, mousse, and hairspray.
Supplements: take one serving of a fiber/green superfood powder (mixed in) or five caplets of a super green formula (swallowed with) twelve-to-sixteen ounces of water or raw vegetable juice. (See the GPRx Resource Guide, pages 346–347, for recommended products.)
Exercise: perform functional fitness exercises for fifteen minutes (three rounds of exercises found in Key #4, pages 138–145) or spend fifteen minutes on the rebounder. Finish with ten minutes of deep-breathing exercises.

Body therapy: get twenty minutes of direct sunlight.

Emotional health: when you face a circumstance that would usually cause you to worry, repeat the following: "Lord, I trust You. I cast my cares upon You, and I believe that You're going to take care of [insert your current situation]." Confess that throughout the day whenever you think about your circumstance.

Breakfast

none (partial fast day)

eight-to-twelve ounces of water

Supplements: take one or two whole food multivitamin caplets and one or two capsules of a probiotic/enzyme blend.

Lunch

none (partial fast day)

eight ounces of water

Supplements: take one or two whole food multivitamin caplets and one or two capsules of a probiotic/enzyme blend.

Dinner

Before eating, drink eight ounces of water.

During dinner, drink hot or iced fresh-brewed tea with honey.

Chicken Soup

cultured vegetables

Oriental Salmon Salad (see appendix A, page 303, for recipe)

Supplements: take one or two whole food multivitamin caplets, one-to-three teaspoons or three-to-nine capsules of high omega-3 cod-liver oil, and one or two capsules of a probiotic/enzyme blend.

Snacks

none (partial fast day)

eight ounces of water

Before Bed

Drink eight-to-twelve ounces of water or hot tea with honey.

Exercise: go for a walk outdoors or participate in a favorite sport or recreational activity.

Supplements: take one serving of a fiber/green superfood powder (mixed in) or five caplets of a super green formula (swallowed with) twelve-to-sixteen ounces of water or raw vegetable juice.

Advanced hygiene: practice advanced hygiene. See page 325 for guidance.

Emotional health (only applicable if there are still people you need to forgive): ask the Lord to bring to your mind someone you need to forgive. Take out a sheet of paper and write the person's name at the top. Try to remember each specific action that person did against you that brought you pain. Write down the following: "I forgive [insert person's name] for [insert the action he or she did against you]." After you fill up the paper, tear it up or burn it, and ask God to give you the strength to truly forgive that person.

Body therapy: take a warm bath for fifteen minutes with eight drops of biblical essential oils added.

Purpose: ask yourself this question: "Did I live a life of purpose today?" What did you do to add value to someone else's life today? Commit to living a day of purpose tomorrow.

Prayer: thank God for this day, asking Him to give you a restoring night's rest and a fresh start tomorrow. Thank Him for His steadfast love that never ceases and His mercies that are new every morning. Pray and confess the following Scripture out loud:

> *Is this not the fast that I have chosen: to loose the bonds of wickedness, to undo the heavy burdens, to let the oppressed go free, and that you break every yoke? Is it not to share your bread with the hungry, and that you bring to your house the poor who are cast out; when you see the naked, that you cover him, and not hide yourself from your own flesh? Then your light shall break forth like the morning, your healing shall spring forth speedily, and your righteousness shall go before you; the glory of the LORD shall be your rear guard. Then you shall call, and the LORD will answer; you shall cry, and He will say, "Here I am."* (Isa. 58:6–9 NKJV)

Sleep: go to bed by 10:30 p.m.

Day 48 (Day of Rest)

Upon Waking

Prayer: thank God because this is the day that the Lord has made. Rejoice and be glad in it. Thank Him for the breath in your lungs and the life in your body. Pray and confess the following Scripture out loud:

> *The LORD is my shepherd; I shall not want. He makes me to lie down in green pastures; He leads me beside the still waters. He restores my soul; He leads me in the paths of righteousness for His name's sake. Yea, though I walk through the valley of the shadow of death, I will fear no evil; for You are with me; Your rod and Your staff, they comfort me. You prepare a table before me in the presence of my enemies; You anoint my head with oil; my cup runs over. Surely goodness and mercy shall follow me all the days of my life; and I will dwell in the house of the LORD forever.* (Ps. 23 NKJV)

Purpose: ask the Lord to give you an opportunity to add significance to someone's life today. Watch for that opportunity. Ask God to use you this day for His intended purpose.

Advanced hygiene: practice advanced hygiene. See page 325 for guidance.

Reduce toxins: open windows for one hour today. Use natural soap and natural skin and body care products (shower gel, body creams, etc.). Use natural facial care products. Use natural toothpaste. Use natural hair care products such as shampoo, conditioner, gel, mousse, and hairspray.

Supplements: take one serving of a fiber/green superfood powder (mixed in) or five caplets of a super green formula (swallowed with) twelve-to-sixteen ounces of water or raw vegetable juice. (See the GPRx Resource Guide, pages 346–347, for recommended products.)

Exercise: do no formal exercise since it's a day of rest.

Body therapies: do none since it's a rest day.

Emotional health: when you face a circumstance that would usually cause you to worry, repeat the following: "Lord, I trust You. I cast my cares upon You, and I believe that You're going to take care of [insert your current situation]." Confess that throughout the day whenever you think about your circumstance.

Breakfast
Turkey Sausage Queen Omelet (see appendix A, page 285, for recipe)
whole grain English muffin
grapefruit or orange
hot tea with honey
Supplements: take one or two whole food multivitamin caplets and one or two capsules of a probiotic/enzyme blend.

Lunch
Before eating, drink eight ounces of water.
During lunch, drink eight ounces of water or hot or iced fresh-brewed tea with honey.
Red Meat Chili (see appendix A, page 305, for recipe)
crackers
Supplements: take one or two whole food multivitamin caplets and one or two capsules of a probiotic/enzyme blend.

Dinner
Before eating, drink eight ounces of water.
During dinner, drink hot or iced fresh-brewed tea with honey.
Marinated Baked Salmon with Capers (see appendix A, page 290, for recipe)
Cinnamon Sweet Potatoes (see appendix A, page 285, for recipe)
green salad
Supplements: take one or two whole food multivitamin caplets, one-to-three teaspoons or three-to-nine capsules of high omega-3 cod-liver oil, and one or two capsules of a probiotic/enzyme blend.

Snacks
Healthy Trail Mix (see appendix A, page 271, for recipe)

berry smoothie mix mixed in eight-to-twelve ounces of water (see the GPRx Resource Guide, page 329, for recommended products)

cottage cheese, honey, and berries

Drink eight-to-twelve ounces of water or hot or iced fresh-brewed tea with honey.

Before Bed

Drink eight-to-twelve ounces of water or hot tea with honey.

Exercise: go for a walk outdoors or participate in a favorite sport or recreational activity.

Supplements: take one serving of a fiber/green superfood powder (mixed in) or five caplets of a super green formula (swallowed with) twelve-to-sixteen ounces of water or raw vegetable juice.

Advanced hygiene: practice advanced hygiene. See page 325 for guidance.

Emotional health (only applicable if there are still people you need to forgive): ask the Lord to bring to your mind someone you need to forgive. Take out a sheet of paper and write the person's name at the top. Try to remember each specific action that person did against you that brought you pain. Write down the following: "I forgive [insert person's name] for [insert the action he or she did against you]." After you fill up the paper, tear it up or burn it, and ask God to give you the strength to truly forgive that person.

Purpose: ask yourself this question: "Did I live a life of purpose today?" What did you do to add value to someone else's life today? Commit to living a day of purpose tomorrow.

Prayer: thank God for this day, asking Him to give you a restoring night's rest and a fresh start tomorrow. Thank Him for His steadfast love that never ceases and His mercies that are new every morning. Pray and confess the following Scripture out loud:

> The LORD is my shepherd; I shall not want. He makes me to lie down in green pastures; He leads me beside the still waters. He restores my soul; He leads me in the paths of righteousness for His name's sake. Yea, though I walk through the valley of the shadow of death, I will fear no evil; for You are with me; Your rod and Your staff, they comfort me. You prepare a table before me in the presence of my enemies; You anoint my head with oil; my cup runs over. Surely goodness and mercy shall follow me all the days of my life; and I will dwell in the house of the LORD forever. (Ps. 23 NKJV)

Body therapy: spend ten minutes listening to soothing music before you retire.

Sleep: go to bed by 10:30 p.m.

Day 49

Upon Waking

Prayer: thank God because this is the day that the Lord has made. Rejoice and be glad in it. Thank Him for the breath in your lungs and the life in your body. Pray and confess the following Scripture out loud:

> *He who dwells in the secret place of the Most High shall abide under the shadow of the Almighty. I will say of the LORD, "He is my refuge and my fortress; my God, in Him I will trust." Surely He shall deliver me from the snare of the fowler and from the perilous pestilence. He shall cover me with His feathers, and under His wings I shall take refuge; His truth shall be my shield and buckler. I shall not be afraid of the terror by night, nor of the arrow that flies by day, nor of the pestilence that walks in darkness, nor of the destruction that lays waste at noonday. A thousand may fall at my side, and ten thousand at my right hand; but it shall not come near me. Only with my eyes shall I look and see the reward of the wicked. Because I have made the LORD, who is my refuge, even the Most High, my dwelling place, no evil shall befall me, nor shall any plague come near my dwelling; for He shall give His angels charge over me, to keep me in all my ways. In their hands shall they bear me up, lest I dash my foot against a stone. I shall tread upon the lion and the cobra, the young lion and the serpent I shall trample underfoot. Because I have set my love upon Him, therefore He will deliver me; He will set me on high, because I have known His name. I shall call upon Him, and He will answer me. He will be with me in trouble; He will deliver me and honor me. With long life He will satisfy me, and show me His salvation.* (Ps. 91 NKJV, in the first person)

Purpose: ask the Lord to give you an opportunity to add significance to someone's life today. Watch for that opportunity. Ask God to use you this day for His intended purpose.

Advanced hygiene: practice advanced hygiene. See page 325 for guidance.

Reduce toxins: open windows for one hour today. Use natural soap and natural skin and body care products (shower gel, body creams, etc.). Use natural facial care products. Use natural toothpaste. Use natural hair care products such as shampoo, conditioner, gel, mousse, and hairspray.

Supplements: take one serving of a fiber/green superfood powder (mixed in) or five caplets of a super green formula (swallowed with) twelve-to-sixteen ounces of water or raw vegetable juice. (See the GPRx Resource Guide, pages 346–347, for recommended products.)

Exercise: perform functional fitness exercises for fifteen minutes (three rounds of exercises found in Key #4, pages 138–145) or spend fifteen minutes on the rebounder. Finish with ten minutes of deep-breathing exercises.

Body therapy: get twenty minutes of direct sunlight.

Emotional health: when you face a circumstance that would usually cause you to worry, repeat the following: "Lord, I trust You. I cast my cares upon You, and I believe that You're going to take care of [insert your current situation]." Confess that throughout the day whenever you think about your circumstance.

Breakfast

Mexican Omelet (see appendix A, page 267, for recipe)
Easy Whole Grain Waffles (see appendix A, page 322, for recipe)
hot tea with honey
Supplements: take one or two whole food multivitamin caplets and one or two capsules of a probiotic/enzyme blend.

Lunch

Before eating, drink eight ounces of water.
During lunch, drink eight ounces of water or hot or iced fresh-brewed tea with honey.
Tuna Tahini Salad (see appendix A, page 279, for recipe)
Supplements: take one or two whole food multivitamin caplets and one or two capsules of a probiotic/enzyme blend.

Dinner

Before eating, drink eight ounces of water.
During dinner, drink hot or iced fresh-brewed tea with honey.
Beef Burgundy (see appendix A, page 322, for recipe)
Blue Corn Posole (see appendix A, page 286, for recipe)
Garlicky Green Beans (see appendix A, page 283, for recipe)
Supplements: take one or two whole food multivitamin caplets, one-to-three teaspoons or three-to-nine capsules of high omega-3 cod-liver oil, and one or two capsules of a probiotic/enzyme blend.

Snacks

baked corn chips with cheese, salsa, guacamole, or hummus
vanilla protein whole food bar (see the GPRx Resource Guide, pages 329–330, for recommended products)
Drink eight-to-twelve ounces of water or hot or iced fresh-brewed tea with honey.

Before Bed

Drink eight-to-twelve ounces of water or hot tea with honey.
Exercise: go for a walk outdoors or participate in a favorite sport or recreational activity.
Supplements: take one serving of a fiber/green superfood powder (mixed in) or five caplets of a super green formula (swallowed with) twelve-to-sixteen ounces of water or raw vegetable juice.
Advanced hygiene: practice advanced hygiene. See page 325 for guidance.
Emotional health (only applicable if there are still people you need to forgive): ask

the Lord to bring to your mind someone you need to forgive. Take out a sheet of paper and write the person's name at the top. Try to remember each specific action that person did against you that brought you pain. Write down the following: "I forgive [insert person's name] for [insert the action he or she did against you]." After you fill up the paper, tear it up or burn it, and ask God to give you the strength to truly forgive that person.

Body therapy: take a warm bath for fifteen minutes with eight drops of biblical essential oils added.

Purpose: ask yourself this question: "Did I live a life of purpose today?" What did you do to add value to someone else's life today? Commit to living a day of purpose tomorrow.

Prayer: thank God for this day, asking Him to give you a restoring night's rest and a fresh start tomorrow. Thank Him for His steadfast love that never ceases and His mercies that are new every morning. Pray and confess the following Scripture out loud:

> *Love is patient, love is kind and is not jealous; loves does not brag and is not arrogant, does not act unbecomingly; it does not seek its own, is not provoked, does not take into account a wrong suffered, does not rejoice in unrighteousness, but rejoices with the truth; bears all things, believes all things, hopes all things, endures all things. Love never fails.* (1 Cor. 13:4–8 NASB)

Sleep: go to bed by 10:30 p.m.

Day 50 (Jubilee Day)

Proclaim liberty throughout all the land to all its inhabitants. It shall be a Jubilee for you.

—Leviticus 25:10 (NKJV)

If you have been faithful to the Great Physician's Rx for the last forty-nine days, then I offer you heartfelt congratulations. This is the day to celebrate your success and renewed physical, mental, emotional, and spiritual health. Treat yourself to any foods you want, except for the Dirty Dozen, of course.

If you still have a little farther to go, however—some pounds to lose, high blood pressure to deal with, some achy joints or unresolved digestive complaints—I encourage you to commit forty more days to take your health to an even higher level by undertaking the forty-day health experience called the Maker's Diet.

If you do not have a copy of *The Maker's Diet,* I would like to offer you a free copy of this revolutionary book as well as an opportunity to receive the Maker's Diet daily newsletter to help you navigate on your road to greater health and wellness. Please log on to www.JordanRubin.com and take your next step on the road to wellness.

If you're happy with your newfound level of health and want to continue on to wellness, I encourage you to log onto www.TheGreatPhysiciansRx.com and embark on the Lifetime of Wellness plan. This plan incorporates all of the principles of *The Great Physician's Rx* with the special three-cheats-a-week bonus meals. The Lifetime of Wellness plan is simply the most doable and effective health plan for you and your family.

I hope you'll let me close by allowing me to pray over you the priestly blessing from Numbers 6:24–26:

> *May the Lord bless you and keep you.*
> *May the Lord make His face to shine upon you and be gracious to you,*
> *May the Lord lift up His countenance upon you and give you peace,*
> *In the name of the Lord Jesus our Messiah,*
> *Amen*

Appendix A

Recipes

Several people whom I greatly admire and appreciate contributed their recipes to the 49–Day meal plan:

- Sally Fallon, founder and president of the Weston A. Price Foundation.
- Richard and James Thomas, owners of R. Thomas Deluxe Grill in Atlanta.
- Sheila Barcelo of Eden's Gourmet, a catering company in Central Florida.
- Mike and Margie Perrin, owners of 11 Maple Street Restaurant in Jensen Beach, Florida.
- My lovely and gracious wife, Nicki, and some of our friends.

Depending on whether you're as handy around the kitchen as Emeril Lagasse or a bit intimidated by the process, I urge you to roll up your sleeves and give these recipes a try. Some are easier than others, so feel free to substitute a more complex recipe for something easier—or tastier. Actually, all these recipes are delicious, so bon appetit!

Sally Fallon

Sally Fallon is the author of the groundbreaking book *Nourishing Traditions* (New Trends Publishing, 1999), from which the following recipes are derived. Mrs. Fallon is a crusader for traditional farming, raw dairy products, fermented foods, and restoring our nation's health.

Oriental Red Meat Salad
Yield: 6 servings

1½ pounds beef flank, or similar cut from lamb or game
½ cup lemon juice
6 tablespoons naturally fermented soy sauce
2 tablespoons extra-virgin olive oil or expeller pressed peanut oil
1 tablespoon toasted sesame oil
1 teaspoon grated fresh ginger
pinch of red pepper flakes
2 tablespoons toasted sesame seeds
½ pound snow peas, steamed lightly and cut into quarters at an angle
1 pound bean sprouts, steamed lightly
1 red bell pepper, seeded and cut into a julienne

Directions:
Using a sharp knife, score the steak across the grain on both sides. Broil 2 to 3 minutes on each side, or until medium rare. Transfer to a cutting board and let stand 10 minutes. Meanwhile, combine the lemon juice, soy sauce, oils, ginger, and red pepper flakes and mix. Cut the meat across the grain at an angle into very thin slices, then cut these slices into a julienne. Marinate with soy sauce mixture for several hours in refrigerator. Mix with sesame seeds and vegetables just before serving.

Basic Omelets
(Various meals)
Yield: 2 servings

4 fresh eggs, at room temperature
pinch of sea salt
3 tablespoons extra-virgin coconut oil or butter

Crack eggs into a bowl. Add a teaspoon of water and sea salt, and blend with a wire whisk. (Do not overwhisk or the omelet will be tough.) Heat coconut oil or butter in a well-seasoned cast iron skillet or frying pan over medium. When foam subsides, add egg mixture. Tip pan to allow egg to cover entire pan. Cook several minutes until underside is lightly browned. Lift up one side with a spatula and fold omelet in half. Reduce heat to medium low and cook another 30 seconds or so—this will allow the egg on the inside to cook. Slide omelet onto a heated platter and serve.

Variation: Mexican Omelet

Add salsa, avocado, sour cream, and jack cheese to omelet just before folding.

Variation: Onion, Pepper, and Goat Cheese Omelet

Sauté 1 small onion, thinly sliced, and ½ red bell pepper, cut into julienne strips, in a little extra-virgin coconut oil or butter until tender. Sprinkle this evenly over the egg mixture as it begins to cook, along with 2 oz. of goat's milk cheddar or feta cheese.

Variation: Garden Herb Omelet

Scatter 1 tablespoon finely chopped parsley, 1 tablespoon finely chopped chives, and 1 tablespoon finely chopped thyme or other garden herb over omelet as it begins to cook.

Variation: Mushroom Swiss Omelet

Sauté ½ pound fresh mushrooms, washed, well dried, and thinly sliced, in extra-virgin coconut oil or butter and olive oil. Scatter mushrooms and grated Swiss cheese over the omelet as it begins to cook.

Blueberry Pecan Pancakes
Yield: 12 pancakes

1½ cups freshly ground or soaked spelt, kamut, or whole wheat flour
¾ cup water mixed with 1 tablespoon of yogurt
1 egg, lightly beaten
½ cup blueberries (fresh or frozen)
½ cup Crispy Pecans (page 270)
1/4 teaspoon sea salt
2 teaspoons baking powder
1 teaspoon vanilla
½ cup extra-virgin coconut oil

Combine flour, water mixture, and egg. Mix well and let stand overnight. Defrost blueberries in refrigerator if frozen. Add blueberries, pecans, salt, baking powder, and vanilla to flour mixture. Heat extra-virgin coconut oil in a skillet or pan over low heat. Increase temperature to moderate heat. Use about three tablespoons of batter for each pancake. Serve with honey, maple syrup, and butter.

Beef & Chicken Fajitas
Yield: 4 to 6 servings

> 6 tablespoons extra-virgin olive oil
> ½ cup lemon or lime juice
> ¼ cup pineapple juice (optional)
> 4 garlic cloves, peeled and mashed
> ½ teaspoon chili powder
> 1 teaspoon dried oregano
> ½ teaspoon dried thyme
> 2 pounds chicken breast (or beef), cut into strips, about 1/4 to 1/2 inch thick
> 1 red bell pepper, seeded and cut into julienne strips
> 1 green bell pepper, seeded and cut into julienne strips
> 2 medium onions, thinly sliced
> extra-virgin olive oil
> 12 sprouted whole wheat tortillas
> melted butter
> crème fraîche or sour cream for garnish
> chismole for garnish
> guacamole for garnish

Combine olive oil, lemon or lime juice, pineapple juice, and herbs and spices. Mix well and add the meat. Marinate several hours. With a slotted spoon transfer to paper towels and pat dry. Put peppers in bowl and marinate. Meanwhile heat a heavy skillet over medium-high heat. Add olive oil and sauté the meat in batches. Transfer to a heated platter and keep warm in the oven. In same skillet sauté vegetables in batches in olive oil and strew over meat. Heat tortillas briefly in a heavy cast-iron skillet and brush with melted butter. Serve meat mixture with tortillas and garnishes.

Chicken Stock
Yield: 6 to 10 servings
By all means, use chicken feet if you can find them: they are full of gelatin. Jewish folklore considers the addition of chicken feet the secret to successful broth.

> 1 whole chicken (free range, pastured, or organic chicken)
> 3 to 4 quarts cold filtered water
> 1 tablespoon raw apple cider vinegar
> 4 medium-sized onions, coarsely chopped
> 8 carrots, peeled and coarsely chopped
> 6 celery stalks, coarsely chopped
> 2 to 4 zucchinis
> 5 garlic cloves

1 teaspoon grated ginger, about a 4-inch piece
2 to 4 tablespoons sea salt
1 bunch parsley

Remove fat glands and the gizzards from chicken cavity. Place chicken or chicken pieces in a large stainless steel pot. Add water, vinegar, onions, carrots, celery, zucchinis, garlic, ginger, and salt. Bring to a boil over high heat and remove foam that rises to the top. Reduce heat to medium low, cover, and cook 12 to 24 hours. The longer you cook the stock, the richer and more flavorful the stock will be. About five minutes before finishing the stock, add parsley. This will impart additional mineral ions to the broth. Remove from heat and take out the chicken. Let cool and remove chicken meat from the carcass. Reserve for other uses such as chicken salads, enchiladas, sandwiches, or curries. (The skin and smaller bones, which will be very soft, may be given to your dog or cat.) Strain the stock into a large bowl and reserve in your refrigerator for use as a base for other soups.

Pepitas
Yield: 4 cups
This recipe imitates Aztec practices of soaking seeds in brine, then letting them dry in the hot sun. They ate pepitas whole or ground into meal.

1 tablespoon sea salt or Herbamare
5 to 6 cups filtered water
4 cups raw, hulled pumpkin seeds
1 teaspoon cayenne pepper (optional)

Dissolve salt in water and add pumpkin seeds and optional cayenne. Soak for at least 7 hours or overnight. Drain in a colander and spread on two stainless steel baking pans. Place in a warm oven (no more than 150 degrees) for about 12 hours or overnight, stirring occasionally, until thoroughly dry and crisp. Store in an airtight container.

Braised Leeks
Yield: 6 servings

6 medium leeks
2 cups Homemade Beef Stock (see page 270)
½ to 1 cup grated Gruyere cheese

Preheat oven to 350 degrees. Trim ends off leeks and split lengthwise. Rinse well and set in a Pyrex pan. Bring beef stock to a boil and pour over leeks. Bake for about ½ hour, or until stock has reduced and leeks are tender. Sprinkle on cheese and melt under broiler for a few minutes. Serve immediately.

Crispy Pecans
Yield: 4 cups

4 cups pecan halves
1 teaspoon sea salt or Herbamare
filtered water

The buttery flavor of pecans is enhanced by soaking and slow–oven drying. Soak pecans in salt and filtered water for at least 7 hours or overnight. Drain in a colander. Spread pecans on two stainless steel baking pans and place in a warm oven (no more than 150 degrees) for 12 to 24 hours, stirring occasionally, until completely dry and crisp. Store in an airtight container. Great for school lunches.

Crispy Almonds
Yield: 4 cups
Blanched or skinless almonds will still sprout, an indication that the blanching process has not destroyed the enzymes. (The skins are probably removed by a machine process.) Many people find that almond skins are irritating to the mouth, even when they have been soaked or sprouted. There is still plenty of goodness in skinless almonds. You can use crispy almonds in numerous dessert recipes.

2 teaspoons sea salt or Herbamare
5 to 6 cups filtered water
4 cups blanched almonds

Combine salt and water and soak the almonds for at least 7 hours or overnight. Drain in a colander. Spread on two stainless steel baking pans and place in a warm oven (no more than 150 degrees) for 12 to 24 hours, stirring occasionally, until completely dry and crisp. Store in an airtight container.

Beef Stock
Yield: 6 to 10 servings
Good beef stock must be made with several sorts of beef bones: knuckle bones and feet impart large quantities of gelatin to the broth; marrow bones impart flavor and the particular nutrients of the bone marrow; and meaty rib or neck bones add color and flavor.

6 to 7 pounds beef marrow and knuckle bones
1 calves foot, cut into pieces (optional)
4 to 5 quarts cold filtered water
5 pounds meaty rib or neck bones

¼ cup vinegar
3 onions, coarsely chopped
3 carrots, coarsely chopped
3 celery stalks, coarsely chopped
2 to 3 sprigs of fresh thyme, tied together
1 teaspoon dried green peppercorns, crushed
1 bunch parsley

Preheat oven to 350 degrees. Place the marrow and knuckle bones and optional calves foot in a very large pot and cover with water. Let stand for 1 hour. Meanwhile, place the meaty bones in a roasting pan and brown in the oven, about 45 minutes. When well browned, add to the pot along with vinegar and vegetables. Discard fat from roasting pan, add a little cold water, set over high heat and bring to a boil, stirring with a wooden spoon to deglaze. Add this liquid to the pot. Add additional water, if necessary, to cover the bones, but the liquid should come no higher than within one inch of the rim of the pot, as the volume expands slightly during cooking. Bring to a boil. A large amount of foam will come to the top, and it is important to remove this with a spoon. After you have skimmed, reduce heat to medium and add thyme and crushed peppercorns. Simmer stock for at least 12 to 72 hours. Just before finishing, add parsley. Let it wilt and remove stock from heat. You will now have a pot of rather repulsive looking brown liquid containing globs of gelatinous and fatty material. It doesn't even smell particularly good. But don't despair. After straining you will have a delicious and nourishing clear broth that forms the basis for many other recipes in this book. Remove bones with tongs or a slotted spoon. Strain the stock into a large bowl. Let cool in the refrigerator and remove the congealed fat that rises to the top. Reheat and transfer to storage containers. Note: Your dog will love the leftover meat and bones.

Healthy Trail Mix
Yield: 5 to 6 cups

1 cup Crispy Pecans (page 270)
1 cup crispy cashews
1 cup raisins
1 cup unsulphured dried apricots, apples, pears, or pineapple cut into pieces
1 cup dried sweetened coconut meat
1 cup carob chips (optional)

Mix all ingredients together. Store in an airtight container.

Blueberry Muffins
Yield: 12 muffins

    1¼ cups freshly ground or soaked spelt, kamut or whole wheat flour
    ¾ cup water mixed with 1 tablespoon of yogurt
    1 egg, lightly beaten
    ¼ teaspoon fine sea salt
    ½ cup extra-virgin coconut oil
    ⅓ cup honey
    2 teaspoons baking powder
    1 teaspoon vanilla
    1 cup blueberries, fresh or frozen

Mix flour with water and yogurt and let stand overnight. Preheat oven to 400 degrees. Add egg, salt, oil, honey, baking powder, and vanilla and mix well. Pour into well-buttered muffin tin about three-quarters full. Place 5 to 7 blueberries on each muffin. Berries will fall partway into the muffins. Bake for 15 to 20 minutes. Note: 1 cup buckwheat flour or cornmeal may be used in place of 1 cup spelt, kamut, or wheat flour.

Variation: Ginger Muffins
Add 1 tablespoon freshly grated ginger and 1 teaspoon ground ginger to batter. Omit vanilla.

Coconut Milk Soup
Yield: 6 to 8 Servings

    1½ quarts homemade fish or chicken stock
    1½ cups whole coconut milk
    1 pound chicken or fish, cut into small cubes
    3 jalapeño chilies, diced, or ½ teaspoon cayenne pepper
    1 tablespoon grated fresh ginger
    2 tablespoons fish sauce (optional)
    2 to 4 tablespoons lime juice
    chopped cilantro for garnish

Combine stock, milk, chicken or fish, jalapeños, ginger, optional fish sauce, and lime juice in a large stockpot over high heat. Bring to a boil. Reduce heat to medium low and simmer until meat is cooked through. Garnish with cilantro.

Five-Grain Porridge
Yield: 4 servings

1 cup five-grain cereal mix (or choose any 5 whole grains, such as wheat, barley, spelt, millet, or quinoa)
1 cup water mixed with 2 tablespoons fermented whey or yogurt
½ teaspoon sea salt
1 cup water
1 tablespoon flaxseeds (optional)

Combine five-grain mixture, water mixture, and salt. Cover and let stand at room temperature for 7 to 24 hours. Bring additional 1 cup of water to boil. Add soaked cereal, reduce heat, cover and simmer several minutes. Meanwhile, grind flaxseed in a mini grinder. Remove cereal from heat and stir in flax meal. Serve with butter or cream thinned with a little water and an organic natural sweetener like Sucanat, date sugar, maple syrup, or raw honey.

Mushroom Soup
Yield: 6 servings
Make sure the mushrooms are fresh!

2 medium onions, peeled and chopped
3 tablespoons extra-virgin coconut oil or butter
2 pounds fresh mushrooms
butter and extra-virgin olive oil
½ cup dry white wine
1 piece toasted whole grain sprouted or sourdough bread, broken into pieces
1 quart homemade chicken stock
freshly ground nutmeg
sea salt or fish sauce and pepper to taste
sour cream or crème fraîche

Sauté the onions gently in extra-virgin coconut oil or butter until soft. Meanwhile, wash mushrooms (no need to remove stems) and dry well. Cut into quarters. In a heavy cast-iron skillet, sauté the mushrooms in small batches in a mixture of butter and olive oil. Remove with slotted spoon and drain on paper towels. Add sautéed mushrooms, wine, bread, and chicken stock to onions, bring to a boil and skim. Reduce heat and simmer about 15 minutes. Purée soup with a handheld blender. Add nutmeg and season to taste. Ladle into heated soup bowls and serve with sour cream or crème fraîche.

Vegetable Frittata
Yield: 4 servings

    1 red pepper, seeded and cut into a julienne
    1 medium onion, peeled and finely chopped
    butter and extra-virgin olive oil
    6 eggs
    ⅓ cup sour cream or crème fraîche
    1 teaspoon finely grated lemon rind
    pinch dried oregano
    pinch dried rosemary
    sea salt and freshly ground pepper
    1 cup broccoli flowerets, steamed until tender and broken into small pieces
    1 cup grated raw Monterey jack cheese

In a cast-iron skillet, sauté pepper and onion in butter and olive oil until soft. Remove with a slotted spoon. Beat eggs with cream and seasonings. Stir in broccoli, peppers, and onion. Melt more butter and olive oil in the pan and pour in egg mixture. Cook over medium heat about 5 minutes, or until underside is golden. Sprinkle cheese on top and place under the broiler for a few minutes, or until the frittata puffs and browns. Cut into wedges and serve.

Variation: Zucchini Frittata
   Omit broccoli, red pepper, and onion and use 3 medium zucchini, cut into a julienne, using the julienne slicer of your food processor. Salt and drain in a colander for ½ hour. Rinse and pat dry. Sauté about 1 minute in olive oil. Proceed with recipe.

All-Day Beef Stew
Yield: 6 to 8 servings

    3 pounds beef stew, cut into 1-inch pieces
    1 cup red wine
    3 to 4 cups homemade beef stock (page 270)
    4 tomatoes, peeled, seeded, and chopped or 1 can tomatoes
    2 tablespoons tomato puree
    ½ teaspoon black peppercorns
    several sprigs fresh thyme, tied together
    2 garlic cloves, peeled and crushed
    2 to 3 small pieces orange peel
    8 small red potatoes

1 pound carrots, peeled and cut into sticks
sea salt and freshly ground pepper

Marinate beef in red wine overnight. (This step is optional.) Preheat oven to 250 degrees. Combine beef, stock, tomatoes, tomato puree, peppercorns, thyme, garlic, and orange peel in an ovenproof casserole dish. Cook for 12 hours. Add carrots and potatoes during the last hour. Season to taste.

Salad Nicoise
Yield: 6 servings

6 4-ounce fresh tuna steaks
extra-virgin olive oil
sea salt and pepper
6 cups baby salad greens or frisé lettuce
6 small ripe tomatoes, cut into wedges
6 small red potatoes, cooked in a clay pot
1 pound green beans, blanched for 8 minutes and rinsed under cold water
2 dozen small black olives
2 cups herb dressing

Brush tuna steaks with olive oil and season with sea salt and pepper. Heat a heavy skillet over high heat. Cook the tuna steaks, two at a time, for about 4 minutes per side. Set aside. Divide salad greens among six large plates. Garnish with tomatoes, potatoes, beans, and olives. Place steaks on top of greens and pour dressing over top.

To make the dressing, pour 1 cup vinegar in a bowl and while whisking add 3 cups extra-virgin olive oil in a slow stream. Add ¼ cup chopped parsley and whisk to combine.

Lentil Salad
Yield: 4 servings

2 cups cooked green lentils
1 cup grated carrots
1 bunch green onions, chopped
2 tablespoons finely chopped parsley
¾ cup salad dressing

Combine all ingredients and mix well. Serve at room temperature.

Salmon and Mixed Greens
Yield: 4 servings

> 1½ pounds fresh salmon filet
> extra-virgin olive oil
> lemon juice
> sea salt and freshly ground pepper
> 2 tablespoons unbleached flour, sifted
> ½ teaspoon paprika
> 6 cups baby lettuces, or mixed greens such as watercress or Mache
> 3⁄4 cup salad dressing
> 1 red bell pepper, seeded, cut into a julienne and sautéed in olive oil
> 1 pound brown mushrooms, washed, dried very well, sliced and sautéed in butter
> and olive oil

Preheat oven to 350 degrees. Brush olive oil on salmon. Squeeze lemon juice over salmon. Combine salt and pepper, flour, and paprika and rub onto salmon. Bake about 10 minutes. Place under broiler for another 2 minutes, or until just lightly browned. Meanwhile mix greens with dressing and divide between four plates. Make a mound of red peppers and mushrooms on each plate, place a portion of salmon on each mound of greens, and pour pan juices on top. Serve immediately.

Simple Beans
Yield: 8 servings

> 2 cups dried black beans, kidney beans, pinto beans, black-eyed beans or white beans
> filtered water
> 2 tablespoons whey
> 1 teaspoon sea salt
> 4 cloves garlic, peeled and mashed (optional)

Soak beans in enough filtered water to cover, whey, and salt for 12 to 24 hours, depending on the size of the beans. Drain, rinse, and place in a large pot and add enough filtered water to cover beans. Bring to a boil and skim off foam. Reduce heat and add garlic if desired. Cover and simmer for 4 to 8 hours. Check occasionally and add more water as necessary.

Lamb Chops
Yield: 4 servings
You will need a very well-seasoned cast iron skillet for this recipe.

8 lamb chops, fat trimmed
freshly ground pepper
½ cup dry red wine
2 to 3 cups homemade beef or lamb stock (page 270)

Heat the skilled over medium-high heat. Season the lamb chops with pepper to tasteSear the pork chops in the pan, in batches if necessary. (No fat is required. Lamb will render its own fat, enough to keep the chops from sticking.) Cook about 3 minutes on each side, or until they are rare or medium rare. Keep in a warm oven if you cook a second batch and while preparing the sauce. Pour the grease out of the pan and return the pan to the stove. Deglaze the pan with the red wine and beef stock. Boil rapidly, skimming off any dirty foam that rises to the top. Reduce to about 3/4 cup. The sauce should have the consistency of maple syrup. Place the lamb chops on heated plates with their accompanying vegetables, and spoon the sauce.

Italian Salad
Yield: 6 servings
Children love this good, basic salad. The secret is to cut everything up small.

1 head romaine lettuce
1 bunch watercress
1 red bell pepper, seeded and julienned
1 cucumber, peeled, seeded, quartered lengthwise, and finely sliced
1 celery heart with leaves, finely chopped
1 small red onion, finely sliced
2 carrots, peeled and grated
1 cup red cabbage, finely shredded
½ cup small seed sprouts
1 cup cooked garbanzo beans
¾ cup garlic-flavored salad dressing

Remove the outer leaves of the romaine, slice off the end and open up to rinse out any dirt or impurities while keeping the head intact. Pat dry. Slice across at ½-inch intervals. Place romaine in a salad bowl. Add the watercress, and chopped vegetables. Sprinkle the sprouts and garbanzo beans over the top for an attractive presentation. Toss with basic or garlic dressing. Serve with grated Parmesan cheese, if desired.

Simple Lentils
Yield: 6 to 8 servings
Excellent with sauerkraut and strongly flavored meats such as duck, game, or lamb.

2 cups lentils, preferably green lentils
filtered water
2 tablespoons fermented whey or yogurt
1 teaspoon sea salt
2 cups beef or chicken stock
2 garlic cloves, peeled and mashed
2 to 3 sprigs fresh thyme, tied together
1 teaspoon dried peppercorns, crushed
pinch dried chili flakes (optional)
juice of 1 to 2 lemons

Soak lentils in filtered water (enough to cover), whey, and salt for several hours. Drain, rinse, and place in a pot and add stock to cover. Bring to a boil and skim. Add garlic, thyme, peppercorns, and chili flakes and simmer, uncovered, for about 1 hour, or until liquid has completely reduced. Add lemon juice and season to taste. Serve with a slotted spoon.

Easy Brown Rice
Yield: 6 to 8 servings

¼ cup extra-virgin olive oil
1 tablespoon butter
2 cups brown rice
4 cups homemade chicken stock or combination of water and chicken stock
½ teaspoon sea salt

Heat the oil in a large pot over medium-high heat. Melt the butter in the hot oil. Stir rice into the butter and oil and sauté about 5 minutes, stirring constantly. Pour in stock, add salt, and bring to a rolling boil. Boil uncovered, for about 10 minutes, until liquid has reduced to the level of the rice. Reduce low heat, cover tightly, and cook for about 1 hour.

Miso Soup
Yield: 6 to 8 servings

1½ quarts homemade fish stock or filtered water
4 tablespoons soy sauce
3 to 4 tablespoons miso

1 onion, sliced
½ green or Chinese cabbage, coarsely shredded
2 tablespoons fish sauce (optional)

Bring stock and soy sauce to a boil, skim and whisk in miso. Add remaining ingredients and simmer gently until vegetables are soft.

Tuna Tahini Salad
Yield: 6 to 8 servings

 2 large cans water packed tuna, drained and flaked
 ¼ teaspoon cayenne pepper
 2 cups tahini sauce (see below)
 4 medium onions, thinly sliced
 ¼ cup melted butter mixed with ¼ cup extra-virgin olive oil
 ⅓ cup toasted pine nuts
 cilantro sprigs for garnish
 sprouted whole grain crackers for garnish

Preheat the oven to 375 degrees. Mix tuna with cayenne pepper and 1 cup of sauce. Arrange the onions on an oiled baking sheet, brush with mixture of melted butter and olive oil, and bake for 30 minutes, or until crispy. Mound tuna on a platter. Scatter onions and pine nuts on top. Garnish with cilantro and serve with crackers and remaining sauce.

Tahini Sauce
Yield: 2 cups

 2 garlic cloves, peeled and coarsely chopped
 1 teaspoon sea salt
 ½ cup tahini
 1 tablespoon unrefined flaxseed oil
 1 cup water
 ½ cup fresh lemon juice

Place garlic in a food processor with the salt. Blend until minced. Add tahini and flaxseed oil and blend. With the top on and the motor running, slowly add the water through the opening. When completely blended, add the lemon juice and blend until smooth. Sauce should be the consistency of heavy cream. If it's too thick, add more water and lemon juice.

James Thomas of R. Thomas Deluxe Grill in Atlanta

R. Thomas Deluxe Grill started as an offbeat burger joint when it opened in the mid-1980s under the direction of Richard Thomas. The restaurant's funky eclectic style captured the hearts of Atlanta natives from day one. A decade ago, the Thomas family added a fresh juice bar and started offering fresh organic carrot juice alongside their burgers. People took notice, and the menu was revamped with high-quality ingredients that honor vegetarians and carnivores with equal respect. Under the instruction of their consulting chef, Donna Gates (nutritionist and author of the *Body Ecology Diet*), the Thomas family came to know the truly healing power of food. With their current team of executive chef John Vo and vice president of operations Cesar Villanaeuva, the R. Thomas Deluxe Grill is poised for an exciting future.

Chicken Piccata
Yield: 1 serving

½ cup clarified butter
¼ cup amaranth flour
1 5½-ounce marinated boneless chicken breast
1 lemon, cut in half
½ cup chopped Italian zucchini
¼ cup cultured vegetables
1 serving Garlicky Green Beans (see recipe on page 283)
1 cup Dijon Hiziki Dressing (see recipe below)
⅛ teaspoon Herbamare

Coat the chicken breast in amaranth flour. Melt the clarified butter in a large sauté pan over medium-high heat. Sauté the chicken breast 1½ minutes to sear on both sides. While searing, add the juice from ½ lemon. Reduce the heat to medium and sauté for about 5 minutes, or until nearly done, turning occasionally to lightly brown. Preheat the oven to 350 degrees. Add the juice from the remaining ½ lemon, zucchini, and the cultured vegetables and finish cooking in the oven, about 10 minutes. While the chicken is cooking, prepare the garlicky green beans as directed. Remove the cooked chicken piccata from the oven and slice diagonally into 5 even strips. Pour the Hiziki dressing over chicken and sprinkle with Herbamare before serving.

Millet Corn Casserole
Yield: 1 serving

⅛ cup coconut oil
3 cups diced yellow onion
⅛ teaspoon crushed red pepper
1 teaspoon ground cumin

2 ounces fajita mix
Herbamare to taste
1¼ quarts hot water
¾ tablespoon sea salt
½ cup grain amaranth
2 cups grain millet
1 cup diced red bell peppers
1 pound corn

Heat the coconut oil in a large pot over medium heat. Add the onion, and crushed red pepper, reduce the heat to low, and simmer until lightly brown. Stir in cumin, fajita mix, and Herbamare and sauté for another 3 minutes. Add the water, salt, amaranth, and millet. Bring to a boil. Stir well, cover and reduce to a simmer. Stir periodically until grains are thick but not lumpy. Rinse the peppers and corn. Preheat the oven to 350 degrees. Fold the peppers and corn into the grain mixture and stir well. Simmer on low heat for about 5 minutes. Remove from the heat and divide the cooked grains evenly into 2 shallow hotel pans. Bake both pans of millet for 30 minutes. Check for doneness and bake for another 30 minutes, or until they have a nice crispy crust. Let the casserole cool before serving.

Soy Ginger Salmon
Yield: 1 serving

¼ cup packed brown sugar
1 tablespoon Dijon mustard
1 tablespoon grated ginger (1 teaspoon ground)
6 ounces salmon
Herbamare to taste
1 serving Garlicky Green Beans (see recipe on page 283)
½ cup quinoa
¼ cup chili sauce
1 tablespoon cultured vegetables

Combine the brown sugar, mustard, and ginger and mix well. Cook salmon on a hot grill to medium rare. Season with Herbamare. When cooked, top the salmon with ginger glaze. Arrange the quinoa near the center of a large plate and heat in the microwave 1 minute. Place the cooked salmon to the right edge of the quinoa, but slightly overlapping. Place the garlicky green beans below the fish and quinoa. Place a 2 oz. ramekin of chili sauce next to the green beans. Place the cultured vegetables above the chili garlic sauce.

Warm Chicken Supreme Salad
Yield: 1 serving

> 1 fluid ounce extra-virgin olive oil
> ⅓ cup chopped fresh green onions
> ⅓ cup chopped carrots
> ⅓ cup chopped red bell peppers
> ⅓ cup chopped apple
> ½ cup cooked and pulled chicken
> 3 tablespoons balsamic honey Dijon dressing
> 1 cup romaine lettuce, chopped
> 1 cup mixed field greens
> ½ cup grated white cheddar cheese
> ¼ cup chopped pecans
> ¼ ounce sunflower sprouts
> 1½ oranges, peeled and sliced for garnish

Preheat the oil in a large sauté pan and sauté the vegetables, the apples, and chicken (sliced ¼-inch thick) for 2 to 3 minutes. Add the dressing and continue to sauté one minute, tossing well. Place the romaine lettuce and the mixed field greens in a large salad bowl. Do not mix. Place the sautéed vegetables and chicken on top of the lettuce. Add cheese and pecans to the top of the vegetables. Arrange orange sliceson the side of the bowl. Sprinkle with sprouts and serve.

Chicken King Omelet
Yield: 1 serving

> 2 tablespoons extra-virgin olive oil
> ¼ cup chopped mushrooms
> ¼ cup chopped zucchini
> ¼ cup chopped cooked chicken
> 3 eggs
> ½ cup grated white cheddar cheese
> 1 slice of 9-grain bread, toasted and buttered
> ½ ounce sunflower sprouts

Heat the oil in a sauté pan over medium heat. Sauté the vegetables and the chicken. Beat the eggs and cook in a separate pan. Place cheese in the center of the eggs. Add the cooked vegetables and the chicken. Fold in the top and bottom edges of the omelet. Fold and roll the sides of the omelet in. Place omelet on a plate with toasted 9-grain bread and garnish with any remaining vegetables and sunflower sprouts.

Southern Range Chicken Dinner
Yield: 1 serving

> 10 ounces whole chicken breast
> Herbamare to taste
> ½ cup smashed red potatoes
> ¼ cup shiitake mushroom gravy
> 2 tablespoons cultured vegetables

Season the chicken with Herbamare and grill over a medium-hot grill for about 7 minutes per side. Heat the potatoes and transfer to a plate. Ladle the gravy over the potatoes, making a well in the center of the potatoes. Place the grilled chicken on the plate. Serve with cultured vegetables.

R's House Salad
Yield: 1 serving

> 2 cups of Bibb lettuce
> 2 ounces mandarin oranges
> ¼ cup chopped pecans
> 2 tablespoons poppy seed dressing (see recipe below)
> ½ ounce sunflower sprouts

Place the lettuce on a medium-sized round plate. Place mandarin oranges, pecans, and dressing on top of the lettuce. Add sprouts.

Garlicky Green Beans
Yield: 1 serving

> 1 ounce extra-virgin olive oil
> 1 teaspoon garlic oil
> 4 ounces fresh green beans
> ⅛ ounce Herbamare

Heat the olive oil in a large sauté pan over medium heat. Add the garlic And sauté for 3 minutes. Add the green beans and sauté for 5 minutes. Add the Herbamare to taste.

Poppy Seed Dressing
Yield: 1 quart

    ¾ cup hot water
    ½ cup Extra-virgin olive oil
    ⅛ cup essential balance oil
    ⅓ cup white vinegar
    ¼ cup honey
    ⅛ cup poppy seeds
    1 tablespoon dry mustard
    ⅛ cup diced red onions
    1 tablespoon Turbinado sugar
    ¼ teaspoon sea salt
    ¼ teaspoon Xanthan gum

Combine all ingredients in order in a large bowl wile mixing with a hand blender. Gradually sift in Xanthan gum last until desired thickness is reached. Cover and refrigerate up to 14 days.

Salmon Lemon Sauté
Yield: 1 serving

    4 tablespoons clarified butter
    ¼ cup amaranth flour
    6 ounces salmon
    1 lemon
    4 ounces quinoa
    ¼ cup Dijon Hiziki (see recipe on page 280)
    2 oz. broccoli and fennel
    ½ cup raw collard kale salad mix
    1 tablespoon cultured vegetables

In a sauté pan, heat the butter. Lightly coat the salmon with the amaranth flour and place in the sauté pan. Squeeze the juice from 1 lemon over the salmon. At the same time, on a large plate, heat the quinoa in the microwave for 1 minute. Place salmon on top of the quinoa, overlapping on the left side. Add Dijon Hiziki to the bottom of the plate. Add the collard green salad above the salmon. Add cultured vegetables to the bottom left of the salmon and serve.

Cinnamon Sweet Potatoes
Yield: 1 quart

   5 pounds sweet potatoes (yams)
   ¼ cup coconut oil
   ¼ tablespoon Herbamare
   ¹⁄₁₆ teaspoon cinnamon spice concentrate
   ¹⁄₁₆ teaspoon ginger spice concentrate

Peel and chop sweet potatoes into 1-inch triangle shapes. Melt the coconut oil and mix with the sweet potatoes in a large bowl. Add Herbamare to taste. Divide the mixture evenly to 3 large sheet pans. Roast the sweet potatoes for 15 minutes in a 350 degree oven. Pull out and stir. Repeat approximately every 10 minutes until the sweet potatoes are soft and brown. Remove sweet potatoes from the pans and place back in the bowl. Mix the cinnamon and ginger extracts with the sweet potatoes by hand. Transfer to a large container, label, and refrigerate.

Turkey Sausage Queen Omelet
Yield: 1 serving

   1 slice of 9-grain bread, buttered
   ¼ cup chopped red onion
   ¼ cup chopped red bell pepper
   2 ounces turkey sausage
   3 fresh eggs
   ¼ cup grated white cheddar cheese
   2 tablespoons shiitake mushroom gravy
   ¼ cup chopped roasted rosemary potatoes
   ½ oz. sprouts

Toast the buttered bread and slice diagonally. Cook the onions, peppers, and turkey sausage (reserve 1 piece of sausage for garnish on top of the omelet) in a sauté pan over medium heat. Beat the eggs and pour into a separate pan over medium heat. Cover and lower the temperature. Cook the covered omelet for 3 to 4 minutes. When the omelet is cooked through add the veggie-sausage mix, mushroom gravy, and cheese. Fold the omelet to the size of the spatula. Place on a plate and garnish with sausage and sprouts.

Blue Corn Posole
Yield: 1 quart

> 3 tablespoons coconut oil
> ½ cup diced yellow onions
> 2 tablespoons garlic oil
> 1 tablespoon chopped fresh oregano
> ½ tablespoon sea salt
> 1 pint blue corn
> 5⅓ cups hot water
> ¼ tablespoon Herbamare

In a pot, sauté coconut oil, onions, garlic, oregano, and sea salt on low heat until the onions sweat. Add blue corn and water. Bring to a boil and reduce to a medium simmer. Stir periodically until the posole is tender, approximately 30 minutes. Water may be added if necessary. Drain off excess water in a colander. Reseason again to desired taste. Let cool. Refrigerate.

Italian Zucchini
Yield: 1 quart

> 1 tablespoon extra-virgin olive oil
> ¼ cup red onion
> 1 teaspoon garlic oil
> ¼ cup chopped fresh oregano
> 1 pint chopped zucchini
> pinch of Herbamare

In a hot braising pan, heat oil. Stir in onions, garlic, and oregano. Sauté the veggies for 3 minutes. Add zucchini and Herbamare and simmer to sweat the zucchini. Remove from the stove and allow to cool. Do not overcook the veggies. Allow to cool completely and refrigerate.

Cajun Sauté Bowl
Yield: 1 serving

> 2 tablesppons extra-virgin olive oil
> 1 tablespoon garlic
> ⅛ teaspoon oregano
> ¼ cup chopped fresh green onions
> ½ teaspoon crushed red pepper (¼ tsp.)

¼ cup chopped red bell peppers
2 tablespoons chopped red onions
3 oz .00 cups cubed roasted rosemary potatoes
⅛ teaspoon sea salt
3 ounces chicken, cooked and pulled
6 ounces marinara sauce
1 cup Blue Corn Posole (see recipe on page 286)
3 tablespoons chopped fresh basil
1 tablespoon sour cream

Heat oil in a large sauté pan. Sauté the garlic, oregano, green onions, and crushed red pepper for 40 seconds. Add the veggies, potatoes, sea salt, and chicken and sauté for 2 minutes. Add the marinara sauce and sauté until heated. In a large bowl, steam the posole in steamer. Top the posole with the sautéed veggies and chicken and garnish with a pinch of fresh basil and sour cream.

Curried Quinoa
Yield: 1 serving

1 serving rosemary quinoa salad
6 tablespoons curry basil sauce

Place the quinoa in a rice steamer and top with the curry basil sauce. Steam for about 10 minutes.

Smashed Potatoes with Shiitake Gravy
Yield: 1 quart

3 tablespoons coconut oil
⅛ cup garlic oil
2 cups diced celery
8 cups diced red potatoes
2 tablespoons sea salt
8 cups hot water
¼ tablespoon Herbamare

Heat the oils in a large pot over medium heat. Sauté the celery until tender. Add the potatoes, salt, and water. Bring to a boil and simmer until potatoes become soft. Strain the potatoes, celery, and garlic and drain for 3 to 4 minutes in a colander. With a hand blender, puree all ingredients. Season with Herbamare and refrigerate.

Shiitake Mushroom Gravy
Yield: 2 quarts

¼ cup coconut oil
¾ cup diced yellow onions
¼ cup garlic oil
1 cup amaranth flour
9 cups hot water
1 tablespoon Herbamare
1 cup dried shiitake mushrooms

In a heavy pot, sauté diced onions with coconut oil until onions are fairly brown. Add garlic in oil and sauté for a bit longer. Add flour and stir frequently until flour is golden brown. Add water, Herbamare, and mushrooms (with stems trimmed, diced). Bring to a boil, reduce the heat, and simmer, stirring well and often, until desired consistency. Be sure to reach the bottom of the pot. Allow to cool and refrigerate.

Warm Smile
Yield: 1 serving

¼ cup quartered roasted rosemary potatoes
¼ cup cooked snow peas
¼ cup cooked curried quinoa
¼ cup sliced cucumbers
1 tablespoon cultured vegetables

Arrange all items prepared appropriately on a large round plate. Place a tablespoon of cultured vegetables in the center of the plate and serve.

Ginger Tamari Bowl with Chicken
Yield: 1 serving

1 ounce extra-virgin olive oil
1 teaspoon garlic oil
¼ cup chopped carrots
3 tablespoons green onions
1 recipe Blue Corn Posole (see recipe on page 286)
1/8 teaspoon sea salt
¾ cup ginger tamari sauce
¼ cup chopped zucchini
3 ounces cooked and pulled chicken

1 cup rosemary quinoa salad
¼ cup Dijon Hiziki (see recipe on page 280)

Wrap Variations:
- Roast Beef with Marinated Cabbage and Unsmoked Provolone Cheese
- Mushroom, Spinach, and Swiss
- Marinated Raw Vegetables with Jack Cheese

In a large sauté pan, heat olive oil and garlic oil. Add the carrots, green onions, posole, and sea salt and sauté for 2 minutes. Add ginger tamari sauce and zucchini and sauté to heat. Add chicken. Heat quinoa in a large bowl in steamer. Heat hiziki in steamer. Spread the sautéed vegetables around the bowl over the quinoa. Place the heated hiziki in the center of the bowl. Top with 1 ounce of ginger tamari sauce.

Tropical Chicken and Vegetable Kabobs
Yield: 4 to 6 kabobs

2 pounds boneless, skinless chicken breast, cut into bite-size pieces
2 tablespoons apple cider vinegar
2 tablespoons paprika
1 tablespoon minced garlic
1 tablespoon onion flakes or powder
1 teaspoon Herbamare
½ cup pineapple juice
2 tablespoons lemon juice
½ cup chicken stock
2 tablespoons extra-virgin olive oil
1 tablespoon honey
2 cups red and green bell peppers, cut into 1-inch squares
1 cup cherry tomatoes
2 cups pineapple, bite-size chunks
Garnish:
2 tablespoons lemon zest

Combine vinegar, paprika, garlic, onion powder, and Herbamare with chicken and marinate for a minimum of 2 hours. Combine pineapple and lemon juices, chicken stock, oil, and honey, and marinate bell peppers, tomatoes, and pineapple. Stir-fry chicken for 20 minutes, or until almost done, then cool until comfortable to skewer. Remove veggies and fruit from marinade, skewer with chicken, pineapple, and red and green bell peppers, with chicken and tomato at the end. Finish under the broiler on the lower rack, or on a grill for 5 minutes, turning once.

Marinated Baked Salmon with Capers
Yield: 4 servings

1 tablespoon chopped fresh rosemary leaves
1 tablespoon chopped chives
1 tablespoon minced garlic
1 tablespoon grated lemon zest
3 tablespoons fresh lemon juice
1 teaspoon Trocomare seasoning
4 6 ounce pieces of skinned salmon
2 tablespoons butter

Combine rosemary, chives, garlic, lemon zest, lemon juice, and Trocomare seasoning. Rub seasoning mixture over salmon well and marinate 2 to 3 hours. Heat butter in a sauté pan. Sear fish on both sides for 2 minutes. Bake 3 to 5 minutes at 385 degrees.

Sauce:

¼ cup orange juice
½ cup apple cider vinegar
1 tablespoon Dulse Flakes
1 tablespoon raw honey
½ cup extra-virgin olive oil
¼ cup pickled ginger
1 tablespoon capers

Blend all ingredients until smooth. Lower blender speed. Slowly pour oil until completely combined. Spoon sauce on hot fish, sprinkle with lemon zest.

Latin Style Orzo Salad
Yield: 4 servings

3 cups chicken or vegetable stock
1 pound orzo pasta, whole grain
½ cup cooked black beans
½ cup raw or frozen corn, thawed
¼ cup red bell peppers, diced
¼ cup green bell peppers, diced
2 tablespoons roasted garlic, crushed
4 stalks green onions, diced

½ cup diced tomatoes, seeded
¼ cup golden raisins
¼ cup vinaigrette dressing
Fresh cilantro for garnish

Bring the stock to a boil. Add the pasta and simmer until liquid is absorbed and pasta is tender. Remove from heat. Add all remaining ingredients, then vinaigrette. Return to low heat until warm. Garnish with fresh cilantro leaves. May be served as a cold salad as well.

Juicy Rosemary Baked Lamb
Yield: 12 to 15 servings

5 to 6 pounds boneless leg of lamb, trimmed
2 tablespoons dried rosemary
1 tablespoon dried marjoram
2 tablespoons dried thyme
4 large garlic cloves, diced
½ cup Spanish onions, finely chopped
2 teaspoons ground cloves
1 teaspoon ground ginger
⅔ cup balsamic vinegar
1 tablespoon Succanet (an organic natural sweetener)
1 teaspoon sea salt
2 cups pineapple juice reduced to sauce consistency
1 large onion, rough chopped
4 stalks celery, rough chopped
3 large carrots, rough chopped
1 cup mixed nuts, finely chopped

Make 1-inch cuts into meat, 3 to 4 inches apart; combine all diced and chopped herbs and spices. Stuff ½ teaspoon of seasoning mix into openings. Rub the meat with the remainder of the seasoning mix. Marinate in the balsamic vinegar, Succanet, sea salt, and pineapple juice covered in refrigerator for 7 hours (preferably overnight).

In a shallow roasting pan, spread out the onion, celery, and carrots. Place the lamb on top of the vegetables and bake in a preheated oven at 325 degrees for 2½ hours or until internal temperature is 155 degrees. During the last 15 minutes of cooking, apply nuts over meat. Allow lamb to rest 15 to 20 minutes before slicing.

Jamaican Style Curried Chicken
Yield: 4 servings

> 2 pounds boneless, skinless chicken (white and dark meat), cut into bite-size pieces
> ½ cup diced onion
> ½ cup diced green bell peppers
> ½ cup diced plum tomatoes
> ½ cup carrots, diced small
> 2 tablespoons thyme
> 1 Scotch bonnet or habanero pepper (whole) or ¼ teaspoon red pepper flakes
> 1 tablespoon coconut oil
> 2 tablespoons curry powder
> 4 garlic cloves, finely chopped
> 2 tablespoons lemon or lime juice
> 1 cup coconut milk

Season chicken and vegetables with all herbs and spices. Marinate for 4 to 5 hours. Remove chicken from vegetables. Heat coconut oil in fry pan over medium heat and stir fry chicken 3 to 5 minutes; add all vegetables, lemon juice, and coconut milk. Lower heat, cover, and allow to simmer on low heat for 12 to 15 minutes or until tender.

Herb Stir-Fried Chicken and Mixed Veggies
Yield: 4 servings

> 2 pounds chicken cut into thin strips
> 2 teaspoons crushed coriander
> 1 tablespoon tamari
> 1 teaspoon ground cumin
> ½ cup thinly sliced carrots
> ½ cup coconut oil
> ½ cup thinly sliced fennel
> 1 cup thinly sliced red and green bell peppers
> 1 tablespoon diced red chilies
> 4 garlic cloves, finely chopped
> ¼ cup Mirin sauce
> 2 tablespoons roughly chopped mint leaves
> 2 tablespoons roughly chopped sweet basil

Season chicken with coriander, tamari, and cumin. Marinate for 3 hours. Stir-fry carrots in coconut oil for 3 minutes. Add fennel andfry for 2 minutes. Add peppers and garlicand fry for 1 minute. Combine chicken and veggies; return to heat and add Mirin sauce. Cook for 3 minutes, or until the chicken is done. Remove from heatAnd add mint and basil leaves. Combine well and serve.

Mushroom and Garden Vegetable Loaf
Yield: 6 to 8 servings

    1 teaspoon oregano
    2 teaspoons cumin powder
    3 teaspoons Trocomare
    2 tablespoons coconut oil
    2 cups diced onion
    2 cups diced carrots
    1 cup diced celery
    ½ cup diced red bell pepper
    ½ cup diced green bell pepper
    2 cups diced tomatoes
    1 pound Portobello mushrooms, diced
    1 pound button mushrooms, diced
    1 tablespoon finely chopped roasted garlic
    4 eggs
    2 tablespoons tamari
    2 cups Kamut or quinoa flakes

Combine oregano, cumin, and Trocomare. Divide herb mixture and sprinkle over each vegetable. Do not combine the vegetables. Preheat coconut oil in sauté pan. Add onions and cook for 2 to 3 minutes. Add carrots and cook until tender. Add celery, peppers, tomatoes, mushrooms, and garlic. Cook for 20 minutes. Whisk eggs slightly and add to cooled mushroom vegetable mixture. Add tamari and fold in flakes. Combine thoroughly. Pour mixture into greased loaf pan. Bake 25 to 30 minutes at 375 degrees.

Blackened Sea Bass
Yield: 4 servings

    2 tablespoons ground cumin
    2 teaspoons ground coriander
    1 tablespoon Dulse Flakes
    1 tablespoon coconut oil
    3 tablespoons tamari
    1 teaspoon Succanet (an organic natural sweetener)
    1 tablespoon capers
    4 6 ounce pieces of fish, covered with blackening spice mix

Heat cumin seed, coriander seed and Dulse Flakes for 1 minute in a small frying pan with coconut oil. Add tamari, Succanet and capers. Blend well. Place fish in a large container and cover with marinade. Cover and place in the refrigerator a minimum of 3 hours. Broilfish 2 minutes on each side.

Stuffed Free-Range Turkey Breast
Yield: 6 to 8 servings

    2 boneless, skinless turkey breasts (preferably organic)
    1 tablespoon Herbamare
    1 tablespoon finely chopped garlic,
    ½ tablespoon oregano
    ½ tablespoon rosemary
    1 tablespoon coconut oil or melted butter
    ½ cup onion, diced
    1 cup mixed green collards and mustards
    ½ cup thinly sliced carrots
    ½ cup red bell pepper, finely chopped
    1 teaspoon Herbamare to season veggies
    2 eggs
    2 tablespoons cold water
    ⅓ cup cornmeal or spelt flour
    ⅓ cup finely chopped mixed nuts
    ½ teaspoon Succanet
    1 cup orange juice
    1 cup chicken stock

Butterfly turkey breasts and place each split breast between plastic wrap. Pound flat with a meat mallet, being careful not to tear the meat. Combine Herbamare, garlic, oregano, and rosemary and season the turkey. Marinate for 2 hours.

While the turkey is marinating sauté the onion, collard greens mixture, carrots, and bell pepper in coconut oil. Season the mixture with Herbamare. Allow to cool. Put 1 tablespoon of sautéed vegetables between each breast and roll the breast. Secure with toothpicks.

Whisk the eggs and cold water to make an egg wash. Dip breasts in egg wash, cornmeal, and nuts. Place on a well-greased baking sheet and bake at 325 degrees for 25 to 35 minutes. Allow the turkey to rest at room temperature for 10 minutes before slicing diagonally. Combine the Succanet, orange juice, and stock pour over the turkey before serving.

Oven-Roasted Kosher Veal
Yield: 4 to 6 servings

    2 pounds boneless veal sirloin steak
    1 tablespoon crushed coriander
    1 tablespoon ground cumin
    1 teaspoon Trocomare
    ½ teaspoon red pepper flakes
    2 tablespoons dried basil

1 tablespoon dried oregano
2 tablespoons coconut oil
1 cup shredded cheese
1½ cups thinly sliced onion
Roasted red pepper sauce

Remove excess fat from meat; place each steak between plastic wrap and pound lightly with meat mallet. Combine the coriander, cumin, Trocomare, red pepper flakes, basil, and oregano and coat both sides of the steaks. In a skillet, heat 1 tablespoon coconut oil; sear steaks 1 minute on each side. Preheat broiler. Cook veal 7 to 10 minutes on the lower rack, turning once. Remove veal, sprinkle with cheese and return to the oven for 1 minute. In a skillet, sauté the onion in 1 tablespoon coconut oil. Top veal steaks with sautéed onions. Serve roasted red pepper sauce on the side.

Thai-Spiced Steak and Vegetables
Yield: 4 servings

1 pound beef fillet
2 teaspoons organic steak seasoning mix
1 large eggplant, cut into 3-inch long thin strips
1 pound Portobello mushrooms, sliced
1 large onion, thinly sliced
1 large red bell pepper, thinly sliced
2 teaspoons Herbamare

Season the beef with steak seasoning mix. Season veggies with Herbamare. Spread beef and veggies on separate shallow baking dishes or sheets. Broil the veggies on the lower oven rackfor 5 to 7 minutes, turning once. On lower oven rack, broil beef for 7 to 12 minutes or until done. Toss hot steak and veggies in sauce recipe below.

Sauce Ingredients:
1 cup beef stock
1 tablespoon tamari
2 tablespoon Mirin sauce
1 tablespoon Hoisin sauce
2 cloves roasted garlic, crushed
¼ teaspoon cayenne pepper
1 large roasted red pepper
1 teaspoon pickled ginger
¼ cup sesame seeds

Blend stock, Mirin and Hoisin sauces, garlic, cayenne, red pepper, and ginger to sauce consistency. Warm sauce in a saucepan over medium-low heat and add sesame seeds. Toss with steak and veggies.

Mike and Margie Perrin of 11 Maple Street Restaurant in Jensen Beach, Florida

Mike and Margie Perrin founded 11 Maple Street twenty years ago with a philosophy that has pretty much stayed the same: start with the best ingredients you can find, then try to enhance them with a little creativity. As you may notice, the following recipes have few exact measurements since the Perrins believe that exact recipes tend to take away the creativeness of cooking. So enjoy!

Filet of Grass-Fed Beef
Yield: 1 serving per beef filet

grass-fed beef filets
salt
black pepper
extra-virgin olive oil
chopped herbs (such as rosemary and thyme)
2 cups port wine
balsamic vinegar
2 teaspoons honey
3 shallots, chopped
2 garlic cloves, chopped
asparagus
porcini mushrooms
soy sauce
black truffle cheese
3 tablespoons whipping cream

Season each filet with salt and black pepper and rub some extra-virgin olive oil mixed with chopped herbs, such as rosemary and thyme. Grill or pan sear to desired temperature and taste. Put 2 cups of port wine in a sauce pan with a good splash of balsamic vinegar, honey, shallots, and garlic. Reduce by 3⁄4 or until slightly thickened. Strain through a sieve if you like. Parboil asparagus in a generous amount of boiling water for 1 to 2 minutes. Shock in a bowl of ice water. Drain. Season with salt and pepper, extra-virgin olive oil, and a little chopped garlic. Chop mushrooms in half and place in a roasting pan with some extra-virgin olive oil, chopped garlic, salt and pepper, and a dash of soy sauce. Roast in a 400 degree oven for 7 to 8 minutes or until browned and soft. Place black truffle cheese in a double broiler with a few tablespoons of cream and warm until melted. Put cooked filets on plates and stack some asparagus next to them. Place some porcini mushrooms on top of the steak, put a spoonful of truffle cheese over steaks, and drizzle on the port wine sauce.

Halibut with Coconut Curry Roasted Nori Rolls
Yield: 1 serving per fish filet

    halibut filets
    flour
    salt
    pepper
    turmeric
    clarified butter or oil
    3 shallots, minced
    fresh ginger, chopped
    lemongrass, choppped
    cilantro, chopped
    jalapeno pepper, chopped
    curry powder
    garlic clove, minced
    2 cans coconut milk
    kefir lime leaves
    basil, rough chopped
    soba noodles
    crushed red pepper
    soy sauce
    extra-virgin coconut oil
    snow peas
    pine nuts
    Nori seaweed sheets
    radish pickles

Dust both sides of the halibut steaks in a mixture of flour, salt, pepper, and turmeric. Sear on both sides in clarified butter or oil. Finish in a hot oven if steaks are thick and still rare. To make coconut curry sauce: cook shallots in a saucepan until soft. Add a little chopped ginger and lemongrass, cilantro, chopped jalapeno pepper, a pinch of curry powder, and garlic. Cook several more minutes. Add coconut milk and simmer until slightly reduced. Toss in several kefir lime leaves, if available, and some roughly chopped basil. Taste for seasoning. Cook soba noodles according to package directions. Drain and season with crushed red pepper, soy sauce, and extra-virgin coconut oil. Add some slivered snow peas and pine nuts. Wrap in Nori seaweed sheets. Place in a roasting pan and roast for about 5 to 10 minutes at 375 degrees. Place 2 Nori rolls in a shallow bowl, put halibut on top, and ladle some coconut curry sauce over the halibut. Garnish with lime leaves, fried shallots, and radish pickles.

Goat Cheese Stuffed Free-Range Chicken Breast
Yield: 1 serving per two chicken breasts

black beans
salt
black pepper
chopped garlic
extra-virgin olive oil
2 free-range chicken breasts
organic flour for dusting
fresh goat cheese
chopped thyme
chopped marjoram
basil pesto (see recipe below)
rhubarb
unsalted butter, melted
½ cup balsamic vinegar
honey
watercress
red onions
Basil Pesto
Kosher salt
2 garlic cloves
Toasted pine nuts
Extra-virgin olive oil
Basil

Soak black beans overnight. Drain. Cook black beans in large pot with a generous amount of water until tender. Drain and season with salt and pepper, a little chopped garlic, and extra-virgin olive oil.

Combine goat cheese with thyme and marjoram. Cut a pocket in the side of each chicken breast and stuff with the goat cheese mixture. Rub inside and out with basil pesto. Dust the chicken breast with flour and pan sear both sides until nicely browned. Check middle to check for pinkness, then finish roasting in a 375-degree oven for 15 minutes, or until done. Wash and cut one rhubarb stalk per person on the diagonal into ½ inch pieces. Peel if stringy. Put in roasting pan, drizzle with unsalted butter until well coated. Add ½ cup of balsamic vinegar and salt and pepper.Drizzle honey over all. Roast in the oven until the rhubarb feels soft and the butter and balsamic vinegar begin to caramelize. Do not stir or pieces will dissolve. Taste for tartness and drizzle more honey if desired. Carefully spoon some rhubarb on each plate and top with a chicken breast. Toss watercress lightly with black beans, sliced red onions, a splash of balsamic vinegar, and extra-virgin olive oil.

To make pesto, grind a good pinch of kosher salt and 2 cloves of garlic in a mortar. Add some toasted pine nuts (or substitute almonds, walnuts, or any other nuts) and a little extra-virgin olive oil. Grind up good. Roughly chop some basil, add to mortar, grind up a little, and finish with more olive oil. Place bean salad on top of chicken and drizzle a little pesto around the plate.

Wood-Grilled King Salmon with Ricotta Gnocchi
Chanterelle Mushrooms and Fava Beans
Yield: 1 serving per salmon filet

> salmon filets
> salt
> fennel seeds, divided
> flat leaf parsley, chopped and divided
> chervil, chopped and divided
> thyme, chopped and divided
> chives, chopped and divided
> basil, chopped and divided
> extra-virgin olive oil
> chanterelle mushrooms
> marjoram, chopped
> rosemary, chopped
> fava beans, shelled and blanched
> garlic clove, chopped
> pepper
> gnocchi
> saffron aioli
> roasted red peppers

Sprinkle salmon filets with salt. Toss some fennel, flat leaf parsley, chervil, thyme, chives, and basil in extra-virgin olive oil in a small bowl and cover. Put a weight on top of the salmon and refrigerate for 12 to 24 hours. Rinse salt off fillets and season with reserved chopped herbs and olive oil. Grill filets over a hot fire until rare. Do not overcook or the salmon will dry out. Wash dirt off of chanterelles and lightly squeeze out excess moisture. Warm extra-virgin olive oil in a sauce pan, toss in chanterelles and cook until soft. Add marjoram, thyme, rosemary, and fava beans. Season with garlic, salt, and pepper. Add more olive oil if desired. Cook your favorite gnocchi recipe and place on plate. Spoon chanterelles and fava beans over gnocchi. Put salmon on top and drizzle the juices from the mushrooms around the plate. Garnish with saffron aioli, chervil, and roasted red peppers.

Pear and Black Currant Sauce

3 to 4 fresh pears, peeled and roughly chopped
clarified butter
1 small leek, chopped
Salt and pepper
2 tablespoons maple syrup
2 cups port wine
2 handfuls black currants
2 cups vegetable stock

In a saucepan, caramelize pears in clarified butter until they **turn golden**. Add leek and season with salt and pepper. Stir for ten minutes, then drizzle with maple syrup. Cook 2 more minutes on medium heat, stirring often. Add port wine and black currants; turn up heat and reduce until mixture starts to thicken. Add vegetable stock and reduce with the port wine.

Rare-Seared Tuna with Brown Rice
Yield: 1 serving per tuna steak

tuna steaks
sake
soy sauce
fresh ginger
cilantro, chopped
clarified butter or grapeseed oil
brown rice
large daikon radish
onion
garlic clove, chopped
jalapeño pepper, chopped
shiitake mushrooms, sliced
salt
pepper
sautéed vegetables
½ cup fish or vegetable stock
3 ounces Cold, unsalted butter
bok choy leaves
wasabi
snow peas
wakame seaweed salad

Marinate each tuna steak in a half-and-half mixture of sake and soy sauce with a little grated ginger and chopped cilantro for at least 1 hour. Heat clarified butter or grapeseed oil in a pan and sear tuna on both sides. If you prefer your tuna medium-rare or medium cook a few minutes longer. Cook your favorite brown rice until tender and place about ⅓ in a Cuisinart or blender and grind coarsely. Using a vegetable peeler make several long strips of a large daikon radish and dip in soy sauce. Cook onions in a saucepan. Add garlic, a small piece of ginger, the jalapeno pepper, and shiitake mushrooms.Cook until soft. Put the ground rice and whole rice in a bowl and season with salt and pepper.Add sautéed vegetables andmix well. Form rice into cakes the size of the tuna steaks, wrap in daikon radish, and sear both sides of rice in a hot pan. In a medium saucepan, warm ½ cup fish or vegetable stock. Add butter and swirl pan until the butter slowly melts. Take off heat and stir in wakame seaweed salad. Put butter sauce on a plate, top with rice cakes, place tuna on top of rice and garnish with stir-fried bok choy leaves, shitake mushrooms, wasabi, and snow peas.

Wood-Grilled Buffalo Tenderloin
Yield: 1 serving per buffalo steak

buffalo steaks
chili powder
honey
olive oil
wild rice
salt
garlic clove, minced
1 handful black currants
pine nuts, optional
1 cup organic milk
1 cup vegetable or chicken stock
Cold milled polenta
whipping cream, optional
Parmesan cheese
Pear and Black Currant Sauce (see recipe below)

Rub each buffalo steak with a mixture of chili powder, honey, and pure olive oil. Grill or pan sear to desired temperature. Cook wild rice according to directions.Drain, and season with salt and garlic, black currants, olive oil, and pine nuts, if desired. Put organic milk and vegetable or chicken stock in a saucepan. Season with salt and bring to a simmer.Slowly stir in polenta until mixture starts to thicken. Turn heat to low and cook, stirring often for about 15 to 20 minutes. If mixture is too thick, thin with some cream or stock. Taste and season with grated Parmesan cheese and salt to taste. Ladle the soft polenta onto each plate with a spoonful of the wild rice. Top with sliced buffalo steak and place some of the Pear and Black Currant compote on the buffalo and around the plate.

Nicki Rubin & Friends

My wife, Nicki, and some of our friends have contributed a number of healthy and tasty recipes that they love preparing. These recipes have been great for entertaining guests at our home.

Cilantro-Lime Sea Bass (or Halibut)
Yield: 2 servings

coconut oil
fresh garlic clove, minced
tomatoes, chopped
cilantro, chopped
2½ pounds sea bass filets (or halibut)

In a pan, melt coconut oil. Stir in garlic and cook for 2 minutes. Stir in chopped tomatoes and cilantro. Cook for another minute. Add filets and cook approximately 10 minutes, turning once.

Garlic Mashed Potatoes
Yield: 4 servings

4 medium potatoes, peeled
⅓ to ½ cup heavy whipping cream
4 tablespoons butter
1½ teaspoons minced garlic
Herbamare or salt and pepper to taste

Cut potatoes into large pieces and boil in salted water for 35 to 45 minutes, or until tender. Drain thoroughly. Mash with a fork. Mix potatoes with cream, butter, garlic, and salt and pepper. Serve immediately.

Easy Spanish Rice
Yield: 8 servings

4 cups cooked brown rice
3 onions, chopped
4 tablespoons olive oil
6 garlic cloves
1 teaspoon mustard powder
3 cups cooked tomatoes (you may use canned)
1 cup grated cheddar cheese
sea salt and pepper to taste
¼ cup chopped red or yellow pepper

Brown onions in oil and combine with remaining ingredients. Pour into well-greased baking dish and bake at 375 degrees for 35 minutes.

Chicken Salad
Yield: 1 to 2 servings

6 ounces chicken, cooked and chopped
1 tablespoon Omega-3 mayonnaise
1 tablespoon flaxseed oil or garlic-chili flax oil
chopped onions
chopped bell peppers
chopped celery
lettuce or toasted sprouted bread, for serving

Combine all ingredients and serve over lettuce or on toasted sprouted bread.

Oriental Chicken (or Salmon) Salad
Yield: 4 servings

3 tablespoons soy sauce
2 teaspoons grated fresh ginger
2 boneless, skinless chicken breasts or salmon filets
5 cups mixed salad greens
1 cup fresh bean sprouts
1 cup fresh snow pea pods, trimmed
½ green bell pepper, thinly sliced
½ red bell pepper, thinly sliced
1 small or medium cucumber, thinly sliced
1 cup sliced green onions
2 teaspoons sesame seeds, toasted for garnish
Oriental Salad Dressing (see recipe below)
Spicy Peanut Sauce (see recipe on page 304)

Combine soy sauce and ginger in a shallow baking dish. Add chicken or salmon. Cover and marinate in refrigerator up to 4 hours. Remove chicken or salmon from marinade and discard remaining marinade. Cook chicken or fish until lightly browned. Combine mixed salad greens with the sprouts, peas, peppers, cucumber, onions, and sesame seeds. Pour ½ cup Oriental Salad Dressing over salad and toss. Arrange cooked chicken or salmon on top and pour remaining salad dressing on top. Serve with Spicy Peanut Sauce.

Oriental Salad Dressing
Yield: 1 cup

4 tablespoons rice vinegar
2 tablespoons soy sauce
2 teaspoons grated ginger
2 teaspoons toasted sesame oil
2 teaspoons finely chopped green onion or chives
2 garlic cloves, peeled and mashed
1 teaspoon raw honey
⅔ cup extra-virgin olive oil
2 teaspoons unrefined flaxseed oil

Place all ingredients in a jar and shake vigorously.

Spicy Peanut Sauce
Yield: 1½ cups

½ cup peanut butter
⅓ cup coconut milk
2 tablespoons soy sauce
1 tablespoon grated fresh ginger
1 tablespoon sesame oil
¼ teaspoon crushed red pepper
¼ cup chicken broth

Combine all ingredients in a bowl and mix well.

Berry Smoothie
Yield: 2 servings

During my healing process, I consumed this smoothie one to two times per day with raw eggs. Contrary to popular belief, eggs from healthy free-range, pastured chickens are often free of dangerous germs. If the egg has an odor, obviously it should not be eaten. Since most of the salmonella infections are caused by germs on the shell, for added protection it is best to wash the eggs in the shell with a mild alcohol or hydrogen peroxide solution or a fruit and vegetable wash. For those who can't stand the thought of consuming raw eggs in their smoothies, you can enjoy healthy smoothies without them, but you should know that the best-tasting ice creams are made with egg yolks.

10 ounces yogurt, kefir, or coconut milk or cream
1 to 2 raw omega-3 eggs

1 tablespoon extra-virgin coconut oil
1 tablespoon flaxseed oil or hemp seed oil
1 to 2 tablespoons raw honey
1 tablespoon goat's milk protein powder (optional)
½ to 1 cup fresh or frozen blueberries, strawberries, raspberries, or blackberries
vanilla extract, optional

Combine all ingredients in a high-speed blender and blend until desired texture.

Lemon Garlic Chicken
Yield: 4 servings

¾ cup honey
¾ cup lemon juice
5 tablespoons soy sauce
3 tablespoons chicken broth
6 garlic cloves, mashed
4 boneless, skinless chicken breasts

Mix honey, lemon, soy sauce, chicken broth, and garlic in a shallow baking dish. Set aside ½ cup of the mixture. Prick chicken breasts several times with a fork and place in remaining mixture. Cover and refrigerate at least 1 hour. Remove chicken and discard remaining marinade. Grill over medium heat 10 to 12 minutes on each side, occasionally basting with the reserved ½ cup marinade.

Red Meat Chili
Yield: 8 servings

1½ pounds ground chuck, venison, or buffalo
48 ounce can tomato juice
1 onion, chopped
3 cans kidney beans, drained and rinsed
1 can Italian style diced tomatoes
chili powder
salt and pepper to taste

Brown meat in a skillet. Bring the tomato juice, onion, kidney beans, and tomatoes to a boil in a large pot. Reduce heat and simmer. Drain meat and add to pot. Add chili pepper, salt and pepper to taste. Cook on low for 30 minutes.

Hobo Potatoes
Yield: 6 servings

> 6 to 8 medium potatoes
> 1 large onion
> 1 stick butter
> Salt and pepper or Herbamare

Fold heavy duty aluminum foil to make cooking area. (Please note that I do not advocate using aluminum foil regularly.) Slice potatoes and onion thinly in order to make layers. A food processor makes this easy. Layer small pieces of butter, potatoes, onions, and salt and pepper. Cover with another sheet of aluminum foil and fold the sides to make a tent over the potatoes. Grill over medium heat for 45 minutes or until tender. Or bake in the oven at 400 degrees for 45 minutes.

Easy Fried Eggs
Yield: 1 to 2 servings

> 4 eggs
> Extra-virgin coconut oil or butter
> 1 tablespoon hot water

Add coconut oil or butter to a preheated pan. Break eggs carefully into a dish and slip into the pan. Add 1 tablespoon of hot water. Cover. Cook slowly until whites are firm and yolks are covered with a thin white film. Add seasonings as you like and serve.

Easy Oatmeal
Yield: 2 servings

> 1 cup rolled oats
> 2 cups water
> 1 teaspoon yogurt
> 1 tablespoon extra-virgin coconut oil or butter
> honey to taste

Soak the oats overnight in 1 cup of water with 1 teaspoon of yogurt added. In the morning, add remaining water. Bring to a boil and simmer for 1 to 2 minutes. Soaked oatmeal cooks *very* fast. Add the oil or butter and honey.

Spaghetti with Meat Sauce
Yield: 6 servings

2 14.5 ounce cans Italian-style diced tomatoes
1 8 ounce can tomato sauce
1 6 ounce can tomato paste
2 teaspoons extra-virgin olive oil
1 teaspoon minced garlic
1 teaspoon dried oregano
1 teaspoon dried basil
½ teaspoon garlic powder
¼ teaspoon thyme
¼ teaspoon crushed red pepper
½ teaspoon salt or Herbamare to taste
½ large onion, chopped
1 cup button mushrooms, washed and quartered, optional
1 tablespoon butter
1 pound ground beef, venison, or buffalo
1½ boxes spelt spaghetti or angel hair pasta (whole wheat is a substitute for spelt)
Parmesan cheese, optional

Combine the diced tomatoes, tomato sauce, tomato paste, olive oil, garlic, oregano, basil, garlic powder, thyme, crushed red pepper, and salt in a medium- or large-sized pot and bring to a slight boil. Reduce to low heat. In the meantime, sauté the onion and mushrooms in butter over medium heat until tender. Brown the meat in a large skillet, stirring until it crumbles. Drain the meat. Add the cooked meat, mushrooms, and onions to the sauce. Prepare the spelt spaghetti or angel hair pasta according to the package directions. (Adding a small amount of olive oil to the boiling water helps the pasta not to stick.) Drain. Top pasta with meat sauce and sprinkle with Parmesan cheese.

Creamy High Enzyme Dessert
Yield: 1 serving

4 ounces goat's milk, plain yogurt, or cultured cream
1 tablespoon raw, unheated honey
1 teaspoon flaxseed oil
½ cup fresh or frozen organic berries

Mix yogurt, honey, and flaxseed oil. Top with berries.

Sweet and Sour Chicken
Yield: 4 servings

1½ cup brown rice
1 tablespoon coconut oil
1 pound boneless chicken, cubed
½ red bell pepper, cut into thin strips
½ green bell pepper, cut into thin strips
1 tablespoon cornstarch
¼ cup soy sauce
1 cup pineapple, cut into small chunks
¼ cup pineapple juice
3 tablespoon vinegar
3 tablespoons Rapadura (a sweetener found in natural health food stores)
½ teaspoon ground ginger
½ teaspoon garlic powder

Prepare brown rice as directed on package. Heat coconut oil in a large skillet and stir-fry chicken until well browned. Add peppers and cook another 2 minutes. Mix cornstarch and soy sauce and pour into the skillet. Add pineapple and juice, vinegar, Rapadura, ginger, and garlic powder. Bring to a full boil. Serve chicken over brown rice.

Mexican Quinoa
Yield: 4 servings

1 tablespoon sesame oil
1 onion, finely chopped
1½ cup quinoa
1 teaspoon minced garlic
8 ounce can diced tomatoes
1½ cups chicken stock, heated
salt and pepper or Herbamare
1 cup frozen peas, thawed and drained
¾ cup fresh cilantro, chopped

Heat oil in a large pot over medium heat. Add onion and quinoa. Cook for 8 to 10 minutes or until lightly browned. Stir in garlic and cook for two more minutes. Add tomatoes and chicken stock and season with pepper or Herbamare. Bring to a boil, cover tightly, and simmer over very low heat for 10 to 15 minutes. Remove from heat and leave covered for 10 minutes or until all the liquid has been absorbed. Stir in peas and sprinkle with cilantro.

Variation:
1 cup of brown rice may also be substituted for 1½ cups quinoa.

Mochachino Smoothie
Yield: two 8 ounce servings

10 ounces yogurt, kefir, or coconut milk or cream
1 to 2 raw omega-3 eggs (optional, see note on page 304)
1 tablespoons extra-virgin coconut oil
1 tablespoon flaxseed or hemp seed oil
1 to 2 tablespoons unheated honey
1 tablespoon goat's milk protein powder (optional)
2 tablespoons cocoa or carob powder
1 tablespoon organic roasted coffee beans
1 to 2 fresh or frozen bananas
½ teaspoon vanilla extract

Combine all the ingredients in a high-speed blender.

Spinach and Goat Cheese Meat Lasagna
Yield: 8 servings

12 spelt lasagna noodles   *4 mins*
1 teaspoon olive oil
1 pound ground chuck, venison, or buffalo
3 cups pasta sauce (or tomato sauce)   *1 can*
3½ cups ricotta cheese
4 ounces crumbled goat or feta cheese   *1/4 cup*
2 eggs, beaten
1 tablespoon chopped fresh basil (or 1 teaspoon dried)
½ cup grated Parmesan cheese
salt and pepper or Herbamare
1 cup shredded mozzarella cheese
4 cups raw baby spinach (or regular chopped spinach)

Preheat oven to 400 degrees. Place lasagna noodles in a large shallow dish and cover with boiling water for 15 to 20 minutes to soften. Cook meat in a large skillet for 10 minutes or until brown, stirring occasionally. Drain fat and return to skillet. Reduce to low heat and add in pasta sauce. Simmer for 5 minutes. In a bowl, mix ricotta and goat cheese, eggs, basil, Parmesan, and salt and pepper or use Herbamare to taste. Spread 1 cup of sauce on bottom of 9 x 13-inch baking dish. Place ⅓ of softened noodles on top of sauce. Add ½ spinach, pressing down to make a flat layer. Spread ½ ricotta mixture as the next layer. Top with meat mixture, and then another ⅓ of noodles. Add remaining spinach as a layer, and then the remaining ricotta mixture as a layer. Top with remaining noodles and last cup of sauce. Bake 45 minutes to 1 hour on the middle rack at 400 degrees. Pour mozzarella cheese over sauce the last 10 minutes of baking. May be prepared and refrigerated up to 24 hours or frozen.

Dirty Eggs
Yield: 1 serving

1 teaspoon butter or coconut oil
2 eggs, beaten
⅛ medium onion, finely chopped
⅛ medium tomato, finely chopped
2 tablespoons cilantro
¼ teaspoon minced fresh garlic
salt and pepper or use Herbamare to taste

Heat butter or oil in pan over medium heat. Mix all ingredients together. Pour into pan, and stir constantly with a wooden spatula until light and fluffy. Serve immediately.

EZ Pizza
Yield: 1 serving

2 pieces sprouted grain bread or 1 sprouted grain English muffin, toasted
pasta sauce
green onions, thinly sliced (optional)
Monterey Jack or cheddar cheese, sliced
Herbamare seasoning

Place bread on a baking sheet. Spoon pasta sauce over bread. Place onions over pasta sauce. Cut slices of cheese and place over onions. Sprinkle with Herbamare and cook in oven for 5 minutes or until cheese melts.

Quick Sprouted Apple Crisp
Yield: 4 servings

4 medium baking apples
1 ounce purified water
1 tablespoon butter
2 tablespoons honey, separated
⅔ cup Ezekiel 4:9 sprouted cereal

Preheat oven to 375 degrees. Peel, core, and chop the apples. Place apples in medium-sized pot with water and butter. Cover and cook on medium heat for 15 minutes or until apples can be mashed with a fork to the consistency of apple sauce. Stir in 1 tablespoon of honey. Pour mixture into a medium-sized baking dish. Pour cereal evenly over apple mixture and press down with a fork. Drizzle with remaining 1 tablespoon of honey. Bake for 15 minutes. Remove from heat, let cool, and serve.

Steak Au Poivre
Yield: 4 servings

4 filet mignons, approximately 6 ounces each
sea salt
2 tablespoons black peppercorns
2 tablespoons butter
1 tablespoon extra-virgin olive oil
⅔ cup whipping cream

Season both sides of steak with sea salt. Crush peppercorns and spread on a plate. Press each side of steak firmly onto the peppercorns until well coated. Melt butter and olive oil in a skillet. When butter is foaming, add steaks and cook over high heat for 2 minutes on each side. Lower heat and continue cooking to desired doneness*. Remove steaks from skillet and keep warm. Pour cream into skillet and add salt and pepper to taste. When sauce is heated, pour over steaks and serve immediately.

*For rare stakes, cook for around 2 minutes per side. For medium steaks, cook around 3 minutes per side. For well-done steaks, cook 4 or more minutes per side.

Sweet Onion Pudding
Yield: 8 servings

2 cups whipping cream
6 tablespoons Parmesan cheese
6 eggs, lightly beaten
3 tablespoons spelt or kamut flour
1 tablespoon honey
2 teaspoons baking powder
1 teaspoon sea salt
½ stick butter
6 medium sweet onions, thinly sliced

Mix whipping cream, Parmesan cheese, and eggs in a large bowl. Combine flour, honey, baking powder, and sea salt. Slowly stir into egg mixture and set aside. Melt butter in a large skillet over medium heat. Add onions, stirring often. Cook 30 to 40 minutes or until onions are caramel colored. Remove from heat. Stir onions into egg mixture. Spoon into a lightly greased 9 x 13-inch baking dish. Bake at 350 degrees for 30 minutes.

Eggs Benedict
Yield: 4 servings

8 slices turkey bacon (which is not a pork product)
2 tablespoons vinegar
4 eggs
2 sprouted grain English muffins
butter

Hollandaise Sauce
2 teaspoons lemon juice
2 teaspoons white vinegar
3 egg yolks, room temperature
8 tablespoons butter, melted
Herbamare or salt and pepper

Cook turkey bacon under the broiler until crisp. Keep warm. Prepare the hollandaise sauce as directed.

To poach the eggs:

Add vinegar to a large pan of boiling water. Lower heat so that water is simmering. Crack eggs and gently slide into water. Discard egg shells. Simmer for about 4 minutes. Remove with a slotted spoon. Toast the muffin halves, butter them, and put onto plates. Place 2 slices turkey bacon and an egg on each muffin and top with sauce. Serve immediately.

To make sauce:

Pour lemon juice and white vinegar into a small glass or metal bowl. Add egg yolks and whisk until light and frothy. Place the bowl over a pan of simmering water and whisk until sauce thickens. Gradually add in melted butter while constantly whisking. Season and keep warm.

Variation:

Spinach is another great variation instead of turkey bacon.

Banana Bread
Yield: 1 loaf

½ cup coconut oil
½ cup honey
½ cup Rapadura (a sweetener found in natural health food stores) or Succanet (an organic natural sweetener)
2 eggs, beaten
5 ripe bananas, mashed
2 cups spelt or kamut flour

1 teaspoon baking powder
½ teaspoon salt
3 tablespoons whipping cream or milk
½ teaspoon vanilla
½ cup chopped walnuts

Preheat oven to 350 degrees. Beat coconut oil, honey, and Rapadura in a large bowl. Add eggs and mashed bananas. Add dry ingredients. Add cream and vanilla. Stir in walnuts. Pour in a greased loaf pan. Bake for 1 hour at 350 degrees.

Italian Turkey Sausage and Peppers
by Jason Longman
Yield: 4 servings

2 tablespoons olive oil
1 large onion, cut in half and sliced
2 green peppers, julienne
1 red pepper, julienne
1 large tomato, diced
4 Italian turkey sausages
sea salt

Heat a heavy saucepan over medium heat. Add olive oil and sauté onions gently for 7 minutes. Add red and green peppers and cook over medium heat until very soft. Meanwhile, cook turkey sausage on the grill or in another pan with a little olive oil. Add tomatoes to the peppers and onions mixture and stir until combined. Cover and reduce heat to low, cookfor 6 to 8 minutes, until tomato is incorporated. Cut up sausage and add to the pepper mixture. Allow the mixture to simmer for a few minutes. Season to taste and serve.

Piña Colada Smoothie
Yield: two 8 ounce servings

10 ounces coconut milk/cream
1 to 2 raw omega-3 eggs (see note on page 304)
1 tablespoon flaxseed oil or hemp seed oil
1 to 2 tablespoons unheated honey
1 tablespoon goat's milk protein powder (optional)
1cup fresh or frozen pineapple
1 fresh or frozen banana
½ teaspoon vanilla extract

Combine the following ingredients in a high-speed blender.

Chicken with Sun-Dried Tomatoes and Spinach
by Jason Longman
Yield: 2 servings

  2 boneless, skinless chicken breasts
  salt and pepper
  2 tablespoons butter
  1 tablespoon olive oil
  ½ cup sliced sun-dried tomatoes
  2 tablespoons capers
  ½ cup white wine
  ½ cup chicken broth
  1 lemon
  1 cup fresh spinach

Cut both chicken breasts into halves. Pound out to 1/4-inch thick. Season both sides with salt and pepper. Heat a large saucepan over medium high heat. Melt 1 tablespoon of butter and add olive oil. Sauté chicken breasts evenly on both sides until done, about 3 minutes per side. Remove chicken and set aside, keeping warm. Add sun-dried tomatoes and capers and let cook for 1 minute. Add white wine, chicken broth, and juice from one lemon. Reduce by half and add spinach, cooking until just wilted.

Tomato Basil Soup
by Jason Longman
Yield: 2 servings

  1 medium onion, halved and sliced
  1 clove garlic, minced
  1 tablespoon olive oil
  2 large cans of diced tomatoes
  ½ cup fresh basil, chopped
  4 cups chicken broth
  2 teaspoons balsamic vinegar
  ½ cups heavy cream (optional)

In a heavy bottomed pan, sauté onions and garlic in oil over medium high heat until soft, being careful not to burn garlic. Add tomatoes, basil, chicken broth, and salt and pepper. Bring to a boil, then reduce heat and simmer for 20 minutes. In a blender, puree the mixture and then strain back into a clean pot. Heat soup and add balsamic vinegar and heavy cream if desired.

Shepherd's Pie
by Jason Longman
Yield: 4 servings

2 sweet potatoes
1 medium onion, diced
1 tablespoon olive oil
1 pound ground bison (or other red meat)
1 cup sliced mushrooms
⅔ cup hummus
1 squash, julienne
1 zucchini, julienne
3 tablespoons butter, plus extra for greasing pan

Heat oven to 350 degrees. Place sweet potatoes in oven and cook for 35 minutes. While sweet potatoes are cooking, sauté onion in olive oil for 2 to 3 minutes over medium heat. Add bison and mushrooms, cooking until done. Stir in hummus and set aside. In another pan, sauté squash and zucchini in 1 tablespoon of butter until just tender. Peel sweet potatoes and mash with 2 tablespoons butter. Grease a 9 x 9-inch casserole dish with butter. Spread the bison mixture evenly in pan. Cover with vegetable mix. Spread mashed sweet potatoes over top. Cover and cook in 350 degree oven for 20 minutes. Uncover and let cook for 5 minutes.

Mocha Swiss Almond Smoothie
Yield: two 8 ounce servings

10 ounces yogurt, kefir, or coconut milk/cream
1 to 2 raw omega-3 eggs (see note on page 304)
1 tablespoon extra-virgin coconut oil
1 tablespoon flaxseed oil or hemp seed oil
1 to 2 tablespoons unheated honey
1 tablespoon goat's milk protein powder (optional)
2 tablespoons cocoa or carob powder and 2 tablespoons raw almond butter or 4 tablespoons chocolate almond spread
1 to 2 fresh or frozen bananas
½ teaspoon vanilla extract

Combine all ingredients in a high-speed blender until desired consistency.

Beef Avocado Salad with Rosemary Dressing
by Keith Tindall of White Egret Farm
Yield: 6 servings

> 2 pounds sirloin steak, cooked medium rare, cut in julienne strips (leftover steak may be used)
> 3 avocados
> 3 tomatoes, ripe but firm
> 1 purple onion, thinly sliced
> 1 bunch watercress, leaves only

Rosemary Dressing ingredients:
> 2 small shallots, chopped
> 1 garlic clove, chopped
> 2 teaspoons parsley, minced
> 1 sprig fresh or ½ teaspoon dried rosemary
> 1½ tablespoons Dijon-style mustard
> ½ cup lemon juice
> 2 teaspoons raw, unheated honey
> 1½ tablespoons vermouth
> ⅔ cup raw wine vinegar
> 1⅓ cup of extra-virgin olive oil
> sea salt to taste
> black pepper, freshly ground

To make the dressing, combine the shallots and garlic. Mix these with the parsley, rosemary, and mustard. Stir in the lemon juice, honey, and vermouth and let this mixture stand for 2 hours (this portion may be done in advance and stored in the refrigerator). Force the dressing through a sieve into a bowl. Add the wine vinegar. Whisk in the olive oil. Season with salt and pepper to taste. Add a portion of the dressing to the beef and stir to coat. (If you are starting with fresh meat, you may also marinate the meat in this dressing before cooking). Peel and chop the avocados and tomatoes. Add the avocados, tomatoes and onion to the dressed beef. Serve on a bed of watercress.

Green Chili
by Jason Longman

> 3 jalapenos, seeded
> 3 bunches green onions
> 1 garlic clove
> 2 tablespoons olive oil
> 1 pound ground turkey
> 1 pound turkey sausage
> 1 large can tomatillos, drained

1 tablespoon cumin
2 tablespoons dried cilantro
2 tablespoons dried parsley
3 ounces green mole (the best comes from Oaxaca, Mexico)
1 cup water
2 cups pinto beans

In a small food processor, blend the jalapenos. If you like a hotter chili, leave the number of seeds that suit your taste. Chop green onions and sauté with blended jalapeno and chopped garlic in olive oil for 3 to 5 minutes. Add ground turkey and turkey sausage and brown. In a food processor, blend tomatillos. Add tomatillos and all spices, simmer for 45 minutes. Bring one cup of water to a boil and add green mole until dissolved. Add mole and pinto beans to turkey mixture and simmer for 30 minutes. Serve with sour cream or crème fraîche.

Cranberry Apple Crunch
Yield: 6 to 8 servings

3 cooking apples (such as Granny Smith) peeled and cut into cubes
1 bag fresh or frozen cranberries
1 cup Rapadura sweetener
coconut oil
1 stick butter, melted
⅓ cup honey
2¼ cups honey oats
1½ cups chopped walnuts

Mix apples, cranberries, and Rapadura and place in casserole dish greased with coconut oil. Mix melted butter, honey, honey oats, and chopped walnuts and pour over apples and cranberries. Bake in a covered dish for 1 hour at 350 degrees.

Easy Scrambled Eggs
Yield: 3 to 4 servings

6 eggs
¼ cup heavy cream
sea salt and pepper
3 tablespoons melted butter or extra-virgin coconut oil
cayenne pepper (optional)

Beat eggs well. Add cream, salt and pepper. Heat butter in skillet or pan and add egg mixture, cooking and swirling slowly. If desired, add one cup of chopped turkey bacon, chicken, beef, or peppers. Season to taste with cayenne pepper if desired.

Easy Lamb Stew
Yield: 6 servings

1½ pounds lamb stew meat
Extra-virgin coconut oil
water
1 teaspoon sea salt
1½ cups diced carrots
1 cup diced celery
¼ cup canned tomatoes
1½ cups diced potatoes
¼ cup chopped onion

Brown the lamb in extra-virgin coconut oil. Cover with water and add salt. Simmer until meat is tender. Add vegetables and cover. Simmer for 30 minutes or until vegetables are cooked.

Nicki's Meatloaf
Yield: 4 to 6 servings

1½ pounds ground chuck, venison, or buffalo
1 egg, beaten
½ teaspoon Dijon mustard
½ cup ketchup
1 onion, finely chopped
½ red or green bell pepper, finely chopped
¼ to ½ cup whipping cream (or milk)
1½ teaspoons salt
½ cup oats
1 cup bread (or torn up buttered sprouted grain toast)
1½ tablespoons Rapadura or Succanet sweeteners

Topping ingredients:
½ cup ketchup
3 tablespoons Rapadura or Succanet (natural sweeteners)
2 teaspoons stone ground mustard
½ teaspoon chili powder

Mix ingredients and bake in loaf pan 1½ hours at 350 degrees. Spoon mixed topping ingredients over loaf the last 10 minutes.

Blueberry Cobbler
Yield: 2 to 4 servings

¼ stick butter
1 cup spelt or kamut flour
½ cup Rapadura sweetener
2 teaspoons baking powder
2 to 2½ cups blueberries

Preheat oven to 375 degrees. Melt ¼ stick butter in 8 x 8-inch dish. Mix dry ingredients and pour on top of melted butter. Pour 2 to 2½ cups berries on top of mixture. Bake at 375 degrees for 35 to 40 minutes.

Variations:
Blackberry, Blackberry & Cherry, Blueberry & Peach

Sweet Potato Pie
Yield: 8 servings

4 medium sweet potatoes
1 teaspoon vanilla
2 well-beaten eggs
½ stick butter, melted
½ cup Rapadura sweetener
¼ cup honey
1 teaspoon coconut oil
Topping (see recipe below)

Boil potatoes with skins on for 25 to 30 minutes, or until tender. Remove from pot, let cool, peel and mash. Mix all ingredients with a fork. Grease a 9 x 13-inch baking dish with coconut oil and pour potato mixture in pan. Sprinkle with topping mixture and bake for 30 minutes at 350 degrees.

1 cup chopped pecans
½ cup spelt or kamut flour
½ cup Rapadura sweetener
¼ cup honey
¾ stick butter, melted

Combine ingredients and sprinkle over potato mixture.

Easy Soft/Hard-Boiled Eggs

Wash eggs and cover with boiling water. Simmer for 4 minutes if you're making soft-boiled eggs, and 12 minutes if you're making hard-boiled eggs. Hard-boiled eggs may be plunged in cold water if you'll be using them in another recipe as sliced additions or garnishes. Hard-boiled eggs may also be made several at a time and then refrigerated for convenient snacking later.

Banana Peach Smoothie
Yield: two 8 ounce servings

   10 ounces yogurt, kefir, or coconut milk/cream
   1 to 2 raw omega-3 eggs (see note on page 304)
   1 tablespoon extra-virgin coconut oil
   1 tablespoon flaxseed oil or hemp seed oil
   1 to 2 tablespoons unheated honey
   1 tablespoon of goat's milk protein powder (optional)
   ½ to 1 cup fresh or frozen peaches
   1 fresh or frozen banana
   ½ teaspoon vanilla extract (optional)

Combine the ingredients in a high-speed blender.

Roasted Pastured Chicken
by Keith Tindall of White Egret Farm
Yield: 4 servings

   1 4 to 5 pound pastured broiler chicken, whole
   1 apple, small
   1 onion, small
   1 stalk celery, plus leaves
   2 to 3 tablespoons olive oil
   1 sprig rosemary
   sea salt
   Freshly ground pepper

Rinse and drain the chicken. If you are starting with a frozen chicken be certain it is completely thawed. Preheat the oven to 350 degrees. Quarter and core the apple. Peel and quarter the onion. Slice the celery into 23-inch lengths. Add about 2 tablespoons of olive oil to the cavity of the bird. Stuff the bird with the apple, celery, onion, and rosemary. Rub the outside of the bird with olive oil. Sprinkle the bird with salt and freshly ground pepper, then rub into the skin. Place the chicken in a baking dish with 2-inch sides. Bake approximately 1½ hours or until meat thermometer reads 180 degrees when pushed into the thigh. Remove the chicken from the oven and allow to rest for approximately 20 minutes before carving. The rest period allows the juices to redistribute and results in more tender meat.

Zesty Popcorn

 3 tablespoons extra-virgin coconut oil
 ⅓ cup popcorn
 2 tablespoons garlic-chili flax
 2 tablespoons melted butter
 Herbamare to taste

Melt coconut oil in a pan over medium heat. Pour popcorn into pan. Cover pan with lid. Cook until popping slows down. Pour popcorn into a large bowl and add melted butter, garlic-chili flax, and seasoning. Mix thoroughly.

Easy French Toast
From the *Lazy Person's Whole Food Cookbook* by Stephen Byrnes
Yield: 4 servings

 2 eggs, slightly beaten
 1 cup plain yogurt
 ¼ teaspoon honey
 ½ teaspoon sea salt
 8 slices sprouted or sourdough whole grain bread
 Extra-virgin coconut oil

Combine eggs, yogurt, honey, and salt in a mixing bowl. Preheat a large pan and add the coconut oil. Dip each slice of bread quickly into the mixture and place in the pan. Brown on each side to desired doneness. Serve with butter and unheated honey, maple syrup or fresh fruit.

Easy Sautéed Greens
From the *Lazy Person's Whole Food Cookbook* by Stephen Byrnes
Yield: 6 to 8 servings

 1 quart spinach or other greens
 Extra-virgin coconut oil
 sea salt and pepper to taste

Wash the spinach or greens in several bowls of water. Remove all stems and brown leaves. Heat extra-virgin coconut oil in skillet. Place leaves in the skillet and cover. Cook until wilted, stirring occasionally. Season as you like.

Creamsicle Smoothie ·
Yield: two 8-ounce servings

> 6 ounces yogurt or kefir
> 4 ounces freshly squeezed orange juice
> 1 to 2 raw omega-3 eggs (see note on page 304)
> 1 tablespoon flaxseed oil or hemp seed oil
> 1 to 2 tablespoons unheated honey
> 1 tablespoon goat's milk protein powder (optional)
> 1 to 2 fresh or frozen bananas
> vanilla extract (optional)

Combine the ingredients in a high-speed blender.

Easy Whole Grain Waffles
From the *Lazy Person's Whole Food Cookbook* by Stephen Byrnes
Yield: 6 servings — make full recipe

> 1 cup water
> 2 tablespoons plain yogurt
> 1⅓ cups whole grain flour (spelt or kamut)
> 2 eggs, separated
> ¾ teaspoon sea salt
> 2 tablespoons unheated honey
> 2 teaspoons non-aluminum baking powder
> 4 tablespoons extra-virgin coconut oil

Combine the water and yogurt and soak the flour in water mixture for at least 7 hours. Beat the egg yolks and add to the flour mixture. Combine salt and honey and add to the flour mixture. Beat the egg whites until they form stiff peaks and then fold them into the mixture. Mix in the baking powder quickly. Grease your waffle iron with coconut oil, pour the batter into the waffle iron and cook according to directions.

Beef Burgundy
by Keith Tindall of White Egret Farm
Yield: 4 to 6 Servings

> 2 pounds lean beef stew meat in small cubes (preferably from pasture-fed beef)
> 2 tablespoons whole grain flour (soaked overnight)
> 1 teaspoon sea salt or Herbamare
> ¼ teaspoon pepper
> 2 tablespoons butter

1 tablespoon olive oil
2 cups brown beef stock
1 cup burgundy wine
8 ounces Crimini mushrooms, sliced
1 medium onion, chopped
2 carrots, sliced
1 garlic clove, minced
1 bay leaf
¼ teaspoon ground thyme
1 tablespoon parsley, snipped

Toss the meat in the flour, salt, and pepper in a brown paper bag. Remove and brown in the butter/olive oil combination. Add the beef stock, wine, mushrooms, onion, carrots, garlic, bay leaf, and thyme. Simmer 2½ to 3 hours, until the meat is tender. Turn the burner off and add the parsley to the hot mixture. If more liquid is needed during cooking, add more stock and wine in the following proportion: 2 parts stock to 1 part wine.

Appendix B

A Refresher on Practicing Hygiene

For hands and nails, jab fingers into semisoft soap four or five times, and lather hands with soap for fifteen seconds, rubbing soap over cuticles and rinsing under water as warm as you can stand. Take another swab of semisoft soap into your hands, and wash your face.

Next, fill basin or sink with water as warm as you can stand, and add one-to-three tablespoons of table salt and one-to-three eyedroppers of iodine-based mineral solution. Swirl water. Dunk face into water and open eyes, blinking repeatedly underwater. Keep eyes open under water for three seconds.

After cleaning your eyes, put your face back in the water, and close your mouth while blowing bubbles out of your nose. Come up from the water, and immerse your nose in the water once again, gently taking water into your nostrils and expelling bubbles. Come up from the water, and blow your nose into facial tissue.

To cleanse the ears, use hydrogen peroxide and mineral-based ear drops, putting two or three drops into each ear and letting stand for sixty seconds. Tilt your head to expel the drops.

For the teeth, apply two or three drops of essential oil based tooth drops to the toothbrush. This can be used to brush your teeth or added to existing toothpaste. After brushing your teeth, brush your tongue for fifteen seconds. (See the GPRx Resource Guide, page 349, for recommended advanced hygiene products.)

THE GPRx
RESOURCE GUIDE

This resource section contains contact information for manufacturers and distributors of products I recommend in the 49-day health plan as outlined in *The Great Physician's Rx for Health and Wellness.*

To the best of my ability, I am suggesting well-established companies whose health goals match up with mine. While I can vouch for these foods, supplements and products, neither I, nor the publisher, can guarantee that these companies subscribe to the same belief system as I do, nor can we be held responsible for any possible consequences relating to the eating or ingestion of foods and/or supplements. A more complete general disclaimer is printed on the copyright page for this health-related book.

You will note that I recommend products with the brand names of Garden of Life and GPRx. In the interest of full disclosure, I founded these companies following my illness when I had trouble finding the nutritional supplements and superfoods that my body needed. Using my knowledge gained from years of studying health and wellness, I set out to create high-quality functional foods, nutritional supplements, and educational resources.

I believe that no matter which company you choose to purchase from in the GPRx Resource Guide, you will be well served on your road to vibrant health. Keep in mind that if you don't find these foods, supplements, or products in your local supermarket, natural food store, or vitamin store, they can be purchased by mail order or through online merchants. Also, if you have any questions, many of these companies can be reached via e-mail, usually through the company's website or by typing info@ plus the company's website. Examples: info@mercola.com or info@gardenoflife.com.

Key #1: Eat to Live

Sprouted/Sourdough Bread

Food for Life Baking Co.
P.O. Box 1434
Corona, CA 92878
(800) 797-5090
www.food-for-life.com
   Food for Life, makers of Ezekiel 4:9 breads, tortillas, pasta, and cereal is by far my favorite supplier of grain products. Easily digestible, well tolerated by many who suffer from digestive ailments and allergies, high in protein and fiber, Food for Life products truly provide the bread of life.

French Meadow Bakery
2610 Lyndale Avenue South
Minneapolis, MN 55408
(877) NO-YEAST (669-3278)
www.frenchmeadow.com
   Food for Life and French Meadow products are found in natural food stores and grocery stores nationwide.

Nature's Path Foods
9100 Van Horne Way
Richmond, BC V6X 1W3, Canada
(888) 808-9505
www.naturespath.com
   Producers of manna-sprouted grain bread.

Pasta

Food for Life Baking Co.
P.O. Box 1434
Corona, CA 92878
(800) 797-5090
www.food-for-life.com

Sprouted pasta, high in protein and fiber. Available in natural food stores and grocery stores nationwide.

Vita-Spelt
Purity Foods
2871 W. Jolly Road
Okemos, MI 48864
(800) 99-SPELT (997-7358)
www.purityfoods.com
   High in protein and fiber with a nutty flavor. Available in natural food and grocery stores nationwide.

Sprouted Tortillas, English Muffins, and Sprouted Cereal

Food for Life Baking Co.
P.O. Box 1434
Corona, CA 92878
(800) 797-5090
www.food-for-life.com
   Sprouted tortillas are great for wraps and fajitas. The English muffins are perfect for personal pizzas, and their sprouted cereal is my favorite dry cereal. Available in natural food stores and grocery stores nationwide.

Whole Grain Cereal

Food for Life Baking Co.
P.O. Box 1434
Corona, CA 92878
(800) 797-5090
www.food-for-life.com
   Ezekiel 4:9 sprouted cereal is my favorite dry cereal. Available in natural food stores and grocery stores nationwide.

Nature's Path Foods
9100 Van Horne Way
Richmond, BC V6X 1W3, Canada
(888) 808-9505
www.naturespath.com

Smoothie Mix/Meal Replacement

Wellness Smoothie by Garden of Life
(800) 622-8986
www.gardenoflife.com
Wellness Smoothies are made with the finest organic ingredients and contain beta glucans from soluble oat fiber, helping to lower serum cholesterol and triglycerides, encourage maintenance of healthy blood sugar levels, support healthy immune function, aid digestive health, and promote maintenance of healthy body weight. Available in natural food stores nationwide or through online merchants.

Living Fuel Rx Super Berry
Living Fuel, Inc.
P.O. Box 1048
Tampa, FL 33601
(866) 580-3835
www.livingfuel.com
A high-quality meal replacement containing berries, protein, fiber, antioxidants, and probiotics.

Food Bars

Whole Food Bars by GPRx
(866) 985-GPRx
www.GreatPhysiciansRx.com
Nutrition Bars—the finest organic nutrition bars available on the market—

are made with organic foods such as sprouted grains and seeds, raw honey, dates, cultured vegetables, nuts, berries, green foods, and coconut. These Bars contain beta glucans from soluble oat fiber, high-quality protein, live probiotics, antioxidants, and more. Whole Food Nutrition Bars are great for all ages and support overall health by lowering serum cholesterol and triglycerides, promoting maintenance of healthy blood sugar levels, supporting healthy immune function, and aiding in maintenance of healthy body weight. Five flavors: Vanilla Protein, Chocolate Protein, Apple Cinnamon Fiber, Antioxidant Berry, and Raspberry SuperGreen.
Available via mail order by calling the toll-free number or online at the web address listed above.

Wellness Bars by Garden of Life
(800) 622-8986
www.gardenoflife.com
The nutritious Wellness Bars are made with the finest organic ingredients and contain beta glucans from soluble oat fiber, helping to lower serum cholesterol and triglycerides, promote maintenance of healthy blood sugar levels, support healthy immune function, and promote digestive health. Available in natural food stores nationwide or through online merchants.

CocoChia Snack Fuel Bars
Living Fuel, Inc.
P.O. Box 1048
Tampa, FL 33601
(866) 580-3835
www.livingfuel.com

CocoChia bars—low in sugar and high in fiber—are made with coconut, almond butter and chia seeds. Available online and via mail order.

Kefir

Amaltheia Dairy
3380 Penwell Bridge Road
Belgrade, MT 59714
(406) 388-5950
www.amaltheiadairy.com
Grade A goat's dairy kefir and cheeses. Available via mail order and in select natural food stores.

Helios Nutrition
214 Main St.
Sauk Centre, MN 56378
(888) 3-HELIOS (343-5467)
www.heliosnutrition.com
Certified organic plain and flavored low-fat kefir. Available in natural food stores nationwide.

Real Foods Market
420 West 800 North
Orem, UT 84057
(866) 284-7325
www.realfoodsmarket.com
Organic raw dairy products from grass-fed cows. Available via mail order.

Coconut Milk

Thai Kitchen Coconut Milk
Epicurean International, Inc.
30315 Union City Blvd.
Union City, CA 94587
(800) 967-8424
www.thaikitchen.com

Native Forest Organic Coconut Milk
Edward & Sons Trading Co.
P. O. Box 1326
Carpenteria, CA 93014
(805) 684-8500
www.edwardandsons.com
Thai Kitchen and Native Forest products available in natural food stores nationwide.

Dairy Products from Cow's Milk

The following companies produce organic milk, butter, cheese, cream, cottage cheese, yogurt, kefir, soft cheese, buttermilk that are either available in natural food stores or by mail order.

Mercola.com
www.mercola.com
Supplies raw cheeses from grass-fed cows. Available online via mail order.

Brown Cow Farm
3810 Delta Fair Blvd.
Antioch, CA 94509
(888) 429-5459
www.browncowfarm.com

Peaceful Pastures
69 Cowan Valley Lane
Hickman, TN 38567
(615) 683-4291
www.peacefulpastures.com

Stonyfield Farm
Ten Burton Dr.
Londonderry, NH 03053
(800) PRO-COWS (776-2697)
www.stonyfield.com

Organic Pastures Dairy Co.
7221 South Jameson Avenue
Fresno, CA 93706
(877) RAW-MILK (729-6455)
www.organicpastures.com

Real Foods Market
420 West 800 North
Orem, UT 84057
(866) 284-7325
www.realfoodsmarket.com

Natural by Nature
P. O. Box 464
West Grove, PA 19390
(610) 268-6962
www.natural-by-nature.com

Organic Valley
One Organic Way
La Farge, WI 54639
(888) 444-6455
www.organicvalley.com

Horizon Organic
WhiteWave Foods Co.
1990 North 57th Court
Boulder, CO 80301
(303) 530-2711
www.horizonorganic.com

Dairy Products from Goat's Milk

The following companies produce organic milk, butter, cheese, cream, cottage cheese, yogurt, kefir, soft cheese, buttermilk that are either available in natural food stores or by mail order.

Destiny Organics
27367 WCR 74
Eaton, CO 80615
(970) 454-9009
www.destinyorganics.com

Organic goat's milk dairy of the highest quality. Easily digestible and rich in protein with probiotics and beneficial fatty acids. Offerings include yogurt smoothies, goat's milk, cheese, and ice cream.

Available via mail order by calling the toll-free number or online at the web address listed above.

Amaltheia Dairy
3380 Penwell Bridge Rd.
Belgrade, MT 59714
(406) 388-5950
www.amaltheiadairy.com

Grade A goat's dairy and cheeses, fresh chevre, flavored chevre, ricotta, and feta.

Meyenberg Goat Milk Products
P. O. Box 934
Turlock, CA 95381
(800) 891-GOAT (4628)
www.meyenberg.com

A variety of goat milk dairy products, including whole, low-fat, evaporated, and powered goat milk.

Peaceful Pastures
69 Cowan Valley Lane
Hickman, TN 38567
(615) 683-4291
www.peacefulpastures.com

Dairy products including milk, cream, butter, buttermilk, whey, kefir, colostrum, and a Pro-Yo-Gurt.®

Eggs

Gold Circle Farms
310 N. Harbor Blvd., Suite 205
Fullerton, CA 92832
(888) 599-4DHA (4342)
www.goldcirclefarms.com
DHA omega-3 eggs. Available in natural food stores and grocery stores nationwide.

Organic Valley
One Organic Way
La Farge, WI 54639
(888) 444-6455
www.organicvalley.com
Certified organic high omega-3 eggs. Available in natural food stores and grocery stores nationwide.

Eggland's Best
860 First Avenue, Suite 842
King of Prussia, PA 19406
(800) 922-EGGS (3447)
www.eggland.com
High omega-3, vitamin E and organic eggs. Available in grocery stores nationwide.

Red Meats

Mercola.com
www.mercola.com
Supplies grass-fed beef. Available online.

Real Foods Market
420 West 800 North
Orem, UT 84057
(866) 284-7325
www.realfoodsmarket.com

Organic grass-fed beef available frozen by mail order.

Brady Ranch Exotic Meats
P. O. Box 536
Okeechobee, FL 34973
(800) 291-9555
www.bradyranchmeats.com
Pasture-fed venison is available via mail order only.

Homestead Healthy Foods
106 Thunderbird Road
Fredericksburg, TX 78624
(888) 861-5670
www.homesteadhealthyfoods.com
Certified organic, grass-fed beef.

Wyoming Natural Products Co.
P. O. Box 962
Newcastle, WY 82701
(800) 969-9946
www.wyomingnatural.com
Grass-fed beef available in select natural food stores and via mail order.

Maverick Ranch Natural Meats
5360 North Franklin Street
Denver, CO 80216
(800) 497-2624
www.maverickranch.com
Natural beef, chicken, lamb, and buffalo. Available in grocery stores nationwide.

Coleman Purely Natural Products
1767 Denver West Marriott Blvd., Suite 200
Golden, CO 80401
(800) 442-8666
www.colemannatural.com

Naturally raised, hormone- and antibiotic-free beef products. Available in natural food stores nationwide.

Peaceful Pastures
69 Cowan Valley Lane
Hickman, TN 38567
(615) 683-4291
www.peacefulpastures.com
Providers of grass-fed and grass-finished beef, lamb, and goat that are all natural and hormone- and antibiotic-free. Ships nationwide.

Baldwin Family Farms
5341 Highway 86 South
Yanceyville, NC 27379
(800) 896-4857
www.baldwinfamilyfarms.com
Grass-fed, all-natural beef.

White Oak Pastures
P. O. Box 98
Bluffton, GA 39824
(229) 641-2081
www.whiteoakpastures.com
Ground beef from free-range, free roaming, and pasture-raised grass-fed cattle without the use of supplemental hormones or antibiotics. USDA approved. Available in select natural food and grocery stores and via mail order.

Northstar Bison
1936 28th Ave.
Rice Lake, WI 54868
(888) 295-6332
www.northstarbison.com
One hundred percent grass-fed and finished bison meat.

Chicken

Oaklyn Plantation
1312 Oaklyn Road
Darlington, SC 29532
(843) 395-0793
www.freerangechicken.com
Free-range chickens and chicken feet (hormone- and antibiotic-free). Available via mail order.

Rosie's Organic Chicken
Petaluma Poultry
P.O. Box 7368
1500 Cader Lane
Petaluma, CA 94954
(800) 556-6789
www.petalumapoultry.com

Shelton's Poultry
204 N. Loranne Ave.
Pomona, CA 91767
(800) 541-1833
www.sheltons.com
Free-range turkey and chicken (hormone- and antibiotic-free).

Bell & Evans
154 W. Main St.
Fredericksburg, PA 17026
(717) 865-6626
www.bellandevans.com
Fresh and frozen natural poultry products. Available in natural food stores and grocery stores nationwide.

Peaceful Pastures
69 Cowan Valley Lane
Hickman, TN 38567
(615) 683-4291
www.peacefulpastures.com

Providers of free-roaming chicken and turkey that are all natural and hormone- and antibiotic-free. Ships nationwide.

Deli Meat

Applegate Farms
750 Rt. 202 South, 3rd Floor
Bridgewater, NJ 08807
(800) 587-5858
www.applegatefarms.com
Packaged meats and deli slices (nitrate- and nitrite-free). Available in natural food stores and grocery stores nationwide.

Frozen Fish

Mercola.com
www.mercola.com
Wild-caught salmon, frozen or canned. Available online for mail order delivery.

Ecofish
340 Central Ave.
Dover, NH 03820
(877) 214-3474
www.ecofish.com
Ocean-caught salmon, halibut, tuna, and other fish. Available in natural food stores and grocery stores nationwide.

Real Foods Market
420 West 800 North
Orem, UT 84057
(866) 284-7325
www.realfoodsmarket.com
Available via mail order and shipped frozen.

Vital Choice Seafood
P.O. Box 4121
Bellingham, WA 98227
(800) 608-4825
www.vitalchoice.com
Available in natural food stores nationwide.

Canned Fish

Crown Prince
18581 Railroad Street
City of Industry, CA 91748
(800) 255-5063
www.crownprince.com
Canned sardines, salmon, tuna and other fish. Available in natural food stores and grocery stores nationwide.

Blue Galleon
260 Boston Post Road, Suite 1
Wayland, MA 01778
(866) 4MY-BELA (469-2352)
www.mybela.com
Tuna and sardines from Portugal. Sardines are canned within two hours of catch.

Waffles

Van's Waffles
Van's International Foods
20318 Gramercy Place
Torrance, CA 90501
(310) 320-8611
www.vanswaffles.com
Organic whole wheat waffles, as well as wheat-free, with flavors such as blueberry, cinnamon apple, and more. Available in natural food stores and grocery stores nationwide.

Almond Milk

Pacific Natural Foods
19480 SW 97th Avenue
Tualatin, OR 97062
(503) 692-9666
www.pacificfoods.com

Honey

Organic Raw Honey by GPRx
(866) 985-GPRx
www.GreatPhysiciansRx.com
This certified organic honey comes from the island of Hawaii. GPRx Organic Raw Honey contains antioxidants, enzymes, vitamins, and minerals, providing all of the benefits that make honey a superfood from the hive. This raw, unheated honey is the original sweetener used for thousands of years and is a superb resource to sweeten smoothies, yogurt, tea, and coffee. This honey is also an important ingredient in many of the delicious recipes you'll find in this book.

Available via mail order by calling the toll-free number or online at the web address listed above.

Wellness Raw Honey Garden of Life
(866) 465-0094
www.gardenoflife.com
This excellent source of organic raw honey is available in natural food stores, online retailers, and mail-order catalogues nationwide.

Sweeteners

Rapadura Whole Cane Sugar
Global Organic Brands

37 W. 20th St., Suite 708
New York, NY 10011
(800) 207-2814
www.rapunzel.com

SweetLeaf Stevia
Wisdom Natural Brands
1203 W. San Pedro St.
Gilbert, AZ 85233
(800) 899-9908
www.sweetleaf.com
Stevia products are believed to be safe for diabetics.

TheraSweet
Living Fuel, Inc.
P.O. Box 1048
Tampa, FL 33601
(866) 580-3835
www.livingfuel.com
TheraSweet is a safe and healthy alternative to the artificial sweeteners on the market today. With a sugar-like taste and texture, TheraSweet is a versatile low-calorie sweetener that dissolves quickly and is heat stable for cooking and baking.

Up Country Organic Maple Syrup
Up Country Organics
1052 Portland St.
St. Johnsbury, VT 05819
(802) 748-5141
www.upcountryorganics.com

Salad Mixes (Prewashed)

Earthbound Farm
1721 San Juan Highway
San Juan Bautista, CA 95045
(800) 690-3200
www.ebfarm.com
Fresh, packaged organic produce.

Available in natural food stores and grocery stores nationwide.

Vegetables (Including Raw Fermented)

Earthbound Farm
1721 San Juan Highway
San Juan Bautista, CA 95045
(800) 690-3200
www.ebfarm.com
Fresh, organic produce available in natural food stories and grocery stores nationwide.

Rejuvenative Foods
P. O. Box 8464
Santa Cruz, CA 95061
(800) 805-7957
www.rejuvenative.com
Rejuvenative Foods produces high-quality raw foods such as sauerkraut, kim-chi, salsas, nut and seed butters, chocolate spreads, raw oils, and more. Available in some grocery and health food stores, and online via mail order.

Native Forest Organic Hearts of Palm
Edward and Sons Trading Co.
P. O. Box 1326
Carpenteria, CA 93014
(805) 684-8500
www.edwardandsons.com

Canned Tomatoes and Asparagus Spears

Bionaturae
5 Tyler Drive
North Franklin, CT 06254
(860) 642-6996
www.bionaturae.com

Bionaturae imports whole tomatoes (peeled, crushed, stewed, and tomato paste) in glass jars from Italy.

Muir Glen
Small Planet Foods
P.O. Box 9452
Minneapolis, MN 55440
(800) 832-6345
www.muirglen.com

Canned Tomato Products, Tomato Sauces, and Salsas

Amy's Kitchen
P.O. Box 7868
Santa Rosa, CA 95407
(707) 578-7188
www.amys.com
Canned tomato products and sauces. Available in health food stores nationwide.

Frozen Fruits and Vegetables

Cascadian Farms
Small Planet Foods
P.O. Box 9452
Minneapolis, MN 55440
(800) 624-4123
www.cfarm.com
Frozen, packaged organic fruits and vegetables, including berries. Available in health food and grocery stores nationwide.

Organic Tomato Sauces and Salsas

Seeds of Change
P. O. Box 15700

Santa Fe, NM 87592
(888) 762-4240
www.seedsofchange.com

Muir Glen
Small Planet Foods
P.O. Box 9452
Minneapolis, MN 55440
(800) 832-6345
www.muirglen.com

Apple Sauce and Fruit Spreads

Cascadian Farms
Small Planet Foods
P.O. Box 9452
Minneapolis, MN 55440
(800) 624-4123
www.cfarm.com
    Organic fruit spreads, but look for fruit juice-sweetened since some have sugar.

Bionaturae
5 Tyler Dr.
North Franklin, CT 06254
(860) 642-6996
www.bionaturae.com
    High quality organic fruit spreads.

Solana Gold Organics
P. O. Box 1340
Sebastopol, CA 95473
(707) 829-1121
www.solanagold.com

Protein Powder (from Goat's Milk)

Primary Protein by GPRx
(866) 985-GPRx
www.GreatPhysiciansRx.com

Primary Protein, the finest protein powder available, contains high-quality protein, probiotics, and enzymes and is the only protein powder currently available that contains omega-3 fatty acids from plant and animal sources. Primary Protein is easily digestible and is great mixed in water, juice, or smoothies.
    For more information, call the toll-free number or visit the website listed above.

Goatein by Garden of Life
(866) 465-0094
www.gardenoflife.com
    Goatein, an exceptional goat's milk protein powder, is a source of eight essential amino acids crucial to good health. Easy to digest, Goatein is well tolerated by those who cannot digest cow's milk. Available in natural food stores, mail-order catalogs, and online retailers nationwide.

Extra Virgin Coconut Oil

Garden of Life
(866) 465-0094
www.gardenoflife.com
    Once thought to be a "bad" fat, coconut oil has been shown to be a stable, healthy saturated fat. In fact, extra-virgin coconut oil is one of the healthiest and most versatile unprocessed dietary oils in the world. Garden of Life Extra Virgin Coconut Oil is an unprocessed culinary oil full of natural coconut flavor and aroma. Available in natural food stores, mail order catalogs, and online retailers nationwide.

Wilderness Family Naturals
P.O. Box 538
Finland, MN 55603
(866) 936-6457
www.wildernessfamilynaturals.com

Virgin Coconut Oil
and Hemp Seed Oil

Nutiva
P. O. Box 1716
Sebastopol, CA 95473
(800) 993-HEMP (4367)
www.nutiva.com

Apple Cider, Organic Balsamic, or
Other Vinegars

Bragg Live Foods
P. O. Box 7
Santa Barbara, CA 93102
(800) 446-1990
www.bragg.com
   Apple cider vinegar made from organically grown apples, as well as other natural products. Available in health food and grocery stores nationwide.

Bionaturae
5 Tyler Drive
North Franklin, CT 06254
(860) 642-6996
www.bionaturae.com

Organic Balsamic Vinegar

Solana Gold Organics
P. O. Box 1340
Sebastopol, CA 95473
(707) 829-1121
www.solanagold.com

Nuts and Seeds

Living Nutz
P. O. Box 11413
Portland, ME 04104
(207) 780-1101
www.livingnutz.com
   Variety of low temperature dried sprouted nuts. Available in select natural food stores and via mail order.

Glaser Organic Farms
19100 SW 137th Avenue
Miami, FL 33012
(305) 238-7747
www.glaserorganicfarms.com
   Extensive supply of organic raw nuts and seeds. Available in natural food stores in Florida or via mail order nationwide.

Nut and Seed Butters

Rejuvenative Foods
P. O. Box 8464
Santa Cruz, CA 95061
(800) 805-7957
www.rejuvenative.com
   The highest-quality, best-tasting raw organic nut and seed butters, including those made from almond, sesame, pumpkin, cashew, and sunflower seeds. Available in some grocery and health food stores, by mail order, or through online merchants.

Maranatha Nut Butters
nSpired Natural Foods
1850 Fairway Drive
San Leandro, CA 94501
(510) 346-3860
www.nspiredfoods.com
   Available in health food stores nationwide.

Macaroons

Jennies Macaroons
Red Mill Farms
290 5th Street
Brooklyn, NY 11211
(888) 294-1164
www.jennies-macaroons.com

Jennies Macaroons, one of my favorite snacks, are made with only three ingredients: coconut, honey, and egg whites. Available in health food and grocery stores nationwide.

Tea

Mount of Olives Treasures
(866) 985-GPRx
www.GreatPhysiciansRx.com

My favorite teas and herbal infusions come directly from the Holy Land, where herbs and spices have been used to enhance wellness since biblical times. High above the ancient walls of Jerusalem, the world's holiest city, stands the Mount of Olives—a revered site with a heritage like no other, a wellspring of purity, serenity, and holiness.

Here amid its sun-splashed olive trees, fragrant plants, and natural herbs, the ancient promise of biblical health and tranquility for body and soul can now be experienced in the Mount of Olives Treasures Teas. Each tea and herbal infusion, whether for the body or soul, has been carefully formulated to offer you the ultimate in soothing and restorative care. The ingredients include antioxidant-rich olive leaves, grape leaves, pomegranate leaves, fig leaves, hyssop and others.

Available via mail order by calling the toll-free number or online at the web address listed above.

Wellness Tea by Garden of Life
(800) 622-8986
www.gardenoflife.com

Certified organic green, black, and rooibos tea delivered in convenient liquid-packs. Wellness Tea is great as hot or iced tea and comes in many flavors: unflavored green tea, raspberry green tea, lemon green tea, peach green tea, and coffee-flavored black and rooibos tea. Wellness Tea is loaded with antioxidants and the exciting compound EGCG.

Available with or without caffeine. Available in natural food stores nationwide and via mail-order catalogues and online retailers nationwide.

Coffee

Pura Vida Coffee
2724 First Avenue South
Seattle, WA 98134
(877) 469-1431
www.puravidacoffee.com

Organic, shade-grown fair trade coffee. All proceeds from sales go to support inner city children's programs in Costa Rica. Available via mail order and at select locations nationwide.

Organic Coffee Co.
1933 Davis Street, Suite 308
San Leandro, CA 94577
(800) 829-1300
www.organiccoffeecompany.com

Green Mountain Coffee Roasters
33 Coffee Lane
Waterbury, VT 05676
(888) TRY-GMCR (879-4627)
www.greenmountaincoffee.com
Certified organic coffees produced worldwide, using sustainable agricultural practices.

Organic Yerba Maté (Similar to Tea)

Guayaki Yerba Maté
P. O. Box 14730
San Luis Obispo, CA 93406
(888) GUAYAKI (482-9254)
www.guayaki.com

Bottled Water

Waiwera Infinity Water
13277 North 101st St.
Scottsdale, AZ 85260
(480) 767-7782
www.waiwera.co.nz
Available in health food stores nationwide.

Mountain Valley Spring Water
150 Central Ave.
Hot Springs, AR 71901
(800) 643-1501
www.mountainvalleyspring.com
Only U.S. water still bottled in glass containers.

Trinity Springs
1101 West River Street, Suite 370
Boise, ID 83702
(800) 390-5693
www.trinitysprings.com
High mineral, alkaline water.

Bottled Fruit Beverages

Apple & Eve
P.O. Box K
Roslyn, NY 11576
(800) 969-8018
www.appleandeve.com
A variety of quality juice products and fruit beverages. Available in select regions; call for availability.

Bionaturae
5 Tyler Drive
North Franklin, CT 06254
(860) 642-6996
www.bionaturae.com
The highest-quality organic bottled juices from Italy. Available in natural food stores nationwide.

Pom Wonderful
11444 W. Olympic Blvd., Suite 310
Los Angeles, CA 90064
(310) 966-5863
www.pomwonderful.com
Producers of pomegranate juice.

Steaz Green Tea Sodas
Healthy Beverage Co.
2865 S. Eagle Road
Newton, PA 18940
(800) 295-1388
www.steaz.com

Trop Coco, Kero-Coco, and H2Coco
Sackel Health Drinks
29 S.W. 5th Street
Pompano Beach, FL 33060
(800) 336-8470
www.sackel.com
Producers of coconut water beverages.

Organic Wine

Frey Vineyards
14000 Tomki Road
Redwood Valley, CA 95470
(800) 760-3739
www.freywine.com

Fetzer Vineyards
13601 Old River Road
Hopland, CA 95449
(800) 846-8637
www.fetzer.com

Organic Beer

Otter Creek Brewery
793 Exchange Street
Middlebury, VT 05753
(800) 473-0727
www.wolavers.com

Eel River Brewery
1777 Alamar Way
Fortuna, CA 95540
(707) 725-2739
www.climaxbeer.com

Sea Salt

Celtic Sea Salt
Grain & Salt Society
Four Celtic Dr.
Arden, NC 28704
(800) 867-7258
www.celticseasalt.com
Celtic Sea Salt (course and fine) and other health products. Available in some health food stores and grocery stores.

RealSalt
P. O. Box 219
Redmond, UT 84652
(800) FOR-SALT (367-7258)
www.realsalt.com
RealSalt is mined in central Utah. Available in health food and grocery stores.

Mercola.com
www.mercola.com
Supplier of Himalayan salt. Rich in naturally occurring minerals.

Seasonings and Other Organic Herbs

Herbamare and Trocomore
Global Organic Brands
37 W. 20th St., Suite 708
New York, NY 10011
(800) 207-2814
www.rapunzel.com
Herbamare and Trocomare seasonings are made with sea salt and organic herbs. Available online or in health food stores and grocery stores.

Simply Organic
Frontier Natural Products
P. O. Box 299
Norway, IA 52318
(800) 669-3275
www.frontiercoop.com
Packaged organic spices in glass jars.

Condiments

Spectrum Organic Products
5341 Old Redwood Hwy., Suite 400
Petaluma, CA 94954

(800) 995-2705
www.spectrumorganics.com
  Healthy, organic omega-3 mayonnaise using expeller-pressed soy and flaxseed oils. Available in some health food stores and grocery stores.

Westbrae Natural Foods
Novelco Distribution
P.O. Box 1346
Downey, CA 90240
(562) 215-4843
www.novelco.com/westbrae/index.htm
  Natural catsup and mustard. Available in some health food stores and grocery stores.

Flaxseed Oil

Barlean's Organic Oils
4936 Lake Terrell Road
Ferndale, WA 98248
(360) 384-0485
www.barleans.com
  Organic high-lignan flaxseed oil and borage seed oil, as well as flaxseed fiber. Available at health food stores nationwide.

Omega Nutrition
6515 Aldrich Rd.
Bellingham, WA 98226
(800) 661-FLAX (3529)
www.omeganutrition.com
  Organic flax oil, olive oil, and garlic-chili flax oil.

Organic Hemp Seed Oil

Manitoba Harvest
15-2166 Notre Dame Ave.
Winnipeg, MB, R3H 0K2

Canada
(800) 665-4367
www.manitobaharvest.com

Nutiva
P. O. Box 1716
Sebastopol, CA 95473
(800) 993-4367
www.nutiva.com

Organic Vegetable Oils

Bionaturae
5 Tyler Drive
North Franklin, CT 06254
(860) 642-6996
www.bionaturae.com
  Organic extra-virgin olive oil.

Raw Almond Oil, Evening Primrose Oil, Sunflower Oil, and Poppy Seed Oil

---

Raw Oils from Rejuvenative Foods
PO Box 8464
Santa Cruz, CA 95061
(800) 805-7957
www.rawoils.com

Bariani Olive Oil
1330 Waller Street
San Francisco, CA 94117
(415) 864-1917
www.barianioliveoil.com

Extra Virgin Olive Oil

Spectrum Organic Products
5341 Old Redwood Hwy., Suite 400
Petaluma, CA 94954

(800) 995-2705
www.spectrumorganics.com

Organic Chocolate Spreads

Rejuvenate Foods
P.O. Box 8464
Santa Cruz, CA 95061
(800) 805-7957
www.rejuvenative.com
Healthy organic chocolate spreads and great for all ages.

Ice Cream

Julie's Organic Ice Cream
885 Grant St.
Eugene, OR 97402
(800) 282-2202
www.oregonicecream.com
Certified organic ice cream.

Laloo's Goat's Milk Ice Cream Company
3900 Magnolia Ave
Petaluma, CA 94952
(707) 763-1491
www.goatsmilkicecream.com
Handmade goat's milk ice cream in a variety of flavors. Available in select natural food stores.

Flaxseed Crackers

Glaser Organic Farms
19100 SW 137th Avenue
Miami, FL 33012
(305) 238-7747
www.glaserorganicfarms.com

Whole Wheat Crackers

Ak Mak Crackers
89 Academy Ave.
Sanger, CA 93657
(559) 875-5511
These popular whole-wheat flat crackers, are available in health food stores.

Baked Corn Chips

Guiltless Gourmet
One Harmon Plaza, 10th Floor
Secaucus, NJ 07094
(201) 333-3700, ext. 2205
www.guiltlessgourmet.com
Baked corn tortilla chips in a variety of flavors.

Baking Products

Simply Organic
Frontier Natural Products
P. O. Box 299
Norway, IA 52318
(800) 669-3275
www.frontiercoop.com
Flavoring extracts also available.

Rapunzel
Global Organic Brands
37 W. 20th St., Suite 708
New York, NY 10011
(800) 207-2814
www.rapunzel.com
Check out the organic dried baking yeast and organic cocoa powder.

Organic Cocoa Powder

Ah!laska Organic Cocoa
nSpired Natural Foods
1850 Fairway Drive
San Leandro, CA 94501
(510) 346-3860
www.nspiredfoods.com
    Certified organic cocoa powder and baker's chocolate.

Organic Dried Baking Powder

Sun Organic Farm
P. O. Box 409
San Marcos, CA 92079
(888) 269-9888
www.sunorganicfarm.com
Carob powder also available.

Food Preparation/Utensils

Mercola.com
www.mercola.com
    Provides food preparation tools such as juicers and convection ovens. Available online.

Vita-Mix Blender
8615 Usher Road
Cleveland, OH 44138
(800) 848-2649
www.vitamix.com
    High-quality durable blender excellent for smoothies and soups. A must-have for every health conscious family.

Lehman's
1 Lehman Circle
P. O. Box 321

Kidron, OH 44636
(888) 438-5346
www.lehmans.com

Country Living Grain Mill
14727 56th Ave. NW
Stanwood, WA 98292
(360) 652-0671
www.countrylivinggrainmills.com

C.F. Resources Fermenting Crock Pots
P. O. Box 405
Kit Carson, CO 80825
(719) 962-3228
www.cfamilyresources.com/fermenting_crock.htm

Salton Yogurt Maker
81A Brunswick
Dollard-des-Ormeaux, QC H9B 2J5, Canada
www.salton.com

Ronco Food Dehydrator
(21344 Superior St.
Chatsworth, CA 91311
(800) 486-1806
www.ronco.com

Green Star Juicer
Tribest Corp.
14109 Pontlavoy Ave.
Santa Fe Springs, CA 90670
(562) 623-7150
www.greenstar.com

For more information
on eating to live, visit
www.BiblicalHealthInstitute.com

Key #2: Supplement Your Diet with Whole Food Nutritionals, Living Nutrients, and Superfoods

Whole Food Multivitamins

Maker's Multi by GPRx
(866) 985-GPRx
www.GreatPhysiciansRx.com

Maker's Multi is a complete whole food vitamin and mineral supplement that delivers essential nutrients to support your demanding nutritional needs. The comprehensive multi-nutrient formula contains whole food vitamins, minerals, antioxidants, and fruits.

Maker's Multi and the nutrients and compounds within the formula provide the following:
• a broad array of nutrients essential for general health and well-being
• superfoods to support your demanding nutritional needs
• nutrients essential for immune system health
• antioxidant-rich protection
• healthy bone and calcium metabolism
• healthy visual function (eye health)
• comfortable pH levels
• normal bone development

This whole food multivitamin also contains beneficial microorganisms (probiotics). Available via mail order by calling the toll-free number or by visiting the website listed above.

Living Multi by Garden of Life
(800) 622-8986
www.gardenoflife.com

Living Multi is a complete vitamin and mineral supplement that delivers superfoods to support your demanding nutritional needs. This comprehensive whole food multi-nutrient formula contains fruits, vegetables, ocean plants, tonic mushrooms, botanicals, and ionic minerals including enzymes, antioxidants, amino acids, and homeostatic nutrient complexes. Living Multi is available in natural food stores, mail order catalogs, and online retailers nationwide.

Omega-3 Cod-Liver/Fish Oil

Omega-3 Cod Liver Oil Complex by GPRx
(866) 985-GPRx
www.GreatPhysiciansRx.com

Available either as a good-tasting liquid and easy-to-swallow liquid-capsules, Omega-3 Cod-Liver Oil Complex is one of nature's richest sources of vitamins A and D, and the omega-3 fatty acids DHA and EPA, which can play an important role in supporting cardiovascular and immune system health. To ensure that its naturally occurring ingredients remain intact, Omega-3 Cod-Liver Oil Complex is always harvested from the pure cold waters of Norway and Iceland and is produced using traditional methods.

Omega-3 Cod-Liver Oil Complex supports:
• normal vision, gene expression, reproduction, embryonic development, growth, and immune function
• healthy vision (eye health)
• normal structure of skin and hair
• healthy immune function
• normal cell proliferation

• normal calcium metabolism helps maintain healthy bone structure
• normal bone density in older women
• normal muscle tone and strength

Available via mail order by calling the toll-free number or by visiting the website listed above.

Olde World Icelandic Cod-Liver Oil by Garden of Life
(800) 622-8986
www.gardenoflife.com

Olde World Icelandic Cod-Liver Oil is one of nature's richest sources of vitamins A and D, which can play an important role in supporting cardiovascular health. To ensure that its naturally occurring ingredients remain intact, Olde World Icelandic Cod-Liver Oil is always harvested from the pure cold waters of Iceland and is cold-processed using traditional methods. Olde World Icelandic Cod-Liver Oil is available in natural food stores, mail order catalogs, and online merchants nationwide.

Living Fuel Rx Omega 3 & E
Living Fuel, Inc.
P.O. Box 1048
Tampa, FL 33601
(866) 580-3835
www.livingfuel.com

Omega 3 & E, antioxidant-protected fish oil caplets, is a powerful combination of omega-3 essential fatty acids EPA and DHA, combined with therapeutic doses of full-spectrum vitamin E to provide antioxidant protection inside the body. Kept in its natural form throughout the production process and rigorously tested to ensure it is free from impurities, Omega 3 & E is one of the safest and healthiest products of its kind.

Living Fuel Rx Pure D & A Sunshine Gel Caps
Living Fuel, Inc.
P.O. Box 1048
Tampa, FL 33601
(866) 580-3835
www.livingfuel.com

Pure D & A Sunshine Gel Caps are a safe and optimum source of vitamin D for everyone in the family. An all-natural dietary supplement made from purified and emulsified fish oil livers, each soft gel capsule contains the same amount of vitamin D and vitamin A found in one teaspoon of commercially available cod-liver oil. Living Fuel Pure D & A is not factory made—it is all natural, derived from mercury-safe fish.

Green Food/Fiber

Organic Fiber Greens by GPRx
(866) 985-GPRx
www.GreatPhysiciansRx.com

Organic Fiber Greens is a combination of organic vegetable juice concentrates combined with whole food fiber sources such as seeds and sprouts as well as live probiotics. Organic Fiber Greens provides broad antioxidant support, sustains healthy gut flora balance, promotes regular bowel function, and supports a healthy immune system.

Fiber Greens defends cardiovascular health, and along with a diet low in saturated fat, may reduce the risks of certain cancers. Fiber Greens supports healthy estrogen metabolism and breast health in women and supports prostate health in men.

Available via mail order by calling the toll-free number or by visiting the website listed above.

Super Greens caplets by GPRx
(800) 985-GPRX
www.GreatPhysiciansRx.com

Super Greens is a highly concentrated green food formula containing green foods, fermented vegetables, seeds, sea vegetables, green tea, and over seventy naturally occurring minerals. Super Greens contains the antioxidant equivalent of over six green salads. Available via mail order by calling the toll-free number or by visiting the website listed above.

Perfect Food by Garden of Life
(800) 622-8986
www.gardenoflife.com

Perfect Food is a green superfood containing organic ingredients, including cereal grass juices, microalgaes, vegetable juice concentrates, sprouts, and seeds. Perfect Food provides antioxidants, enzymes, chlorophyll and trace minerals. Available in natural food stores and through online retailers.

SuperSeed by Garden of Life
(800) 622-8986
www.gardenoflife.com

SuperSeed is a whole food fiber blend containing organic ingredients including sprouted and fermented seeds, grains, and legumes. SuperSeed is available in natural food stores, mail order catalogs and online retailers nationwide.

Living Fuel Rx Super Greens
Living Fuel, Inc.
P.O. Box 1048
Tampa, FL 33601
(866) 580-3835
www.livingfuel.com

Probiotics and Enzymes

Probio-Enzyme by GPRx
(866) 985-GPRx
www.GreatPhysiciansRx.com

Probio-Enzyme is a high-potency, room-temperature stable probiotic and enzyme supplement containing a naturally occurring blend of minerals and trace elements in an organic matrix that promotes overall wellness.

The Probio-Enzyme blend supports healthy gut flora balance, regular bowel function, and a healthy immune system as well as enhancing your body's ability to properly utilize minerals such as zinc, magnesium, and iron. The hardy probiotics in Probio-Enzyme are resistant to acidic conditions in the stomach and the harsh effect of bile acids in the intestine.

Available via mail order by calling the toll-free number or online at the web address above.

Primal Defense
(800) 622-8986
www.gardenoflife.com

Primal Defense contains probiotics, green grass juices, and a naturally occurring blend of minerals and trace elements. This whole food probiotic blend promotes overall wellness and is available in natural food stores, mail order catalogues and online retailers nationwide.

Omega Zyme by Garden of Life
(800) 622-8986
www.gardenoflife.com

Omega Zyme is a whole food digestive enzyme blend that supports gastrointestinal health, carbohydrate digestion, and normal bowel function. Available in natural food stores, mail order catalogs, and through online retailers.

Energy Formulas

CS Energy by GPRx
(866) 985-GPRx
www.GreatPhysiciansRx.com

CS Energy is designed to support overall health and wellness, manage stress and promote energy, and promote stamina and mental clarity as well as concentration. CS Energy contains whole food B-vitamins to support healthy cardiovascular function, herbal adaptogens to manage stress, and extracts from beverages to promote energy.

The ingredients in CS Energy are believed to:
• help increase resistance to fatigue, stress, tension, and irritability
• help promote emotional well-being
• help regulate and balance body organs for increased physical and mental rejuvenation
• help support blood sugar levels already within the normal range
• help support healthy cardiovascular function
• help restore and sustain energy levels
• help promote better sleep
• help support the body's natural antioxidant defense system

• help slow the effects of aging by inhibiting oxidative damage to cells and tissues
• help support the body's immune defenses
• help enhance focus and mental stamina
• help promote healthy weight management by controlling overeating triggered by stress.

Available via mail order by calling the toll-free number or online at the web address above.

Clear Energy by Garden of Life
(800) 622-8986
www.gardenoflife.com

Clear Energy is a botanical adaptogenic formula that supports overall health and wellness, promotes a healthy mood, and supports energy and stamina. Available in natural food stores, mail-order catalogs, and through online retailers.

Antioxidant Fruit Product

Fruits of Life by Garden of Life
(800) 622-8986
www.gardenoflife.com

Fruits of Life blends more than twenty-one nutrients, including antioxidant food concentrates of blueberries, raspberries, strawberries, and blackberries. Using a unique blend of minerals and enzymes from goat's milk that support beneficial flora in the gastrointestinal tract, Fruits of Life provides a wide range of health benefits, such as neutralizing free radicals and protecting against oxidative stress in the body. Available in natural food stores, mail order catalogs, and through online retailers.

Radical Fruits by Garden of Life
(800) 622-8986
www.gardenoflife.com

Radical Fruits is a comprehensive blend of antioxidant-rich fruit extracts and alkalinizing minerals that provide a wide range of health benefits. Radical Fruits is available in natural food stores, mail order catalogs, and through online retailers.

Frutaiga
(800) 803-7505
www.russianhealthbeverage.com

A functional food beverage containing precise amounts of active, health-enhancing compounds.

> For more information on supplementing your diet with whole food nutrition, living nutrients, and superfoods, visit www.BiblicalHealthInstitute.com

Key #3: Practice Advanced Hygiene

Advanced Hygiene Products

Advanced Hygiene System by GPRx
(866) 985-GPRx
www.GreatPhysiciansRx.com

Advanced Hygiene System supports vibrant health by thoroughly cleansing the areas of your body most vulnerable to germs: hands, eyes, mouth, ears, and nose. This advanced hygiene product reinforces overall health and well-being, promotes clear skin, and refreshes teeth and gums. Call the toll-free number or visit the website for more information.

Bausch & Lomb
One Bausch & Lomb Place
Rochester, NY 14604-2701
(585) 338-6000
www.bausch.com

Bausch & Lomb Eye Wash and Eye Irrigating Solution flushes away foreign objects, chlorine, and other eye irritants. Available in supermarkets and drugstores nationwide.

Xlear
P.O. Box 970911
Orem, UT 84097
(877) 599-5327
www.xlear.com

All natural, drug-free nasal wash. Available in natural food stores nationwide.

Clay Neti Pots
By the Planet
5111-A NW 13th St.
Gainesville, FL 32609
(888) 543-9294
www.bytheplanet.com

Helpful in relieving sinus and nasal passage congestion.

> For more information on the practice of advanced hygiene, visit www.BiblicalHealthInstitute.com.

Key #4: Condition Your Body with Exercise and Body Therapies

Functional Fitness Video

Functional Fitness DVD by GPRx
(866) 985-GPRx
www.GreatPhysiciansRx.com

Experience the energizing, enjoyable world of functional fitness exercise. Functional exercise teaches you to train whole body movements, not just isolated muscles. Increase fitness, coordination, flexibility, and agility. Decrease your chances of injury during daily activity. Featuring fun and easy routines that can be performed anywhere and anytime, functional fitness is great for people of any age or skill level.

Call the toll-free number or visit the website for more information.

Aromatherapy

Purifying Biblical Oil by Mount of Olives Treasures from GPRx
(866) 985-GPRx
www.GreatPhysiciansRx.com
Mount of Olives Treasures Purifying Biblical Oil is a moisturizing oil, bath oil, and fragrant perfume oil made from ingredients harvested in the Holy Land. This biblical oil contains herbs and spices including frankincense, myrrh, and olive oil.

Call the toll-free number or visit the website for more information.

Oshadhi
1340-G Industrial Ave.
Petaluma, CA 94952
(888) OSHADHI (674-2344)
www.oshadhiusa.com
Undiluted organic essential oils.

Rebounders

Optimum Performance Systems
438 NW 13th Street
Boca Raton, Florida, 33432
(561) 393-3881
www.opsfit.com
Exercise videos, books, and programs for recreational, amateur, and professional athletes.

Rebound Air
993 North 450 West
Springville, UT 84663
(888) 464-JUMP (5867)
www.reboundair.com
Supplier of rebounders, which are great for low-impact exercise.

Lympholine
Life Source International
1112 Montana Ave., Suite 125
Santa Monica, CA 90403
(310) 284-3565
www.lympholine.com
The Lympholine rebounder activates the lymphatic system to purify the body.

Needak Manufacturing
P.O. Box 776
O'Neill, NE 68763
(800) 232-5762
www.needak-rebounders.com

Music Therapy

"Faith Is a Place" Music Video from GPRx
(866) 985-GPRx
www.GreatPhysiciansRx.com

For more information on conditioning your body with exercise and body therapies, visit www.Biblical HealthInstitute.com

Key #5: Reduce Toxins in Your Environment

Skin and Body Care

Miessence by GPRx
(866) 985-GPRx
www.GreatPhysiciansRx.com

Miessence is the world's first extensive line of certified organic skin, body, hair, and oral care products. All Miessence products are made with real ingredients from natural and organic sources. Miessence produces dozens of products, including cosmetics, skin care, body care, hair care, soaps and cleansers, and tooth-paste. Miessence is the only product line of its kind that meets my standard for body care and supports the healthy reduction of toxins in your environment.

For more information, call the toll-free number or visit the website.

Aubrey Organics
4419 N. Manhattan Ave.
Tampa, FL 33614
(813) 877-4186
www.aubrey-organics.com

Aubrey Hampton, the founder of Aubrey Organics, has been formulating and manufacturing skin and body care products for thirty years. Aubrey produces hundreds of products, including skin care, hair care, soaps and cleansers, tooth-paste, natural hair color, and perfumes and colognes.

MyChelle Dermaceuticals
P. O. Box 1
Frisco, CO 80443
(800) 447-2076
www.mychelleusa.com

MyChelle Dermaceuticals utilizes innovative fruit, vegetables, and enzymes in their products to deliver outstanding results for men and women.

Miracle Distributors
P.O. Box 2455
Matthews, NC 28106
(866) 567-2326
www.miracledistributors.com

Nontoxic soaps and cleansers great for hair, skin, and home.

Kiss My Face
P. O. Box 224
Gardiner, NY 12525
(800) 262-KISS (5477)
www.kissmyface.com

Try Kiss My Face's olive oil bar soaps.

Extra Virgin Coconut Oil by Garden of Life
(800) 622-8986
www.gardenoflife.com
E-mail: info@gardenoflife.com

Coconut oil has been traditionally used by tropical cultures to condition skin during and after sun exposure. Available in natural food stores and through online retailers.

Cosmetics

Miessence by GPRx
(866) 985-GPRx
www.GreatPhysiciansRx.com

Miessence is the world's first extensive line of certified organic skin, body, hair, and oral care products. All Miessence products are made with real ingredients from natural and organic sources. Miessence produces dozens of products, including cosmetics, skin care, body care, hair care, soaps and cleansers, and toothpaste. Miessence is the only product line of its kind that meets my standard for body care and supports the healthy reduction of toxins in your environment.

For more information, call the toll-free number or visit the website.

Peacekeeper Cosmetics
350 Third Avenue #351
New York, NY 10010
(866) 732-2336
www.iamapeacekeeper.com

In addition to quality ingredients, the company donates all profits, after taxes, to support women's health advocacy and human rights issues.

Toothpaste

Miessence by GPRx
(866) 985-GPRx
www.GreatPhysiciansRx.com

Miessence is the world's first extensive line of certified organic skin, body, hair, and oral care products. All Miessence products are made with real ingredients from natural and organic sources. Miessence produces dozens of products, including cosmetics, skin care, body care, hair care, soaps and cleansers, and toothpaste. Miessence is the only product line of its kind that meets my

standard for body care and supports the healthy reduction of toxins in your environment.

For more information, call the toll-free number or visit the website.

Jason Natural
3515 Eastham Dr.
Culver City, CA 90232
(877) JASON-01 (527-6601)
www.jason-natural.com

Tom's of Maine
302 Lafayette Center
Kennebunk, ME 04043
(800) FOR-TOMS (367-8667)
www.tomsofmaine.com

Cleaning Supplies

PerfectClean Ultramicrofiber Mops, Wipes, & Dusters
www.SixWise.com

As discussed earlier, indoor pollution has become one of the leading causes of disease. A main health risk is dust, which commonly contains over twenty toxins such as heavy metals, PCBs, viruses, bacteria, and allergens. I urge you to throw away your typical mops, sponges, and wipers, which do a remarkably poor job of eliminating dust and biological contaminants. These products also require the use of chemical cleaners, which only introduce more toxins into your environment.

Instead, I recommend the PerfectClean line of mops, wipes & dusters, which are available exclusively at one of my favorite websites, www.SixWise.com. PerfectClean's innovative "ultramicrober" construction means that with just the use of water—no chemical cleaners required—the surfaces in your home will become clean down to the microscopic level, eliminating even the biological contaminants that no other cleaning tool or solution can touch. PerfectClean lasts for hundreds of uses, so it's also economical.

PerfectClean products are available online at www.SixWise.com

Bi-O-Kleen
P.O. Box 820689
Vancouver, WA 98682
(800) 477-0188
www.bi-o-kleen.com
Try Turbo Plus Ceramic Laundry Discs and Flora Brite papaya enzyme laundry additive and whitener.

Orange TKO
3395 S. Jones Blvd. #221
Las Vegas, NV 89146
(800) 995-2463
www.tkoorange.com
All-purpose cleaner, stain remover, and odor remover made from organic orange oil.

Seventh Generation
212 Battery St., Suite A
Burlington, VT 05401
(800) 456-1191
www.seventhgeneration.com

Air Purifiers

Pionair
813 Pavilion Ct.
McDonough, GA 30253

(866) PIONAIR (746-6247)
www.pionair.net
The Pionair air purification system enhances the quality of air in the home and reduces harmful toxins such as yeasts, molds, bacteria, and debris. Available in select health stores and via mail order.

Water Purifiers

New Wave Enviro Products
P.O. Box 4146
Englewood, CO 80155
(800) 592-8371
www.newwaveenviro.com
Water purifiers and shower filters remove harmful toxins, including chlorine.

Produce Wash

Veggie Wash
Beaumont Products
1560 Big Shanty Dr.
Kennesaw, GA 30144
(800) 451-7096
www.citrusmagic.com
Made 100 percent with natural ingredients derived from citrus fruit, corn, and coconut, Veggie Wash aids in the removal of pesticides, germs, and toxins from fruits and produce.

Paper Products

Seventh Generation
212 Battery Street, Suite A
Burlington, VT 05401

(800) 456-1191
www.seventhgeneration.com
    Unbleached paper towels, napkins,
toilet paper, and tissue.

Feminine Products

Organic Essentials
822 Baldridge St.
O'Donnell, TX 79351
(800) 765-6491
www.organicessentials.com
    Also producers of organic cotton
balls and cotton swabs.

Natracare
14901 E. Hampden Ave., Suite 190
Aurora, CO 80014
(303) 617-3476
www.natracare.com

Life-Flo
11202 N. 24th Avenue
Phoenix, AZ 85029
(888) 999-7440
www.life-flo.com

Organic Clothing

Under the Canopy
3601 North Dixie Hwy., Bay 1
Boca Raton, FL 33431
(888) 226-6799
www.underthecanopy.com
    World's largest source of modern
and sophisticated organic fiber fashions
for women, men, and children.

Organic Bedding

Heart of Vermont
P. O. Box 612
Barre, VT 05641
(800) 639-4123
www.heartofvermont.com
    Great selection of handmade organic
futons, blankets, sheets, and other
organic bedding.

Sleep Systems

Tempur-Pedic
1713 Jaggie Fox Way
Lexington, KY 40511
(800) 886-6466
www.tempurpedic.com

Natura Bed Systems
Nirvana Safe Haven
3441 Golden Rain Rd., Suite 3
Walnut Creek, CA 94595
(800) 968-9355
www.nontoxic.com/natura
    Wide selection of organic mattresses
and futons.

Nontoxic Paint

Oshadhi
1340-G Industrial Ave.
Petaluma, CA 94952
(707) 763-0662
www.oshadhiusa.com

*Nontoxic Carpeting and Other Building
Materials*
Natürlich Flooring and Interiors
7120 Keating Ave.

Sebastopol, CA 95472
(707) 829-3959
www.natauralfloors.net

Nontoxic Wool Carpets and Other Flooring

Building for Health
P. O. Box 113
Carbondale, CO 81623
(800) 292-4838
www.buildingforhealth.com
   Nontoxic carpets and other nontoxic building materials.

For more information on reducing toxins in your environment, visit www.BiblicalHealthInstitute.com

Key #6: Avoid Deadly Emotions

For information on avoiding deadly emotions, visit www.BiblicalHealthInstitute.com.

Key #7: Live a Life of Prayer and Purpose

For information on living a life of prayer and purpose, visit www.BiblicalHealthInstitute.com.

Notes

Introduction
1. National Center for Disease Control study, "Prevalence of Overweight and Obesity Among Adults: United States, 1999–2002," www.cdc.gov/nchs/products/pubs/pubd/hestats/obese/obese99.htm.
2. *Archives of Internal Medicine,* October 13, 2003, archinternmed.com.
3. Jeffrey Krasner, *Boston Globe,* "Diabetes Therapy Deal," 16 March 2005.
4. *Purdue News,* March 1998, http://news.uns.purdue.edu/html4ever/9803.Ferraro.fat.html.

Key # 1
1. Rex Russell, *What the Bible Says About Healthy Living* (Ventura, CA: Regal, 1996), 62–63.
2. Ibid., 63.
3. U.S. Department Agricultural Research Service, "What We Eat in America," NHANES 2001–2002.
4. Stephen Byrnes, *The Myths of Vegetarianism,* originally published in the *Townsend Letter for Doctors & Patients,* July 2000, revised January 2002.
5. M. L. Burr and P. M. Sweetnam, "Vegetarianism, Dietary Fiber, and Mortality," *American Journal of Clinical Nutrition,* 1982, 26:873.
6. Sally Fallon, *Nourishing Traditions* (Washington, DC: New Trends Publishing, Inc., 2001), 27.
7. Ibid., 28.
8. Gary Farr, "What Are Fats?" *Nutrition Week,* 22 March 1991, 21:12:2–3, http://www.becomehealthynow.com/ebookprint.php?id-39.
9. Mireille Guiliano, *French Women Don't Get Fat: The Secret of Eating for Pleasure* (Westminister, MD: Knopf, 2004).
10. United States Department of Agriculture Fact Book, 2001–2002, Chapter 2, "Profiling Food Consumption in America," http://www.usda.gov/factbook/chapter 2.htm.
11. "Dairy Industry Shows Impressive Gains in Reducing N and P Excretion in Manure," *Better Farming,* April 2004, http://www.betterfarming.com/nov99/apr04-2.htm.
12. *MSN Encarta Encyclopedia,* http://encarta.msn.com/encyclopedia_761578951/Liver.html.
13. Don Colbert, *Fasting Made Easy* (Lake Mary, FL: Charisma House, 2004), 22.

14. F. Batmanghelidj, M.D., *You're Not Sick, You're Thirsty!* (New York: Warner Books, 2003), 225–226.

15. Richard and Rachael Heller, *Carbohydrate Addict's Diet* (New York: Signet), 96–97.

Key # 2

1. Joseph Mercola's website, Mercola.com, "Should You Take Vitamin Supplements?" http://www.mercola.com/2002/jul/10/vitamin_supplements.htm.

2. Council for Responsible Nutrition article "The Benefits of Dietary Supplements," and Johns Hopkins Bloomberg School of Public Health article "Vitamins: More May Be Too Many" by Gina Kolata, http://www.jhsph.edu/CHN/Resources/vitaminwarning.html.

3. *Forbes* magazine, "None a Day?" June 27, 2003.

4. *Encyclopedia of Natural Healing* (Burnaby, BC, Canada: Alive Publishing Group, Inc., 1997), 198–199.

5. "Maternal Supplementation with Very-Long-Chain n-3 Fatty Acids During Pregnancy and Lactation Augments Children's IQ at 4 Years of Age" *Pediatrics*, Vol. 111, No. 1, January 2003, e39-e44.

6. "Grass as a Food: Vitamin Content," a paper presented by G. Kohler, W. Graham, and C. Schnabel on April 10, 1940, at the 99th meeting of the American Chemical Society.

7. Niki Gratrix, "Wheat Grass," How Alive Ltd., at http://www.alexhoward.me.uk/research/wheatgrass.html.

8. Rolf Benirschke, *Alive & Kicking* (Firefly Press, revised 1999), 282.

9. *Enzyme Nutrition* (Garden City Park, NT: Avery Publishing Group, 1995).

Key # 3

1. From a 2003 study sponsored by the American Society of Microbiology as part of its "Take Action: Clean Hands Campaign," http://www.asm.org/Media/index.asp?bid=21773.

2. Dr. S. I. McMillen and Dr. David Stern, *None of These Diseases: The Bible's Health Secrets for the 21st Century* (Grand Rapids, MI: Fleming H. Revell, rev. ed. 2000), 11.

3. Gerald Ensley, "Carting Around More Germs Than Groceries," *Tallahassee Democrat,* 16 January 2005.

Key # 4

1. Dr. James B. Maas, *Power Sleep* (New York: Perennial Currents, 1999).

2. From "Adolescent Sleep Needs and Patterns," National Sleep Foundation research report and resource guide (2002), www.sleepfoundation.org.

3. "Lack of Sleep Alters Hormones, Metabolism, Simulates Effects of Aging,"

University of Chicago Hospitals press release, October 21, 1999, http://www.uchospitals.edu/news/1999/19991-21-sleepdebt.php.

4. "Aging Alters Sleep and Hormone Levels Sooner Than Expected," University of Chicago report, August 15, 2000.

5. Quoting Dr. Eve Van Cauter, a sleep researcher at the University of Chicago, *20/20* (ABC), February 18, 2005.

6. S. I. McMillen and David Stern, *None of These Diseases* (Grand Rapids, MI: Fleming H. Revell, rev. ed. 2000) 194.

7. *The Encyclopedia of Natural Healing* (Burnaby, BC, Canada: Alive Publishing Group, Inc., 1997), 348.

Key # 5

1. "Body Burden: The Pollution in People," Environmental Working Group report, January 2003. (A complete rundown of this landmark 2003 study can be found at www.ewg.org/reports/bodyburden/es.php.)

2. Jeanie Pyun, ed., and staff, "How to Stay Healthy," *Organic Style* magazine, May 2004, http://www.organicstyle.com/feature/0,8028,sl-37-0-0-593,oo.html.

3. Jennifer Davis, "Business in a Bottle," *San Diego Union-Tribune,* January 16, 2005.

4. From the online article, "The Real Cost of Bottled Water," on Dr. Joseph Mercola's website, www.mercola.com. Also available at http://www.mercola.com/2001/may/23/bottled_water.htm.

5. "Researcher Dispels Myth of Dioxins and Plastic Water Bottles," Johns Hopkins Bloomberg School of Public Health News Center, June 24, 2004, http://www.jhsph.edu/publichealthnew/articles/Halden_dioxins.html.

6. Interior Landscape Plants for Indoor Air Pollution Abatement," National Aeronautics and Space Administration study, September 15, 1989.

Key # 6

1. Richard Swenson, *Margin: Restoring Emotional, Physical, Financial and Time Reserves to Overloaded Lives* (Colorado Springs, CO: NavPress, 1995).

2. Dr. Carl Thoresen and Dr. Fred Luskin, "Psychological Effects of Forgiveness Training with Adults," part of the Stanford Forgiveness Study, 1999.

Key # 7

1. Germaine Copeland, *Prayers That Avail Much* (Tulsa, OK: Harrison House, 1997) 17.

2. Ibid., 121.

3. Joseph Mercola, "The Power of Prayer," posted on his website, www.mercola.com, available at http://www.mercola.com/2001/jun/30/prayer.htm>.

4. Daisy Maryles, "No Room at the Top," *Publishers Weekly,* March 28, 2004, http://publishersweekly.reviewsnews.com/article/CA512903.

5. About.com's section on Quotes: Achievement, http://quotations.about.com/cs/inspirationquotes/a/Achievements27.htm.

6. *Super Size Me* was a documentary film released in 2004, and more info is available at www.supersizeme.com.

INDEX

About the Authors

Jordan Rubin has dedicated his life to transforming the health of God's people one life at a time. He is the founder and chairman of Garden of Life, Inc., a health and wellness company based in West Palm Beach, Florida, that produces organic functional foods, whole food nutritional supplements, and personal care products. Rubin is also founder and CEO of GPRx, Inc., a biblically based health and wellness company providing educational resources, small group curriculum, and wellness services.

He and his wife, Nicki, are the parents of a toddler-aged son, Joshua. They make their home in West Palm Beach,

Contributing author Dr. David Remedios is a bi-vocational pastor, general practitioner, and general surgeon who is also a decorated veteran. Among other awards, he has received the Bronze Star Medal for his USAF Services in Desert Shield/Storm and the Meritorious Medal of Honor of the United States Air Force. He is a member of the Southeastern Surgical Congress and the Society of American Gastrointestinal Endoscopic Surgeons and is a part of the Major Medical Corps of the United States Air Force. In his work as a bi-vocational pastor, he has taken missionary trips to Romania and Santa Cruz, Bolivia, where he performed medical services and taught an ACLS course to 200 doctors and nurses, as well as provided translations. He and his wife Yvonne have five children. He enjoys hunting and fishing and has an interest in ornithology.

Acknowledgments

Even though my name is in bold letters on the cover of this book, many others have played important roles in *The Great Physician's Rx for Health and Wellness:*

- Mike Yorkey, my writer and editor, is one of the best in the business. He's quickly become a trusted friend and co-laborer in this awesome mission to bring health and hope to a lost and dying world.

- I would like to thank Sam Moore, Chairman of the Board of Directors of Thomas Nelson, and his wife, Peggy, for being faithful in providing biblical content to the world for many years and putting their trust in me.

- The executive leadership at Thomas Nelson—Mike Hyatt and Jonathan Merkh—believed in me and made me feel a part of the Nelson family, as did Victor Oliver.

- Tina Jacobson, my literary agent, publicist, and media specialist, helped me tremendously with her wisdom and experience.

- Kristen Parrish, a Thomas Nelson editor, displayed great skill and flexibility, especially on the last-minute changes.

- My friend David Remedios, M.D., and a senior pastor, is prepared to take the message of the *Great Physician's Rx* into the Spanish-speaking community and beyond.

- To my pride and joy Joshua Michael, I want you to know that all those times Daddy has to go bye-bye to share the message contained in this book, it breaks my heart to be away from you.

- To my beautiful wife, Nicki: I can never thank you enough for allowing me to spread my wings and go where God has called me, even when it's thousands of miles away.

- And finally, I'd like to thank the Great Physician, my Lord and Savior Yeshua Ha Mashiach, Jesus the Messiah, who was and is and is to come. I only ask that You breathe on the project and show us a glimpse of Your glory. Any chance of success this book has rests upon You.

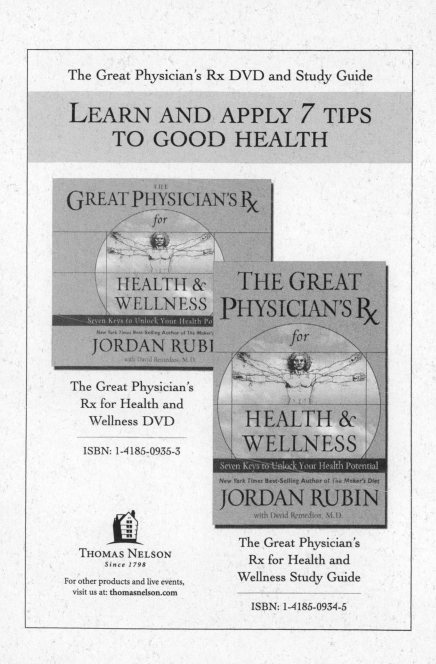

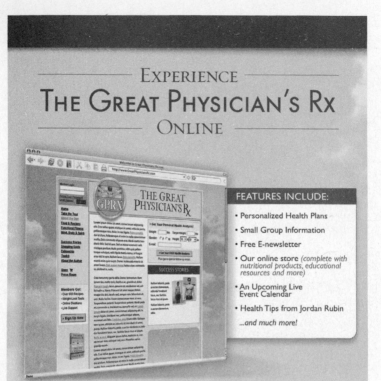
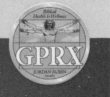

BHI
BIBLICAL HEALTH
INSTITUTE

The Biblical Health Institute (www.BiblicalHealthInstitute.com) is an online learning community housing educational resources and curricula reinforcing and expanding on Jordan Rubin's Biblical Health message.

Biblical Health Institute provides:

1. "101" level **FREE**, introductory courses corresponding to Jordan's book The Great Physician's Rx for Health and Wellness and its seven keys; Current "101" courses include:

   * "Eating to Live 101"

   * "Whole Food Nutrition Supplements 101"

   * "Advanced Hygiene 101"

   * "Exercise and Body Therapies 101"

   * "Reducing Toxins 101"

   * "Emotional Health 101"

   * "Prayer and Purpose 101"

2. **FREE** resources (healthy recipes, what to E.A.T., resource guide)

3. **FREE** media--videos and video clips of Jordan, music therapy samples, etc.--and much more!

Additionally, Biblical Health Institute also offers in-depth courses for those who want to go deeper.

Course offerings include:

   * 40-hour certificate program to become a Biblical Health Coach

   * A la carte course offerings designed for personal study and growth (launching late April 2006)

   * Home school courses developed by Christian educators, supporting home-schooled students and their parents (designed for middle school and high school ages—launching in August 2006).

**For more information and updates on these and other resources go to
www.BiblicalHealthInstitute.com**

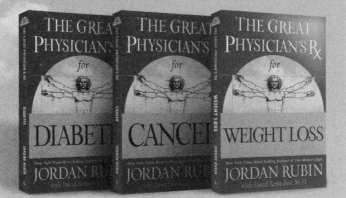
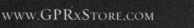
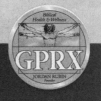

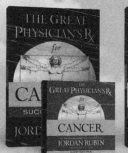
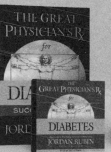
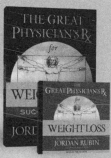

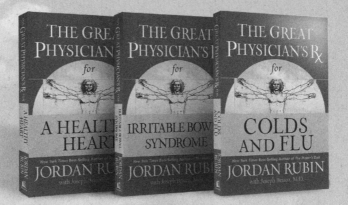
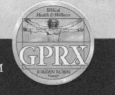

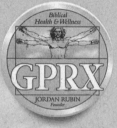

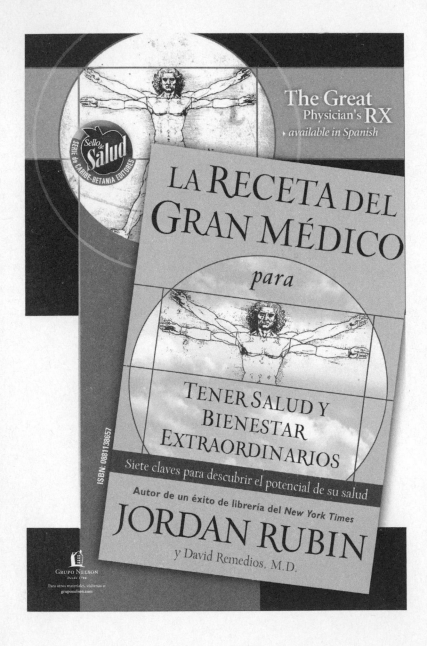